Barts and The London
Queen Mary's School of Medicine and Dentistry
WHITECHAPEL LIBRARY, TURNER STREET, LONDON E1 2AD
020 7882 7110

ONE WEEK LOAN

Books are to be returned on or before the last date below, otherwise fines n

Representing Health
Discourses of Health and Illness in the Media

Edited by

**Martin King and
Katherine Watson**

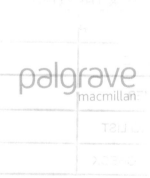

First published 2005 by
PALGRAVE MACMILLAN
Houndmills, Basingstoke, Hampshire RG21 6XS and
175 Fifth Avenue, New York, N.Y. 10010
Companies and representatives throughout the world

PALGRAVE MACMILLAN is the global academic imprint of the Palgrave Macmillan division of St. Martin's Press, LLC and of Palgrave Macmillan Ltd. Macmillan® is a registered trademark in the United States, United Kingdom and other countries. Palgrave is a registered trademark in the European Union and other countries.

ISBN 0–333–99787–5 paperback

This book is printed on paper suitable for recycling and made from fully managed and sustained forest sources.

A catalogue record for this book is available from the British Library.

A catalog record for this book is available from the Library of Congress.

10   9   8   7   6   5   4   3   2   1
14   13   12   11   10   09   08   07   06   05

Printed in China

Contents

PART III   UNRULY BODIES AND THE MEDIA

PART IV   MORALITY AND HEALTH: DISCOURSES OF GOOD AND EVIL IN HEALTH TEXTS

List of Figures

Acknowledgements

Thanks go to Jon J. Reed and Magenta Lampson at Palgrave Macmillan, and to Sandra Coughlan and Esme Dodson for administrative support.

Notes on the Contributors

Andrea Beckmann is Lecturer in Criminology at the University of Lincoln.

Solange Davin is a freelance researcher.

Yumiko Doi is Researcher in Social Medicine, University of Manchester.

Philip Guy is Lecturer in Addictions in the Faculty of Health and Social Care at the University of Hull.

Michael Hardey is Senior Lecturer in Sociology in the School of Geography, Politics and Sociology at the University of Newcastle.

Angela Kershaw is Lecturer in the School of Languages and European Studies at Aston University, Birmingham.

Martin King is Senior Lecturer in the Department of Health Care Studies at Manchester Metropolitan University.

Anthony Pryce is a Reader in the Sociology of Sexual Health and Honorary Research Fellow at the University of Kent.

Clive Seale is Professor of Sociology in the Department of Human Studies, Brunel University.

Clare Street is Senior Lecturer in the Department of Health Care Studies at Manchester Metropolitan University.

Katherine Watson is Senior Lecturer in the Department of Health Care Studies at Manchester Metropolitan University.

Stephen Whittle is Reader in the School of Law at Manchester Metropolitan University.

Alison Wilde is a Researcher in the Centre for Disability Studies at the University of Leeds.

Introduction

Martin King and Katherine Watson

In the introduction to this text we aim to unpack the key concepts which feature in the title of the book. The introduction is therefore divided into three sections – 'Health and Illness', 'Mass Media' and 'Representations'. In these sections we will explore some of the debates, key issues and themes relating to each of these three key concepts. In doing this we will explain why we think that texts on the representation of health and discourses of health and illness in the mass media are a vital part of the study of 'health' and also an important development for media and cultural studies, given the growth in 'health TV' at the end of the twentieth and the beginning of the twenty-first century.

Health and illness

This book analyses some of the ways in which notions of 'health', 'illness' and the 'body' are mediated through the media. In our experience, as academics teaching a variety of core health studies modules to students either studying on a generic health studies degree or completing 'professional' qualifications in the nursing field, we have found that various media (print media, TV and film) are used to form ideas of health and illness and as a source of health information (and misinformation). Interestingly, however, the notion of entering the field of media studies to interrogate these issues has yet to be fully adopted by health educators and the health studies field itself.

The popularity of stories about the NHS in the print media and its central place in political debate, the rise in popularity (and, therefore, production) of medical soap operas (*ER, Holby City,* etc.), hospital docudramas (*Jimmy's*), and dedicated satellite health channels (*Channel Health*), together with the high proportion of health and lifestyle items on daytime TV (and increasingly, popular talk shows such as *Trisha* and *Ricki Lake*), as well as the more traditional public health and health education media campaigns and the increase in health-related sites on the internet, have created a huge health 'agenda' for the mass media. In

1

short, it seems that we cannot escape a 'daily diet' of health advice, or representations of therapy, illness and medicine, as long as we have access to any forms of media.

The chapters presented in this text, therefore, reflect the breadth of current work being done in the field, but from a wide range of disciplines, illustrating not only just how pervasive the study of media is, but also how notions of health and illness traverse interdisciplinary boundaries. Whilst media studies as a 'discipline' is now well established (if not always well regarded), there has been relatively little so far that has attempted to bring together ideas about the ways in which narratives of health and illness get shaped by, and echo in, various media genres (sometimes obviously, sometimes more subtly).

Context

Since McLuhan's (1964) seminal work on the future of mass media in society, the recognition of its role and influence has grown and a field of academic study, intertwined with the field of cultural studies, has developed to explore the relationship between media, culture and society. Cultural studies has traditionally resisted classification as an academic 'discipline' primarily because its concerns, such as identity, subjectivity, language etc., could be positioned as relevant to the study of all disciplines. Instead of occupying a boundaried space of study, therefore, cultural studies could instead be seen as a mobile, adaptive 'strategy' (Bennett, 1998), a 'tool' to be used in a transdisciplinary fashion. Media studies, similarly, whilst having a notion of *what* to study (in terms of its artefacts), have found their way into nearly every disciplinary area in the last ten years.

This is an important point in relation to 'health studies', as we have discussed elsewhere (King and Watson, 2001), as this field of study on the one hand has no clear disciplinary boundaries (i.e. it draws from a variety of theoretical and applied areas) and yet has been 'disciplined' in order to occupy a 'legitimate' academic space. In reality, 'health studies' (even in their most applied forms, such as nursing) are naturally hybrid studies (Turner, 1993) and these are not (or should not be) easy to define. Historically, however, 'hybrid' degrees have tried to claim legitimacy by drawing on other disciplines subject to legitimising criteria (such as scientific or pseudo-scientific disciplines). The result of this process is a marginalising of 'reluctant disciplines' such as cultural studies (Bennett, 1998). Media studies have suffered a similar fate, as we have experienced in our attempts to bring these issues into the remit of 'health studies' (King and Watson, 2001).

If we view cultural/media studies as mobile and adaptive intellectual strategies (Bennett, 1998), then their application to the study of health seems self-evident.

Rather than viewing cultural and media studies as discrete disciplines with fixed boundaries, we would advocate the use of the strategies associated with media and cultural studies to 'interrogate' health issues. One of the other central issues has been the debate about 'low' and 'high' culture and the concomitant 'disciplines' associated with each. Traditionally, media studies have been seen as a 'low'-status discipline concerned with the study of 'low' culture (i.e., popular culture, devoid, in some peoples' opinion, of any higher content of meaning). We would argue, however, as others have, that it is necessary to engage with the study of media as a field that is immensely influential in its use and scope, is richly productive of message and content and is inherently reflective of contemporary discourses. In this respect, the study of 'health' discourses is no less important than any other constructions and representations.

Theorists such as Karpf (1989), Lupton (1998), Moody and Hallam (1998) and Seale (2003) have all acknowledged the contribution cultural and media studies can bring to the study of health, illness and medicine and there is a burgeoning body of work located at the public health/media interface that has focused on issues of discourse and audience around a variety of issues (Bunton, 1997; Lyons and Willmot, 1999; Southwell, 2000). In addition, many theorists from a variety of disciplines have been interested in health issues in relation to the media (Baudrillard, 2002; Gilman, 2001, 1995; Lury, 1998). The study of 'health' and the media is thus a vibrant field of study with many possibilities and it is our hope that this text can contribute to the emerging debates in the field.

How we interpret notions of 'health' and 'illness', and how we construct notions of therapeutic interventions, have been the subjects of years of sociological theorising and ideas that underpin health promoting philosophies. That 'health' belies strict definition should give us some insight into the myriad ways in which we may interpret its entry into media sites.

Mass media

It is a truism that Mass Media have a decisive political, social and cultural importance. Mass Media have lost and won wars (Vietnam and the Gulf), removed and elected political leaders (Nixon and Berlusconi), and generally contributed to the manufacturing of consent. Mass Media are also engaged in the production of the fabric of everyday life as they organize our leisure time, shape our social behaviour and provide the material out of which our very identities are constructed in terms of class, role, nationality, sexuality, and distinctions between 'us' and 'them'.   (Torfing, 1999, p. 210)

This chapter will explore some of the issues outlined in the quotation above. Torfing (1999, p. 216) outlines his view of what mass media actually are:

Mass Media comprises television, radio, film, music, print media and computers that privilege either sound or sight, or any mix of the two. Mass Media culture is an industrial culture, and the predominant regime of accommodation is that capitalist mass production (Fordism).

Devereux (2003, p. 9) conceptualises the mass media in a number of different ways:

- as a means of communication between 'senders' and 'receivers';
- as industries and organisations;
- media texts as commodities produced by media industries;
- media texts as cultural products with social, cultural and political significance;
- as agents of social change and globalisation;
- as agents of socialisation and powerful sources of social meaning.

Marshall McLuhan's (1964) work on the mass media provided an analysis of the growing power of the media in the late 1950s and early 1960s and outlined the possibilities in terms of its global reach. However, his often quoted idea that 'the medium is the message' (McLuhan, 1964, p. 7) provided an analysis of the self-perpetuating and consuming nature of media products.

Forty years later, Baudrillard takes up these themes:

> McLuhan's formulation can be seen to be absolutely brilliant: the medium has swallowed the message and it is this, the multi-medium which is proliferating in all directions. And we are, indeed, seeing terrestrial and cable channels and services proliferating, while actual programme content is disappearing and melting away.   (Baudrillard, 2002, p. 188)

Baudrillard characterises television as the predominant global medium of the twenty-first century. He argues that despite predictions that it offered possibilities for education, information and multiple viewpoints it has become 'conformist and servile' (Baudrillard, 2002, p. 188).

Thompson (1995) argues that the globalisation of the mass media has resulted in the concentration of the production of media products in a small number of transnational media conglomerates in an increasingly deregulated environment. He argues, like Baudrillard, that this has resulted in homogenisation and standardisation and that this is inevitably bound up with consumerism and capitalism. Fiske (1987) and Bourdieu (1998) have examined the results of this globalisation in the ways in which journalism and news reporting operates. Bourdieu talks of 'economic censorship'. He claims that it is important 'to know that NBC is owned by General Electric...that CBS is owned by

Westinghouse, and ABC by Disney . . . and that these facts lead to consequences through a whole series of mediations' (Bourdieu, 1998, p. 16).

Gripsrud (2002) advances the view that the globalised media are also important in the production of identity:

> The media contribute significantly to the definition of the world around us and thereby also to the definition of ourselves. They present ways to understand the world, to represent the world, in images, sounds and writing. They suggest ideas of what is important and what isn't, what is good and bad. . . . They present parts and dimensions of the world that we ourselves have not experienced directly and may never come to experience directly. (Gripsrud, 2002, p. 5)

Gripsrud argues that this influences the way in which we locate ourselves and decide who we are and what we would like to be. These ideas are also explored further later in the chapter.

Silverstone (1994) has written extensively on the role of television (as one dominant form of mass media) as a domestic medium, shaping and ordering our lives, and how TV provides a link between public and private spheres. Gripsrud takes up this argument:

> Television has its place in the interplay between individuals' ongoing construction of identity on the one hand and the general 'macro' functions of society on the other. . . . Television is, as the most central of all media, part of the very fabric of everyday life. (Gripsrud, 2002, p. 25)

Some argue that the plethora of channels now available via cable and satellite have diluted the concept of television as a shared experience (Baudrillard, 2003; Gripsrud, 2002). However, others, such as Dayan and Katz (1992), argue that television still acts as a master of ceremonies for ceremonial events – where a global audience sets aside other activities to take part in the ritual watching of an event or a global shared experience. This would include events such as the moon landing, the funerals of President Kennedy and Princess Diana, or sporting events such as a World Cup or the Olympics.

Bourdieu (1998), though, claims that events such as the Olympics, rather than being a global spectacle and sporting contest between nations, have become one more capitalist consumer product. He argues that the original ideas (promoting international trust and understanding, equal competition, coming together)

> are transformed by the market and the field of journalism into both a war by other means and a vast commercial enterprise (both of which pay nothing but lip service to Olympic

ideals). In other words, the games have been taken from the participants and sold to the market.   (Webb et al., 2002, p. 193)

This section has provided an introduction to the concept of the mass media and some of the debates about its power and influence. This will be taken up in the chapters that follow. We will now take this further by examining, in more depth, the various debates around power and the ways in which the media represent and re-present reality.

Representations

Representation is the process by which members of a culture use language (broadly defined as any system which deploys signs, any signifying system) to produce meaning. Already this definition carries the important premise that things – objects, people, events, in the world – do not have in themselves any fixed, final or true meaning. It is us – in society, within human cultures – who make things mean, who signify.   (Hall, 1997, p. 61)

Hall's definition of representation sets out some of the key issues to be addressed. There are a number of debates about how the mass media represent or re-present reality and a number of theories drawn from the disciplines of psychology, linguistics and media and cultural studies, which seek to explain the relationship between the mass media and society. Here we will attempt to outline some of these debates and demonstrate that the inter-disciplinarity inherent in this area of study means that theories and positions on 'representation' are not necessarily mutually exclusive.

So how are groups or issues represented in the mass media? Do the media reflect or construct reality? Branston and Stafford (1996, p. 78) claim that the 'reality' represented in the mass media is 'always a construction, never a transparent window'.

Kellner (1995, p. 157) states: 'Media culture reproduces existing social struggles and discourses, articulating the fears and suffering of ordinary people while providing materials to produce identities and make sense of the world.'

Hall (1997) explores the relationship between meaning, language and culture and distinguishes between three accounts: the reflective, the intentional and the constructionist approaches.

Does language simply reflect a meaning which already exists out there in the world of objects, people and events (reflective)? Does language express only what the speaker or writer or painter wants to say, his or her personally intended meaning (intentional)? Or is meaning constructed in and through language (constructionist)?   (Hall, 1997, p. 15)

It is the final category which has become a central area of study in the field of media and cultural studies and it is the constructionist approach we wish to focus on here.

Semiotics

There are two key elements to this approach – semiotic approaches which grew from linguistics and, in particular, the work of Saussure (1960) and Barthes (1972), and discursive approaches, which grew mainly from sociology/psychology and, in particular, the work of Michel Foucault (1973; 1977; 1980).

Saussure developed a concept which has become key to the analysis of media texts – the idea of language as a system of signs (these can include written words, images, paintings, photographs) that communicate ideas which can be understood in a particular cultural context. The actual form – word, image etc. – he called the signifier, which acts as a trigger for a concept in the head – the signified. 'Both are required to produce meaning but it is the relation between them, fixed by our cultural and linguistic codes, which sustains representation' (Hall, 1997, p. 31). Thus the letters d – o – g on a page trigger off the idea of a four-legged animal that barks (but also a non-PC term for an unattractive woman). This last comment is not mere flippancy but illustrates the fact, as later critics of Saussure have pointed out, that meanings are not fixed, and meanings and language shift. Hall (1997) gives the example of the reclaiming of the term 'black' as a word with positive connotations ('black is beautiful') rather than its common negative usage (dark, evil, devilish).

Saussure's work was developed by others, in particular Barthes (1972), to become semiotics – the study of signs and the social production of meaning through sign systems. Semioticians introduced the concept of the referent – the actual thing referred to.

> The underlying argument behind the semiotic approach is that, since all cultural objects convey meaning, and all cultural practices depend on meaning, they must make use of signs and in so far as they do, they must work like a language works and be amenable to an analysis which basically makes use of Saussure's linguistic concepts. (Hall, 1997, p. 36)

Thus, semioticians developed the idea that meaning is contained not only in language but also in film, television, photographic images, clothing and many other visual signs. Signs are said to denote, for example the word 'red' refers to part of the colour spectrum, and also to connote, for example the colour red is linked to other ideas or concepts – romance, passion, danger (Branston and Stafford, 1996). In this sense, signs are said to be polysemic, which goes back to Hall's (1997) point about lack of fixed meanings.

Ellis (1975, pp. 79–80) points out, though, that our ability to 'decode' texts depends very much on our understanding of the codes at work:

> The distribution of codes necessary for the interpretation of texts is unequal: some codes are not known by almost all of the working and lower middle classes... codes are not units of meaning, they are areas of connotation that are occupied differently by different classes and even class fractions, complicated by other factors such as region and sex, as well as the whole cultural experience of the viewer.

These methods and concepts are by no means uncontested. There have been many criticisms of linguistic and semiotic approaches used to analyse media texts, the main one being that they do not take any account of the notions of power relations in society. For example, Greg Philo and David Miller from the Glasgow Media Group have been highly critical of what they see as the apolitical work of media and cultural studies practitioners. They say:

> the division between language and reality is a false dichotomy... language is formed in a world of relationships and objects and is part of the measurable reality of that world... judgements and expectations about what is true and what occurs are necessarily measured against the flow of actions and events in the world... we might for example ask for evidence of the view that meaning is constituted by the encounter between the reader and the text (i.e. there are no intrinsic meanings which can be objectively measured).   (Philo and Miller, 2000, p. 5)

Foucault and Gramsci

While the semiotic approach broadened out Saussure's work to look at language in a cultural context it is towards Foucault's (1980) work on discourse and Hall et al.'s (1980) work on cultural Marxism that we need to look to explore the ideas of knowledge and power in media and cultural studies.

Foucault (1980) was concerned with the production of knowledge (rather than just meaning) in society through discourse (rather than just language). Focusing on the human and social sciences and their obsession with 'true' meaning, he developed the concept of discourse related to ideas of power and knowledge, and the question of the subject.

Rejecting grand narratives such as Marxism, which claimed to explain power relations in terms of social class, and linguistic and semiotic approaches which focused on language and dialogue, Foucault developed the idea of discourse as a system of representation:

Here I believe one's point of reference should not be to the great model of language (langue) and signs, but to that of war and battle. The history which bears and determines us has the form of a war rather than that of a language: relations of power not relations of meaning. (Foucault, 1980, pp. 114–15)

Foucault's concept of discourse is outlined by Hall (1997, p. 291):

> a group of statements which provide a language for talking about – a particular topic at a particular historical moment.... Discourse is about the production of knowledge through language. But... since all social practices entail meaning, and meanings shape and influence what we do – our conduct – all practices have a discursive aspect.

Foucault's concept of discourse links language and practice. Discourse defines what and how things are talked about, influences ideas and is used to regulate, ruling in and ruling out different ways of talking about ourselves, the world, relations between groups (Hall, 1997). The concept of discursive formations refers to the way in which different statements, texts or actions come together. Foucault argues that knowledge and meaning are produced through these discursive formations. This is a key concept when analysing media texts. Geertz (1983) has developed this idea in looking at the notion of 'common-sense' as a populist concept and raising awareness of its ideological and political dimension:

> As a frame of thought, and a species of it, commonsense is as totalising as any other. No religion is more dogmatic, no science more ambitious, no philosophy more general. Its tonalities are different and so are the arguments to which it appeals, but like them – and like art and ideology – it pretends to reach past illusion to truth, to, as we say, things as they are. (Geertz, 1983, p. 84)

There are many similarities, we would argue, between Foucault's concept of discursive formations and Gramsci's (1971) concepts of hegemony. The defining difference between the two is the idea of *location* of power – Gramsci takes a Marxist perspective on power, seeing it as being top–down, state produced and controlled, whereas Foucault sees power as located in various relationships within society, such as gender, race relations – not just social class.

Foucault's idea that nothing has meaning outside of discourse has often been misinterpreted by his critics, who claim that he denied that things exist outside of discourse. It is this sort of semantic argument that critics such as Philo and Miller (2000) have picked up on.

However, Foucault's works on madness (1973), punishment (1977) and sexuality (1978) have been highly influential in demonstrating how talking about certain topics is regulated, gains authority, produces subjects which personify the discourse (the madman, the criminal), becomes 'the truth' and produces actions to deal with the subjects of the topic area based on the discourse itself.

Foucault advanced the contentious notion that there is no historical continuity in the way that discourses operate:

> Things meant something and were 'true' he argued, only within a specific historical context. Foucault did not believe that the same phenomena would be found across different historical periods. He thought that, in each period, discourse produced forms of knowledge, which differed radically from period to period, with no necessary continuity between them.   (Hall, 1997, p. 46)

Knowledge (and resultant practices), according to Foucault, are historically and culturally specific. He later developed these ideas around the way in which this knowledge and resultant power are used to regulate behaviour. Foucault's linking of the concepts of knowledge and power is central to the universe of his work in his notion that the application of knowledge produced through discourse becomes true – has the power to make itself true (Hall, 1997). Analysis of the 'good versus evil' discourses around war in the tabloid press or, similarly, of coverage of paedophilia provides a good illustration of Foucault's work. His concept of a regime of truth is often to be seen at work in the tabloid newspaper and TV environment of the twenty-first century.

> it may or may not be true that single parenting inevitably leads to delinquency and crime. But if everyone believes it to be so, and punishes single parents accordingly, this will have real consequence for both parents and children and will become 'true' in terms of its real effects, even if in some absolute sense it has never been conclusively proven. (Hall, 1997, p. 48)

As previously mentioned, the other unique feature of Foucault's work is his conception of power as something which circulates, rather than being top–down. He sees power relations as existing within various societal institutions – the family, the workplace, the law, political spheres – rather than monopolised at the centre. His work on the body (1977) gives examples of the way in which the body becomes the site around which these power relations operate – in the context of crime and punishment and sexuality, for example.

Foucault's ideas on 'the subject' also set him apart from other theorists of representation. In Foucault's work the subject no longer has a privileged, autonomous position in the production of meaning through language, but rather subject positions are produced through discourse.

This approach has radical implications for a theory of representation. For it suggests that discourses themselves construct the subject-positions from which they become meaningful and have affects. Individuals may differ as to their social class, gendered, 'racial' and ethnic characteristics (among other factors), but they will not be able to take meaning until they have identified with those positions which the discourse constructs, subjected themselves to and hence become the subjects of its power/knowledge.   (Hall, 1997, p. 56)

This is where Mulvey's (1975) idea of the 'male gaze' in viewing visual texts comes from – the idea that women in film, for example, are always viewed from a male subject position. This is another contested concept and is a theme that emerges in later chapters.

The British Cultural Studies movement, developed at the Birmingham Centre for Contemporary Cultural Studies under Richard Hoggart in the 1960s and later under Stuart Hall in the 1970s, is, we would argue, another key player in this field. In rejecting the Frankfurt School's view of low and high culture and limited scope for social and political change they developed a new approach to media studies which focused on culture in relation to power and knowledge. This had a particular focus on class relations but, within that, the notions of gender and race were explored within the overall power relationship.

Not only did the scholars attached to the Birmingham Centre for Contemporary Cultural Studies reject the notion of mass culture for being elitist and contemptuous on the masses; they also invoked Gramsci to produce critical studies of the cultural mediation of social antagonisms, primarily concerned with relations of power and resistance and how they are shaped in and through mass media.   (Torfing, 1999, pp. 211–12)

Hall (1997, p. 48) explains Gramsci's theory of hegemony:

Gramsci's notion was that particular social groups struggle in many different ways, including ideologically, to win the consent of other groups and achieve a kind of ascendancy in both thought and practice over them. This form of power Gramsci called hegemony. Hegemony is never permanent, and is not reducible to economic interests or to a simple class model of society. This has some similarities to Foucault's position, though on some key issues they differ radically.

In looking at the work of Saussure, Barthes, Foucault and Hall et al. we are, we would argue, going back to source – to trace the historical development of the ideas around representation which have informed an interdisciplinary process in examining media texts. Hall (1997, p. 6) describes these as 'a set of complex, and as yet tentative ideas in an unfinished project.'

The work of the Centre for Contemporary Cultural Studies, therefore, provides a text-centred analysis linked to notions of power and resistance. Over the years its work has covered a broad range of media and cultural studies topics including methodology (Hall et al., 1980), working-class youth and resistance (Willis, 1977), youth subculture (Hebdidge, 1978) and audience reception studies (Morley, 1980).

This introduction has provided an outline of some of the key concepts and debates around the mass media, its power and influence, and the increasing interest of the mass media in health and illness. The chapters that follow, therefore, take up some of these debates in relation to specific examples and case studies.

Organisation of the book

The book is divided into four parts. Part I groups together three audience reception fieldwork studies. This section has a preamble which traces the development of studies that examine the relationship between the media and audience and outlines some of the key issues and debates in this particular area of research. This includes a continuum of perspectives ranging from the audience as cultural dopes to the audience as media literate and aware of the polysemic nature of media texts.

The three featured studies provide an interesting insight into the ways in which audiences read and interpret three different types of media text; a medical drama, a health promotion radio campaign and soap operas. The studies share key findings concerning the need to understand the complex ways in which media-literate audiences interact with visual and audio texts.

Part II groups together three studies which use the methodology of content/discourse analysis, one that looks at the internet as an increasingly popular health site, and the following two examining discourses of health and illness in the print media. The preamble to the section picks up on some of the key debates around representation and discourse featured in this introductory section. The three chapters all examine the ways in which the media frame debate and construct discourses around a variety of health issues: childhood cancer, the BSE crisis of the 1980s and 1990s, and professional representations of health and illness.

All address key questions about the role of the media in constructing particular discourses around health and illness and draw conclusions about the importance of understanding the impact this has on the way that audiences – which includes policy makers – interpret and use these discourses in practice.

Thus, these three chapters all make links between representations of health and the consequences of such representations on individuals and on the shaping of social policy.

Part III continues to examine the eruption of discourse in media texts, but this time in relation to unruly or 'grotesque' bodies; i.e. bodies that have been positioned, through biomedical or cultural discourses, in opposition to the 'good', 'healthy' body. Drawing on the burgeoning field of sexuality studies, the authors in this section attempt to illustrate the ways in which media texts both construct and reinforce the discourse of 'heteronormativity' (see Part III Glossary). The first chapter looks at the ways in which health promotion texts of the 1940s and 1950s dealt with sexually transmitted infections. Certain bodies were clearly positioned as 'dangerous' or 'polluting' in these texts, and ultimately a heteronormative message, emphasising the 'purity' of marriage, is encoded in the images and text. The second chapter (utilising a method similar to some earlier chapters) analyses a range of print media in relation to body modification and, in particular, focuses on the various narratives that construct transsexuality in the news. The authors illustrate the ways in which certain transsexual identities are seen to be more 'deserving' than others, and analyse the underpinning discourses that frame body modification. The final chapter in this section continues the theme of unruly bodies, by comparing discourses of disability and 'sadomasochism' in advertising. The author invites us to engage with an alternative narrative: one which is spoken through the voices of her research participants, all of whom were involved in bodily practices.

The preamble to this section, therefore, sets the scene by rehearsing some of the important developments in the field of sexuality studies in recent years. As we discuss later, the construction of sexual bodies and their representation is a (fairly recent) example of enlightenment medico-scientific thinking which has had an enormous influence on the ways in which individuals experience their bodies and identities.

Part IV brings together two chapters which examine discourses of morality around health, illness and health-related behaviours. One chapter looks at the portrayal of drug use and drug users in twentieth-century cinema, the other at literary constructions of illness in late nineteenth-century and early twentieth-century literature. Despite their very different subject matter, both examine a number of texts to uncover the morality discourses at work. Key conclusions emerge from both chapters about the ways in which illness, or health-threatening behaviours, are used in media texts as markers of good and evil or of societal approval and disapproval. 'Bad' behaviours include illegal substance use, membership of a counterculture or homosexuality – all, the authors point out, punishable within the narrative of the text: usually by death – both chapters provide a number of examples of this.

The preamble to the chapter looks at a number of works in this developing area of media and cultural studies, making links with some of the debates around lifestyle regulation and morality and examining how discourses of morality and judgementalism are present in media texts as varied as those featured in this section, as well as in the new 'lifestyle TV' programming of the late twentieth and early twenty-first centuries.

A glossary of key terms is included to highlight some of the concepts often referred to impicitly by the authors.

REFERENCES

Barthes, R., *Mythologies* (London: Jonathan Cape, 1972).

Baudrillard, J., *Screened Out* (London: Verso, 2002).

Bennett, T., 'Cultural Studies: a Reluctant Discipline?' *Cultural Critique*, 12:4 (October 1998), pp. 528–45.

Bourdieu, P., *On Television* (Cambridge: Polity Press, 1998).

Branston, G. and Stafford, R., *The Media Student's Book* (London: Routledge, 1996).

Bunton, R., 'Popular Health, Advanced Liberalism and *Good Housekeeping* Magazine', in S. Peterson and R. Bunton (eds), *Foucault, Health and Medicine* (London: Routledge, 1997), pp. 223–48.

Dayan, D. and Katz, E., *Media Events: The Live Broadcasting of History* (Cambridge, MA: Harvard University Press, 1992).

Devereux, E., *Understanding the Media* (London: Sage, 2003).

Ellis, J., 'Made in Ealing', *Screen*, 16:1 (1975), pp. 78–127.

Fiske, J., *Television Culture* (London: Routledge, 1987).

Foucault, M., *The Birth of the Clinic* (London: Tavistock, 1973).

Foucault, M., *Discipline and Punish* (London: Tavistock, 1977).

Foucault, M., *The History of Sexuality* (Harmondsworth: Penguin Books, 1978).

Foucault, M., *Power/Knowledge* (Brighton: Harvester, 1980).

Geertz, H. C., *Local Knowledge* (New York: Basic Books, 1983).

Gilman, S., *Health and Illness: Images of Difference* (London: Harvester Wheatsheaf, 1995).

Gilman, S., *Making the Body Beautiful: A Cultural History of Aesthetic Surgery* (Princeton, NJ: Princeton University Press, 2001).

Gramsci, A., *Selections from the Prison Notebooks* (London: Lawrence & Wishart, 1971).

Gripsrud, J., *Understanding Media Culture* (London: Edward Arnold, 2002).

Hall, S., Hobson, D., Lowe, A. and Willis, P. (eds), *Culture, Media, Language: Working Papers in Cultural Studies, 1972–79* (London: Hutchinson, 1980).

Hall, S. (ed.), *Representation: Cultural Representations and Signifying Practices* (London: Sage, 1997).

Hebdidge, D., *Subculture: The Meaning of Style* (London: Methuen, 1978).

Karpf, A., *Doctoring the Media* (London: Routledge, 1989).

Kellner, D., *Media Culture: Cultural Studies, Identity and Politics, between the Modern and Postmodern* (London: Routledge, 1995).

King, M. and Watson, K., 'Transgressing Venues: Health Studies, Cultural Studies and the Media', *Health Care Analysis*, 9 (2001), pp. 401–16.

Lupton, D., 'Medicine and Health Care in Popular Media', in A. Peterson and C. Waddell (ed.), *Health Matters* (Oxford: Oxford University Press, 1998).

Lury, C., *Prosthetic Culture: Photography, Memory and Identity* (London: Routledge, 1998).

Lyons, A. C. and Willmot, S., 'From Suet Pudding to Superhero: Representations of Men's Health for Women', *Health*, 3:3 (1999), pp. 283–382.

McLuhan, M., *Understanding Media: The Extensions of Man* (Massachusetts: MIT Press, 1964).

Moody, N. and Hallam, J., *Medial Fictions* (Liverpool: Liverpool John Moores University, 1998).

Morley, D., *The Nationwide Audience* (London: British Film Institute, 1980).

Mulvey, L., 'Visual Pleasure and Narrative Cinema', *Screen*, 16:3 (1975), pp. 6–18.

Philo, G. and Miller, D., *Cultural Compliance and Critical Media Studies*, www.gla.ac.uk/departments/sociology/cultural.htm, accessed 03/04/04 (2000).

Saussure, F., *Course in General Linguistics* (London: Peter Owen, 1960).

Seale, C., *Media and Health* (London: Sage, 2003).

Silverstone, R., *Television and Everyday Life* (London: Routledge, 1994).

Southwell, B., 'Audience Constructions and AIDS Education Efforts: Exploring Communication Assumptions of Public Health Interventions', *Critical Public Health*, 10:3 (2000), pp. 314–19.

Thompson, J. B., *The Media and Modernity: A Social Theory of the Media* (Cambridge: Polity Press, 1995).

Torfing, J., *New Theories of Discourse, Laclau, Mouffe and Žižek* (Oxford: Blackwell, 1999).

Turner, B., *Citizenship and Social Theory* (London: Sage, 1993).

Webb, J., Schirato, T. and Danahar, G., *Understanding Bourdieu* (London: Sage, 2002).

Willis, P., *Learning to Labour* (Farnborough: Saxon House, 1977).

Part I

Audience Reception Studies

A key issue in the field of media and cultural studies is the relationship between the mass media and its audience. This section of the book examines some of these debates and presents three new studies in the field.

There are a number of different models advanced by researchers in this area. The first of these is the *effects* model, developed by the Frankfurt School in the 1930s. The Frankfurt School were a group of left-wing German Jewish intellectuals – including Adorno and Marcuse – whose initial work was based around 1930s Nazi propaganda (Branston and Stafford, 1996). They developed what became known as critical theory, which examined the power of capitalism and its control over the media. The media were assumed to be all-powerful, imposing the views of the government on subservient masses. This idea of 'cultural doping' has been criticised since (Fiske, 1987; Morley, 1993), as later researchers began to examine the complexity of the relationship between 'the message' and its reception.

However, the effects model was a dominant force for several decades. The power of the media in the political arena – inspired by the work of Lazarsfield et al. in the 1940s (Lazarsfield et al., 1944) – became a key area of research. John F. Kennedy's success in winning the US Presidency in 1960 (particularly his victory in a TV debate with Richard Nixon) is often attributed to his media-friendly looks and persona (Hayward and Dunn, 2001).

The National Viewers' and Listeners' Association, established in the UK in the 1960s (Branston and Stafford, 1996), was a response to concerns about the effects of an increasingly liberal TV agenda on the viewing public. The work of behavioural scientists was also drawn into the field and the issue of television violence as an influence on behaviour was raised.

> A now much-criticised piece of research was called the 'Bobo Doll Experiment' (Bandura and Walters, 1963). It showed children some film of adults acting aggressively towards a 'Bobo Doll' then recorded children acting in a similar way when left alone with it. The implication was then extended to violent media content, which was asserted to have similar effects on children.   (Branston and Stafford, 1996, p. 311)

These ideas emerged again in the 1970s – around the concept of the media and 'moral panics' (Cohen, 1972); in the 1980s – in relation to video nasties (O'Sullivan et al., 1994); and again in the 1990s – Philo's (1990) work on the miners' strike in the 1980s found that in retrospect audiences forgot important details but remembered key media phrases such as 'picket-line violence'.

The *uses and gratifications* model developed in the USA in the 1940s was based on the idea of viewers and users of the media as 'consumers', with the media providing certain satisfactions (Morley, 1986). The implications of free access, choice and empowerment inherent in this term have since led to criticisms of this approach (Strinati, 1995).

The work of the Centre for Contemporary Cultural Studies (discussed in the Introduction) has many implications for the relationship between audience and media texts. Much of this work argues that audiences are involved in decoding media texts. Morley's (1980) work on 'the Nationwide Audience' (viewers of an early-evening national news programme) used Gramsci's (1971) work combined with Hall's (1980) work on coding to assert that there are different types of audience readings of texts: dominant–hegemonic, where an audience recognises the 'preferred' dominant message and broadly agrees; oppositional, where the audience rejects the dominant message on cultural, political or ideological grounds; or negotiated, where the audience may accept, reject or refine elements of a text, depending on previously held views. Kitzinger's (1998) empirical study on the reception of HIV/AIDS messages adds weight to the concept of negotiated readings and resistance.

Ideas about single preferred meanings and the concept of the media as a conveyor belt for messages have also been questioned subsequently by Morley (1993) himself. This body of work raises some interesting ideas about the relationship between audience and texts and has paved the way for more empirical work and audience reception studies.

The idea of an active audience has, however, been subjected to criticism from some quarters. Philo (2000), for example, raises questions about how many different interpretations audiences can make of a message.

There are a number of other interesting areas of audience research which need to be mentioned here. The domestic context – where and how we consume media texts (Gray, 1992) – is a burgeoning research area.

Bourdieu's (1984) work on 'cultural competence', which examined the concepts of high and low culture in relation to class and education, has since been applied to TV soaps, looking at the skills and knowledge viewers require to engage with so-called 'low'-status programming.

Jane Shattuc's (1997) work on audiences and American TV chat shows – from the more traditional 1980s *Oprah* to the more extreme 1990s versions such as *Jerry Springer* and *Ricki Lake* – engages with a number of debates about the 'audience as spectacle', exploitation vs visibility of certain 'minority' groups in such shows, and the positive nature and uses of internet chat rooms associated with the shows.

Thus, audience research, as with the whole field of mass media research, is ever expanding and developing – a complex unfinished project (Hall, 1997).

Solange Davin's chapter, on *ER*, adds to the body of audience reception studies, supporting the view that audiences are not dumb but discerning, complex, postmodern, 'media-literate analytical spectators'. Davin found that her respondents saw docu-dramas such as *ER* as trustworthy and as providers of health information, learning about welfare state structures and the effects of a profit culture.

Audiences are also, however, well aware of what enhances or fractures the 'realism' of the programmes. One of the key points raised by Davin is that we all learn about real life from fiction: 'the line which separates television from reality is no longer clear-cut'. Davin's research supports the view that texts are polysemic and that meaning is produced 'in the encounter between contingent texts and nomadic viewers'.

Yumiko Doi's chapter also reflects the media literacy of audiences. In a study of the reception of a health promotion radio campaign which aimed to raise awareness and change behaviours within a minoritised ethnic group, Doi emphasises the 'reality gap' between a media-literate audience and campaign planners. Examining the literature concerning health promotion work with ethnic minority communities and drawing on the results of her own study she reiterates the need for prior knowledge and understanding of target audiences when conducting health promotion campaigns via the mass media.

Doi states that when working with ethnic minority communities on health issues, ethnocentric ideas have had the result that 'the emphasis is on enumerating pathologies rather than understanding the cultural, social and economic conditions which impact upon health'. She also emphasises the limitations of mass media-based campaigns and questions the use of 'primitive' methods, such as radio: 'informants at the Pakistani Advice Centre in Sheffield laughed when they were asked the question "Do you listen to the radio?"' In addition, she raises the key issue of the dangers of not giving the audience enough attention, leading to negative outcomes, due to a lack of cultural competence and understanding of those planning campaigns.

Alison Wilde's chapter contrasts the social and medical models of disability, where the social model, as defined by Barnes (1990) and Oliver (1990), 'designates disability as the social oppression of people with accredited impairments'. Using TV soap operas as a case study she examines the representation of disability on television, and, through her own audience reception study, explores the soap-viewing pleasures (Mulvey, 1975) of people with and without disabilities. Her findings produce conclusions about the way the representation of disability in the media is received by audiences. The polysemic nature of texts and the ability of viewers to take on multiple viewing positions are key themes. Wilde also draws conclusions about the negative representation of disability on television.

REFERENCES

Bandura, A. and Walters, R., *Social Learning and Personality Development* (New York: Holt, Rinehart & Winston, 1963).

Barnes, C., *Cabbage Syndrome: The Social Construction of Dependence* (London: Falmer, 1990).

Bourdieu, P., *Distinction: A Social Critique of the Judgement of Taste* (London: Routledge, 1984).

Branston, G. and Stafford, R., *The Media Student's Book* (London: Routledge, 1996).

Cohen, S., *Folk Devils and Moral Panics* (Oxford: Martin Robertson, 1972).

Fiske, J., *Television Culture* (London: Routledge, 1987).

Gramsci, A., *Selections from the Prison Notebooks* (London: Lawrence & Wishart, 1971).

Gray, A., *Video Playtime: The Gendering of Leisure Technology* (London: Routledge, 1992).

Hall, S., 'Encoding and Decoding', in S. Hall, D. Hobson, A. Lowe and P. Willis (eds), *Culture, Media, Language: Working Papers in Cultural Studies, 1972–79* (London: Hutchinson, 1980).

Hall, S. (ed.), *Representation: Cultural Representations and Signifying Practices* (London: Sage, 1997).

Hayward, A. and Dunn, B., *Man about Town: The Changing Image of the Modern Male* (London: Octopus Publishing, 2001).

Kitzinger, J., 'Resisting the Message: the Extent and Limits of Media Influence', in P. Miller, J. Kitzinger, K. Williams and P. Beharrell (eds), *The Circuit of Mass Communication* (London: Sage, 1998), pp. 192–212.

Lazarsfield, P., Berelson, B. and Gaudet, H., *The People's Choice* (New York: Duell, Sloane & Peace, 1944).

Morley, D., *The Nationwide Audience* (London: British Film Institute, 1980).

Morley, D., *Family Television, Cultural Power and Domestic Leisure* (London: Comedia, 1986).

Morley, D., 'Active Audience Theory: Pendulums and Pitfalls', *Journal of Communication*, 43:4 (1993), pp. 13–19.

Mulvey, L., 'Visual Pleasure and Narrative Cinema', *Screen*, 16:3 (1975), pp. 6–18.

Oliver, M., *The Politics of Disablement* (Basingstoke: Macmillan 1990).

O'Sullivan, T., Hartley, J., Saunders, D., Montgomery, M. and Fisk, J., *Key Concepts in Communication and Cultural Studies* (London: Routledge, 1994).

Philo, G., *Seeing and Believing: The Influence of Television* (London: Routledge, 1990).

Philo, G., *Media Effects and the Active Audience*, www.gla.ac.uk/departments/sociology/effects.htm, 03/04/03 (2000).

Shattuc, J., *The Talking Cure: TV Talk Shows and Women* (London: Routledge, 1997).

Strinati, D., *Introduction to Theories of Popular Culture* (London: Routledge, 1995).

Public Medicine: the Reception of a Medical Drama*

1

Solange Davin

Introduction

Medical dramas have been a staple of British networks since the early days of television. From *Dr Kildare, Emergency Ward 10* and *Dr Finlay's Casebook* through *Angels, Peak Practice* and *St Elsewhere* to *Cardiac Arrest, Chicago Hope* and *ER*, they have been enthusiastically received by the public, whose interest shows no sign of fading. *Casualty*, the flagship BBC1 medical drama, first aired in 1986, continues to draw over eleven million viewers, and its off-shoot, *Holby City*, also on BBC1, nine million, according to figures published in the television magazine *Radio Times*. *ER* attracted a record thirty-five million fans in its first season in the USA (Pourroy, 1996) and rapidly acquired a quasi-cult status in many countries, including Britain, where it has a following of over four million, a respectable rating for Channel 4. Yet scholars have paid scant attention to the genre and, apart from Buckingham's (1997) chapter on young *Casualty* spectators and an early telephone survey of American *ER* viewers (KFF, 1997), how these substantial audiences respond to medical dramas remains unexplored. This chapter begins to fill the void by reporting on a reception study of *ER*.[1]

The study

Following Ang's (1991) methodology in her reception study of the American soap opera *Dallas*, an advertisement was circulated in television magazines.

---

*In this chapter, *italics* are verbatim quotes from informants.

Its wording was open[2] – simply asking viewers to explain why they watch *ER* – in order to allow respondents to express themselves in their own terms and to address issues of interest to them rather than topics pre-selected by the researcher. The aim was to generate rich respondent-focused data.

This chapter is based on almost two hundred letters received in answer to this message. Women and men[3] aged between 12 and 84 and from very diverse backgrounds (unemployed, doctors, students, clerks, teachers etc.) replied. After repeated readings, the letters were submitted to an open coding procedure (Strauss and Corbin, 1990) which enabled the *post-hoc* emergence of thematic categories from the data. This initial classification was further analysed and divided into a number of sub-categories (and sub-sub-categories when and as appropriate) according to similarities, to differences, to contradictions etc. in the informants' statements (Deacon et al., 1999). The limitations of the study are acknowledged – the respondents were self-selected and more women than men took part in the study.

The findings demonstrate, first, that viewers use *ER*, a popular entertainment show, as a reliable source of knowledge, from which they gather information through emotional and/or ludic strategies. Secondly, viewers trust this information primarily because they perceive *ER* as realistic. But their concepts of realism go well beyond a simple television–reality comparison: they see the programme as a transparent representation of the world and yet as constructed; they disagree as to which elements decrease or increase realism, with some items described as doing both, depending on perspective; consensus about the realistic properties of a component may conceal underlying discrepancies; informants write of realism of details, or of blanket realism; the American origins of *ER* can reinforce or hinder realism or may be erased altogether; and television and reality overlap.

Thirdly, the intricacy of interpretations[4] stems from the fragmentation of the postmodern individual into an array of dynamic identities, including health and illness, which, in spite of being fundamental identity segments, have been obscured by the academic preoccupation with factors like gender or socio-economic levels, and which need further examination.[5] Finally, the study illustrates that real viewers are astute and insightful, which undermines perennial stereotypes of dumb audiences.

ER – a medical documentary?

Conceived in the 1970s by Michael 'Jurassic Park' Crichton and based on his own training on casualty wards as a medical student, *ER* is a fast-paced drama which follows the trials and tribulations of a group of health professionals in the emergency department of a Chicago hospital. Well-known actresses/actors (e.g. Julianna Margulies, George Clooney) and directors (e.g. Quentin Tarantino) have contributed to the serial.

Unsurprisingly, viewers see *ER* as outstanding entertainment. They like its broken rhythm where action and emotion, chaos and calm, happiness and sadness follow each other in quick succession. They look forward to their weekly rendezvous with their favourite characters, whose lives they compare to those of the actors who embody them (Figure 1.1). They enjoy guessing the content of the next episodes, rewriting the scenarios, imagining happy-ever-after endings.

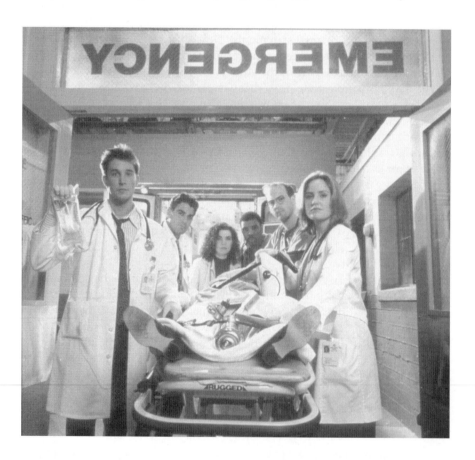

Figure 1.1   Viewers look forward to their weekly rendezvous with the cast of *ER*

But many also describe *ER* as a trustworthy source of information, sometimes as, literally, a documentary:

If you remove the humour, it is like a documentary, things which happen round the clock and rather gloomy. [Michelle]

When I watch ER *it is more like watching a documentary.* [Jean]

What do informants report learning from the serial? First, they assimilate medical details about physiology, symptoms and syndromes, diagnoses, operations etc.:

It teaches you about diseases, like in one episode a woman had Alzheimer's disease. [Laurence]

It gives you the opportunity to learn more about medical knowledge and knowledge of your own body. [Lillian]

Secondly, *ER* is said to impart health promotion advice:

We learn all sorts of things, what damage a car crash can do, the consequences of taking drugs or drinking. [Christopher]

It does help with health promotion when it can. It warns about glue sniffing, drug abuse, smoking. [Gwen]

This echoes the findings of a 1997 US telephone survey (www.kff.org/content/archive/1358/ers.html) where just over half the subjects interviewed had improved their knowledge of health care by watching *ER* and 12 per cent recalled consulting a doctor after being worried by an episode. The date-rape narrative was estimated to have informed five million viewers about emergency contraception.

Such responses are not limited to *ER*. According to Kingsley (1995), millions of viewers have acquired medically-related information from *Casualty*, and some fans have used the data given in the show to make a self-diagnosis. My own (Davin, 1999) reception study of the serial confirmed that its followers learned about diseases, about high technology, about emergency procedures, and, as Buckingham (1997) found in his work with adolescents, that the show helps viewers to prepare themselves for a possible involvement in a real emergency.[6]

Nor is it only medical dramas which provide useful medical data. Other entertainment broadcasts, such as soap operas, have proved to be a valuable resource.[7] A spectator gave *All my Children*, where she heard about ovulation prediction kits, credit for her getting pregnant (Rogers, 1995) and some fans of *The Young and the Restless* lost weight alongside the main character (Cassata, 1985). Viewers learnt about amniocentesis from *Dallas* (Rapp, 1988) and about mental illness from *Brookside* (Philo, 1996). Melodramatic serials have also been an efficient device for the dissemination of health promotion material in developing countries (Singhal and Rogers, 1999).

That continuous serials act as a pool of knowledge should not be surprising since some of their producers have regarded their remit at least in part as one of information-provider.[8] The *Casualty* team try to include helpful medical and first-aid advice in their storylines, and their scenarios are overseen by medical experts whose motto is to 'educate as well as entertain' (Kingsley, 1995, p. 86). The producer of the British soap opera *Crossroads*, Jack Barton, was committed to 'using the soap-opera form for bringing to the notice of the audience the problems of the disabled, the need for kidney donors, and many more issues of social concern' (Hobson, 1982, p. 47). Likewise, the BBC soap *EastEnders* was intended to help raise awareness of social problems and has featured many, from racism to rape, including a range of health topics – vaccination, cot death, drugs, alcoholism, infertility, cancer, HIV/AIDS, spina-bifida, mental illness (depression, schizophrenia) etc. – often championed by 'teacherly' characters such as the local nurse or GP (Buckingham, 1987, p. 84); the creator of *Brookside* had similar ambitions (see Gottlieb, 1993, p. 40). Even science-fiction can have pedagogic objectives (see Cull, 2001, on *Dr Who*).

On the other hand, although the *ER* production team was keen to ensure 'that the finalized script interprets the medicine correctly and that, once shot, it remains authentic', it refused to 'pander to viewers medically' (Pourroy, 1996, pp. 18–24). Nevertheless, *ER* possesses many attributes commonly associated with documentaries: the medical storylines are based on real emergency cases sent by health professionals from all over America, medical consultants supervise the script-writing and filming stages, some of the actors are acquainted with real hospital procedures, the technological equipment is authentic, the Steadycam cameras are indicative of factuality (Pourroy, 1996).

ER – a socio-political drama?

While many viewers are fascinated by the medical angle of *ER*, some are also attentive to its social aspects. First, they gather socio-medical information about the organisation of health care. They compare the welfare state structures with which they are familiar with the American privatised health market, where, apart from a few underfunded and overcrowded hospitals, public provision for those without private insurance is almost non-existent. These respondents conclude that the public-service egalitarian ethos is far superior to the no-payment-no-treatment consumerist model, which they condemn as a harmful manifestation of an overarching for-profit culture.

Secondly, because *ER* takes place in one of these rare state hospitals, it also serves as a refuge to many homeless and/or unemployed people in time of sickness or accident, and it is therefore ideally situated to reveal the flip-side of the American dream – a utopian land where all aspirations can be achieved through hard work and resilience – portrayed in some Hollywood-style serials. Some viewers praise this *non-PC approach* [Lisa], which exposes the climate of violence, of poverty, of exclusion, with which the less privileged are confronted:

> *We keep seeing patients who need social workers, who cannot afford care, children with bodies full of gunshots, abused children etc. It seems to me that* ER *is a rich and realistic portrait of American society.* [Sylvia]

These viewers find such depictions of a country in chronic crisis shocking and alarming, and the underlying *laissez-faire*, profiteering and consequent lack of compassion and of support for those most in need unacceptable. These political comments reflect those made in other studies: both the Russian interviewees in Liebes and Katz's (1993) cross-cultural research on *Dallas* and the young fans of *EastEnders* (Buckingham, 1987) interpreted the shows in an ideological framework even where it was not made explicit within the programme itself.

How do *ER* viewers learn?

Two approaches to learning, one ludic and one emotional, are prevalent in this study. The first is the transformation of *ER* into a quiz, a detective story, whereby spectators join in the investigations and try to predict which diagnosis, test(s) and treatment(s) will be given to each patient, if possible before the screen medics:

> *We record it so we can stop the tape and guess the diagnosis once we know the symptoms. Some of our friends even play games to guess which tests they are going to carry out for each patient.* [Elizabeth]

The second strategy is identification. *ER* fans identify particularly with medical students because of the affinity of a (perceived) common position of novice:

The student is the beginner prototype, to whom everything happens, who is ignored or patronised, but who evolves. I really like him. He resembles the spectator. [Jean-Paul]

We see the ward through the student's eyes. [Laurent]

Viewers empathise with the ups and downs of students' training, sharing their joy when they succeed and their sadness when they fail or make mistakes. These future medics become the 'open sesame' which unlocks the doors of the strange hospital universe to viewers, which enables them to discover the intricacies of the casualty department and to engage in a virtual course in emergency medicine. This corroborates previous evidence that 'emotional' tactics foster learning (e.g. Brown and Basil, 1995; Poole-Hayward, 1997).

Thus informants re-genre an entertainment programme as a quasi-factual broadcast from which they extract information through sentimental or playful tactics. Being in apparently incompatible viewing modes – cognitive/emotional, distant/close, critical/involved – echoes both the 'edutainment' trend and the 'travelling' or 'growing' theories of learning which juxtapose 'desk' and 'couch' metaphors (involved concentrated viewers and relaxed easy-going viewers) (MacMahon, 1997, pp. 88–91), and where the objectives of the broadcast are to entice viewers into exploring a topic (Meyer, 1997). *ER* certainly is inspiring:

ER *makes me feel like finding out more. I'd like a doctor to comment on the gestures and the words.* [Carol]

My daughter has just started studying medicine partly because of the series and she is not the only one [Eileen].

While 'top–down' transfer of knowledge (intentional or otherwise) does occur in *ER*, its audiences are by no means the proverbial blank slates waiting to be injected with information, but media-literate, analytical spectators evaluating programmes in the light of their considerable pre-existing knowledge and experiences. This resonates with health promotion campaigns using melodramatic serials in developing countries, whose efficacy was largely due to the acknowledgement not that viewers are sponges ready to unthinkingly absorb all television images, but that they are simultaneously serious and playful, sentimental and critical, detached and involved, educating and enjoying themselves. It is by enabling individuals to empathise with characters, to assess the pros and cons of various solutions, to discuss the questions raised in the narratives with friends and families, that advice seems to be best disseminated (see Davin, 2000), rather than through information-processing approaches where direct influence is inferred between message and behaviour (e.g., being made aware that their actions are potentially dangerous should lead rational receptors to modify their conduct).

The transformation of *ER* into a reservoir of medical information is of particular importance since it is known, first, that medical subjects top the public's list of interests (Wellcome Trust, 2000), and secondly, that television has long been a prime source of medical information (e.g. Karpf, 1988; Kitzinger, 1998). By their very content, medical dramas are therefore likely to play a key role in this search for knowledge; all the more so since, when consulted, viewers have repeatedly articulated their preference for hybrid broadcasts which amuse them while addressing their problems (e.g. Elkamel, 1995). When the radio soap *The Archers* was created in 1950 to disseminate agricultural advice, the format was chosen by the farming community (Kingsley, 1988). More recently, adolescents have requested that safe-sex issues be included in soap operas (BAC, 1999). Furthermore, in a study on the reception of parallel illness storylines in fictional and factual programmes, interviewees, in a somewhat counter-intuitive fashion, expressed scepticism about documentaries, which they criticised for being selective, incomplete and artificial, and contended that continuous serials are a better support for the communication of (medical) data because they have massive followings, their multiple plots render distressing narratives less upsetting, they promote identification and they allow repetition (Davin, 2003).

Realism(s)

Viewers give a number of reasons for trusting the data imparted by *ER*. Some have read (p)reviews in magazines and newspapers praising its authenticity or have heard about it from friends or acquaintances involved in health care. But the most widespread argument is the realistic quality ascribed to the *ER* images and storylines, which is mentioned in almost all letters. Informants make 'referential statements' (in Liebes and Katz's (1993) terms): they connect fictional situations and/or characters to real life:

> *I have been to casualty and it reminds me of the atmosphere and the gestures so typical of this ward.* [Jane]

> *In Benton's lack of realism about his mother and his verbal violence I can see my own father and my grandmother.* [Sue]

But respondents' conceptions of realism go well beyond basic dichotomies whereby television mirrors reality (with varying degrees of accuracy). Just as

Hagen's (1992) informants described news bulletins as a transparent reflection of the world and yet as fabricated, and in spite of their repeated affirmations that *ER* does *show what really happens in casualty*, viewers are, like Pasquier's (1999) adolescents, well acquainted with the 'manufactured' aspect of television and cite many factors likely to raise or to detract from the impression of realism. The Steadycam cameras, which have long been associated with *cinéma-vérité*, enhance realism because *they move around a lot as if the viewer IS the camera looking all over the place. It makes it look very real* [Didier]. Conversely, actors' outside commitments may hinder realism. As one person asks:

> *In episode one, Susan meets a psychiatrist who vanishes. Did the actor have a contract somewhere else?* [Janine]

Financial constraints and the quest for ratings may also compromise realism. The first can lead to the numerous romances between characters being mostly confined to the group of medics (*this way, they have fewer actors to pay* [Monica]). The second compels producers to maximise audiences, even if realism suffers in the process:

> *The medicine is fairly real but not to the point of putting people off.* [Liz]

> *Most of the cast are good-looking, which is not the case in hospitals. But I know that they have to do this so that more people will watch.* [Anna]

This viewer is not alone in perceiving the characters as better looking than average:

> *Most characters are attractive and slim, not as in a normal hospital.* [Dorothy]

But when informants write about this subject, antagonistic criteria begin to appear as some perceive the characters as 'deglamourised':

> *The actors are not all cute with lots of make up, they are just everyday people.* [Justin]

> *They are not all good-looking as in some other American series.* [Didier]

This is in line with the remit of casting officers and make-up artists to have plain, tired, sickly-looking characters to match the hospital setting:

ER takes place in Chicago, which is filled with people who have come from all over the world, who are too tall and too short, too fat and too thin – and who look like hell because they are sick. Or feel like hell because somebody they care about is sick. None of us are at our stylish best when we're in *ER*. That's not the story we are after. (Casting director John Levey, quoted in Pourroy, 1996, p. 42)

Equally controversial is the question of the speed at which the patients are brought in, assessed and treated, which is taken, on the one hand, as evidence of realism:

Everything is done at breakneck speed just as in my everyday work. Everything happens so fast. [Janet, nurse]

and, on the other, as a mark of unrealism:

In the hospital I know there is no such speed. [Camilla]

Speed is a fundamental and recurrent feature of *ER* and essential to its sense of urgency and excitement, as is the endless cortège of seriously injured patients arriving on the ward, and respondents are very aware of these implausibilities. Yet they discount them and persist in asserting that *ER* is very realistic, because they are fully *au courant* that such excesses are neither accidental nor due to mistakes, sloppiness or deception, but deliberately included in the scenario to heighten the tension that a quality drama requires:

A series needs drama hence everything happens in the same place. [Maria]

Although it is rare for a casualty to have so many disasters, the fiction requires it! [Andrew]

Gibbs (a physician) and Ross (1996), in their book on *ER* and its medicine, concur that most of the unrealistic details which they spotted in the episodes – students never going to the library, residents being on call on the ward rather than at home, etc. – are explainable by the imperatives of dramatic stimulation. The *ER* script-writers do not deny that realism occasionally has to be sacrificed to the demands of drama: 'From the beginning we decided to take liberties when necessary. We knew there would be times when scenes would not depict exactly the way emergency medicine is practised. But *ER* is a dramatic show...' (medical consultant Dr Gentile, quoted in Pourroy, 1996, p. 26).[9]

Moreover, *ER* is not exempt from minor medical errors, and manifestations of this 'approximate realism', often expressed in 'it's realistic but…' formulas, are most frequent in the replies of physicians, who are in a good position to detect them:

> *The medical terms ring true, and it shows the problems of being an intern, but there are too many intubations and reanimations which work. It shows electric shocks as miraculous, which is far from being true.*   [Catherine, gynaecologist]

> *There is a good medical realism except that the reanimation scenes are shortened too much, and the doctor who goes out of the reanimation room, removes his gown and simply gets on with something else is not very realistic.*   [Jerry, GP]

Other informants, however, are not concerned with technical or medical minutiae and concentrate instead on blanket links to reality:

> *It is real, the decoration, the people waiting, running all over the place, worrying. It is real in its facts, that is, the person arrives, she has a problem; this follows real life. Outside too, things are real, like they take the tube.*   [Tony]

That evaluation of realism happens at various levels and is exemplified by the following quotes about the episode 'Love's Labour Lost', with its string of mistakes and difficulties leading to the death of a young patient. At the micro-level, the intern *would not have made such basic errors of judgement, having delivered a couple of hundred babies* [Charlotte]. But, in a more general way, *'Love's Labour Lost' put things back in place, things are not always great* [Lucy].

Not only can viewers disagree on whether a particular item reinforces or decreases realism, as seen above, but when they do agree, this consensus sometimes conceals underlying discrepancies. Thus there is no doubt in many respondents' minds that the medical jargon which peppers *ER* is realistic. For some, failing to understand this vernacular is a guarantee of realism:

> *The universe of the hospital is well represented with its language which is incomprehensible to outsiders.*   [Lisa]

> *The medical jargon makes the situations more real. I mean, how many times have you been to the doctor's or to the hospital and not known what on earth they are talking about!*
> [Helen]

This is what the *ER* executive producer hoped to achieve. He claims that unlike other dramas, where

> you hear characters saying a lot of ridiculous things like 'it's time to do the laparotomy! Joe get that tube so we can see if there's blood in his stomach!' when, clearly, everybody in the scene would know what a laparotomy was . . . [w]e allowed the audience to feel as if they'd stepped into a real hospital.   (John Wells, quoted in Pourroy, 1996, p. 18)

But, again, their efforts are not entirely successful and some viewers (outside health professionals) do understand the medical expressions and take this as a proof of realism:

> *The doctors talk in such a way that the patients understand, so we can understand as well.*
> [Michelle]

> *I think that what makes it realistic is the expressions, the use of medical terms. It gives an impression of competence. And some of them we already know so we know they are real.*
> [Robert]

The complexities of respondents' notions of realism are perhaps best illustrated by their constant to-and-fro oscillations when they write about the American-ness of *ER*. The origins of the show are sometimes foregrounded when, as above, the US and UK health care systems are contrasted. For example, some informants point out that many non-urgent patients would not be in casualty in the UK because they would have attended their local GP surgery instead. In this sense, *ER* is 'their' reality, that is, *it is reality made in the US, it is different from here* [Jonathan]. Nevertheless, for some, *ER* may be a worrying preview of the future as 'their' reality threatens to become 'ours', and the serial thus has a potentially realist dimension: they fear that a US-style two-tier medical system may be implemented in their own country and that the social problems which plague America may soon reach their shores. Likewise, some young viewers of news bulletins read images of violence in the United States as a warning of what may happen in Britain, and voice their unease about the growth of crime through comparisons with the US: ' "We are just going to be like New York" [or] "I feel lucky that I don't live in America" ' (Buckingham, 1997, p. 195).

On the other hand, *ER*'s made-in-America label contributes to its realism, first, because medical experts supervise the making of the show while, as a number of viewers complain, *many of our programmes lack medical advisers*, and secondly, because American broadcasts are believed to be less censored than European ones and to have more latitude to handle issues which may be avoided or inadequately covered on their side of the Atlantic:[10]

> *I never know why British audiences have to be protected from all unpleasantness, it makes the programmes so bland.... Why is UK entertainment sanitized to the extent that they* [sic] *fail to grasp the imagination?* [Moira]

The American-ness of *ER*, then, manifests itself in idiosyncrasies, which lower realism but which give rise to a potentially closer realism, and an added veracity and openness which enhance it. At other times the foreign roots of the serial disappear altogether behind the (perceived) universality of biomedicine, of emergency procedures and of high technology. The casualty department, which in the previous discourse was typically American, remote, different, now becomes one of many identical casualty wards, a global, familiar, realistic location:

> *Everything seems true, it is universal. We are in America and the equipment is new but it is in all the ERs in the world.* [Gwen]

We saw how viewers sometimes establish parallels between *ER* and their lives. But they also assess realism by contrasting the elements of different broadcasts:

> *The pace of* Casualty *is so slow and unreal compared to* ER. [Julia].

Moreover, fictional programmes may be a reference point to which factual ones are compared. Thus *ER* can be taken as the blueprint for the documentary *The Real ER*, filmed at County Cook Hospital in Chicago and believed to be the model for *ER*:

> The Real ER *is the same hospital as* ER. *The real doctors resemble the* ER *doctors.* [Jean]

> *If I did not know that* The Real ER *is a documentary I would think that it is another* ER. *The characters look like* ER *characters. At the beginning, it's Dr Greene, and the nurse could be Carol.* [Avril]

The juxtaposition of programmes can be so ambiguous that the inside and the outside, critical distance and suspension of disbelief, reality and television are inextricable:

In Chicago Hope, *I did not get the impression that they were concerned. They were in a film, while in* ER *you feel that they are real doctors, because they are on call, they get woken up, they are constantly in this milieu, facing all sorts of problems, and we feel that we are in a hospital when it is a series.*   [Carol]

Such overlaps and reversals are only to be expected since much of our *savoir*, our knowledge, is, has always been, in some way, mediated, derived not from direct acquaintance with facts or with events but from hearsay, from friends, from books, from magazines, from newspapers, from the radio, from films, from television, from CDs, from the internet (or, in days gone by, from posters or from the town crier), particularly when the subject matter is outside the daily routine of most people, as Gerbner and Gross (1976, p. 179) underline:

How many of us have ever been in an operating room (awake), a criminal courtroom, a police station, jail, penthouse, corporate boardroom, movie studio, or other staples of television locales? Yet how much do we 'know' about such places, about what goes on in them, about the people who live and work in them? How much, indeed, of our images of the real world has been learned from fictional worlds?

We live in a 'pseudo-environment', as Lippman wrote as early as 1921, and we learn about real life from fiction:

In my family everybody watches. They are delighted to have an insight into what I do. [Jude, nurse]

Thanks to fiction, we can go in the parts of the hospital which are prohibited to the public and to families, operating theatres and others.   [Brian]

Thus reality can be interpreted through the media: patients' expectations of (and disappointments about) their therapy were partly based on media representations (O'Keefe, 1999) and one of Seiter's (1994, p. 390) interviewees described his malaise by recollecting a favourite drama: 'I was rushed to hospital in an emergency. So then all the General Hospital things that went on, that I had seen, sort of become real to me. I could not believe that I was in hospital playing the part of a very sick man.'

Sometimes the media can be more potent, more compelling – more real – than experience, and it is on the screen that events are 'real-ised' (see Fiske, 1995): some of Philo's (1996) informants trusted media information on mental illness over their own experience. In *The Cosby Show*, Clare Huxtable as a lawyer and the Cosby family as 'middle-class' were deemed more representative than those met by viewers in real life (Press, 1991, pp. 110–11). For Woolley (1993, p. 195), who was at the site of the Clapham rail accident, it was nevertheless on the screen that 'the event happened'; his own experience had a 'lower meaning'. Along similar lines, a police officer changed his testimony in the 'Rodney King trial' after seeing a videotape to which he too attributed a 'higher truth' than he accorded to his experience (Fiske, 1995, p. 130). And some spectators seem puzzled when reality fails to match fiction, as one informant ponders:

> *People say to my wife* [a nurse]: *Why don't you wear a green jacket? Why is your husband an engineer and not a doctor as on television?* [Timothy]

Television, then, is not the legendary window on the world. In our intertextual postmodern world, the line which separates television from reality is no longer clear-cut. The two endlessly deconstruct, construct, reconstruct themselves and each other. Viewers compare television to reality, programme to programme, reality to television. Attempting to disentangle them is a thankless (and pointless) task because

> The media do not impart a slice of reality.... Reality consists of that which has been mediated both by the media and by other things, and is constantly constructed anew. The content of television radiates out into the rest of reality, which therefore cannot be separated from it. (Bausinger, 1984, p. 350)

It is 'the dissolution of TV into life, of life into TV...a sort of fantastic telescoping, of collapsing of one into the other of two traditional poles... implosion' (Baudrillard, 1981, pp. 54–5).

Attempting to evaluate programmes unambiguously as un/realistic is therefore over-simplistic. In informants' letters, form and content interact, contradictions and ambiguities abound, television and life are intertwined, and *ER* remains realistic regardless of errors, of implausibilities, of excesses, of artificiality, of American hallmarks:

> *We really feel as if we were in the hospital with its disorder, its fauna. In short, we believe it.* [Carol]

This suggests that it may be fruitful to replace the reel/real dichotomy by a continuum which can accommodate degrees and levels of realism, overlaps, incongruities, approximations, antagonisms, ambivalence, conflicting perceptions and criteria, etc. Understanding audiences' notions of realism is important not solely for media studies but also for health promotion because realism is a crucial requirement for people's willingness to accept advice and to take it on board (Elkamel, 1995).

Health and illness identities

Audiences who are capable of reading television in such an intricate and fluctuating fashion cannot be divided *a priori* into pre-set groups, cannot be expected to produce bounded, distinctive interpretations according to the category to which they have been ascribed, a not uncommon approach in media studies (and in other social sciences disciplines). In his seminal Nationwide Study, for example, Morley (1980) endeavoured to establish links between subjects' socio-economic levels and interpretations. Instead he found that 'social position in no way directly correlates with decodings' (Morley, 1980, p. 137)[11] and he later suggested that we should

> try and reinstate the notion of persons actively engaged in cultural practice. To put the point another way, one cannot conclude from a person's class, race, gender, sexual orientation and so on, how she or he will read a given text... [because] the same man may be simultaneously a productive worker, a trade union member, a supporter of the social Democratic Party, a consumer, a racist, a home owner, a wife beater and a Christian. (Morley, 1991, p. 43)

While Morley's stance befits the multiple subjectivities of the postmodern 'screenager',[12] a conspicuously missing component in his list is health and illness identities. Health and illness are fundamental identity segments (Crawford, 1994), and, although they are usually taken for granted and have therefore remained invisible (partly because they have been obscured by the academic focus on some of the sociological variables mentioned by Morley, such as gender, class, ethnicity), they are likely to contribute to the shaping of interpretations, especially when programmes include medical themes.

Health and sickness, however, are not a straightforward matter of biology, whereby each disorder can be explained by a particular underlying pathology, but fluid concepts created at the interface of the material and social/cultural realms. Accordingly, they have a range of meanings. Health, for instance, has been equated to an absence of illness, to a reserve of health, to self-care, to vitality, to equilibrium, to mental well-being, to the ability to carry out everyday tasks. Moreover, the line between health and sickness is hazy: countless people are suspended in a limbo state, in between health and ill health, by recurring but benign aches and pains; some ailments are 'normal', healthy even (children's diseases, colds), and even a serious condition need not prevent patients from describing themselves as being in good health (e.g. Robinson, 1971). Likewise, illness has a variety of meanings, from destructive to liberating; recovery can be of minimal concern or it can monopolise patients' time and efforts and develop into a new way of life.[13]

Any alteration of health status can engender anxiety and an erratic sense of-identity. Sickness, especially if it is life-threatening, chronic or disabling, profoundly affects our self-consciousness and our world-view, as Duff (1994, pp. 9–11), who has Chronic Fatigue Syndrome, vividly describes:

> I find it difficult to reconcile the contrary visions of health and illness, or even hold them in my mind at the same time. They slip away from each other, like oil and water.... There is, perhaps rightly so, an invisible rope that separates the sick from the well, so that each is repelled by the other, like magnets reversed. The well venture forth to accomplish great deeds in the world, while the sick turn back onto themselves and commune with the dead; neither can face the other very comfortably, without intrusions of envy, resentment, fear or horror. Frankly, from the viewpoint of illness, healthy people seem ridiculous, even a touch dangerous, in their blinded busyness, marching like soldiers to the drumbeat of duty and desire.

The removal of this invisible rope was one of the objectives of some early medical documentaries, whose producers hoped that their programmes might help lower the 'barrier which too often isolate healthy people ... from the sick' (Barrère, Desgraupes and Lalou, 1976, pp. 94).

A particular disease, however, need not give rise to a unique, immutable identity segment. Any disorder can create a number of identities in sufferers (and in non-sufferers, see below), as shown, in the case of asthma, by Adams, Pill and Jones (1997),[14] who uncovered different relations to the illness: 'accepters' acknowledge asthma as part of their lives, 'deniers' develop strategies to hide it, and a few redefine their asthma as acute rather than chronic. To all these patients several sickness subjectivities are available, and these may guide interpretations of (medical) narratives in varied ways: an asthmatic viewer may not interpret an episode – especially if it features asthma – as would non-asthmatics, but an 'accepter' may produce different readings from those of a 'denier'. Furthermore, conceptions of asthma fluctuate across time and place (Gabbay, 1982) (as is the case for many diseases, whose changing constructions are well documented in the medical humanities), and illness identities would fluctuate accordingly. It is also important to note that such identities have no necessary link to biology or to diagnosis, and are not the prerogative of patients. In the previously mentioned study of fictional and factual sickness narratives, it emerged that a number of healthy respondents had incorporated an illness segment in their otherwise healthy identities after prolonged contact with seriously ill relatives or friends, and that many of their responses differed markedly from those of viewers who had had little or no contact with disease.

Incidental findings show that sickness identities can affect interpretations and viewing practices. For example, the respondents in Cumberbatch and Negrine's study (1992) read media texts according to their illness experience. A woman who had had breast reduction read the *Roseanne* episode dealing with the subject in a more critical way than did others (Crowther, 1998). Tulloch's (1990) older informants watched the Australian 'medical soap opera' *A Country Practice* because they found its medical items relevant and were eager to find out more. Experience of ill health can also make viewers hesitate before watching:

> *I watch sometimes, but with moderation. The reason is simple: after a few 'minor life accidents' (car crash, beginning of cancer), I ended up in hospital several times. I know hospitals well enough and it is not a pleasure I enjoy when I want to escape in front of the screen.* [Eric]

Such memories can have a lasting impact: a couple disapprove of the use of ill health for entertainment because of their daughter's lengthy stay in hospital over twenty years previously. However, the impact can be mitigated by other identities, as suggested by this college pupil, who explains how the same accident led to different responses to *ER*:

> *My friend had an operation for her foot and since that she has stopped watching. She said that it was so horrible that she does not feel like watching anymore. I too had surgery on my foot but it made no difference! I too broke my foot at Christmas, but maybe I still like ER because I want to work in a hospital setting and she does not.* [Nadia]

Furthermore, curiosity can overcome caution:

> *The medical milieu is not really 'my thing' because it reminds me of bad childhood memories. But I said to myself: 'don't stay ignorant, watch' and I watch.* [Sue]

And *ER* can have 'medicinal' qualities which counterbalance disturbing recollections:

> *I was myself admitted to A&E several times. Before ER I could never watch medical programmes where you are shown operations (blood, flesh...). This series helps me not to feel concerned by the physicians' aggressive gestures.* [Jill]

Health and illness identities, then, are flexible and dynamic. They intersect and interact with other identities[15] and colour interpretations in multiple ways. Reciprocally, they may be shaped by television representations.[16] These processes need further scholarly attention.

Conclusion

The skills and intelligence of television viewers have too often been under-estimated in media studies. Time and time again research agendas have assumed, more or less explicitly, a one-way linear model of communication which reduces reception to the regurgitation of fixed narratives transmitted by an omnipotent media to a naive, gullible public with little agency (e.g. the viewer-in-the-text, information-processing etc.) – a mere referendum, complains Barthes (1970, p. 10). But there exists no necessary correspondence between sent and received messages. Meaning is not inscribed 'in the text' but generated in the encounter between contingent texts and nomadic viewers. Recent qualitative reception studies (Baudin, 2001; Buckingham, 1997; Hill, 1999; Pasquier, 1999; Turnock, 2000) illustrate that real audiences are media-literate, insightful, astute, that they read, reread, modify, extend, analyse, assess, play with, learn from, and variously use broadcasts in unexpected, sometimes idiosyncratic, possibly contradictory ways according to their frames of reference, to their moods, to their situation, to their dominant identities, at a given moment.

The sophistication of viewers is manifest in this study, where they re-genre a popular entertainment show as a reliable (medical, social, political) pedagogic broadcast – a documentary – and collect data from the episodes through sentimental or recreational tactics of identification or game-playing. They trust this information largely because they consider *ER* to be realistic – despite conflicting viewpoints, despite dissent on which elements heighten or reduce this sense of reality and why, despite unconvincing excesses and implausible details, despite its American roots, which may be highlighted or disregarded. Their evaluations rest not merely on their own *vécu*, their lived experience, but on their substantial knowledge of production practices, on friends' opinions, on the written press and on other programmes, as the media and real life increasingly overlap and merge into a transtextual, global hyper-reality. In spite of its limitations, this research demonstrates that viewers are neither cultural dopes nor witless dupes, that they do not resemble traditional caricatures of innocent simpletons, that their multiple subjectivities – including health and illness identities – promote complex contextual readings. More attention needs to be given to the reception of (medical) broadcasts, with or without pedagogic ambitions, if the elaborate information-gathering and meaning-making processes viewers engage in are to be fully comprehended. This calls for more qualitative audience research and for theories grounded in their findings.

NOTES

1. The project began as a cross-cultural study of British and French viewers. The rationale was less national differences *per se* than the disparity in the number of, and enthusiasm for, medical dramas between the two countries. However, no cross-cultural difference emerged at analysis (see my article at http://wjfms. ncl.ac.uk/ER.htm). For full details of the study, see Davin (forthcoming, 2004).

2. This openness can be seen in the fact that six detractors of *ER* replied.

3. Almost a third of the respondents were men, who answered mostly by email. Some stated that it was the technology which had enticed them to do so. This indicates that men do watch broadcasts with an allegedly 'feminine' content – romance, health, illness – and that they may come forward given appropriate means and incentives.

4. 'Interpretation' is used here in its largest sense – as including denotation, connotation and evaluation (see Palmer, 1995, chapter 3).

5. Another reason for the diversity of interpretations is that texts have many blanks (without which television would be impossible), which viewers who are knowledgeable about media grammar, routinely fill in (for instance, unless this is part of the plot, characters are not usually shown going from one place to the next, yet the public know that some travel has occurred) (see Iser, 1995).

6. It would, however, be hasty to conclude that all medical dramas are equal: one informant trusts *Peak Practice* more than *Casualty*, another is more confident if a helpline number is given at the end of the broadcast (Davin, 1999). In terms of health promotion, such questions have to be attended to at the formative research stage.

7. Soap operas have an ambivalent status. They started on American radio in the 1930s, sponsored by domestic cleaning products manufacturers eager to target housewives (hence their name). Replete with sentimental and familial storylines, they earned a reputation of being 'women's programmes', of triviality. In Britain soaps were part of the public service ethos and as such had a duty to inform and educate as well as to entertain (see Anger, 1999; Buckman, 1999). Nevertheless, the stigma endures: *I despise Casualty because it is a soap and not a medical drama* [Helen].

8. Two meanings of 'information' need to be distinguished: 'pedagogic' ('learning that') and 'instrumental' ('learning how to'). Whether television is an adequate medium through which to 'learn how to' do first-aid, for example, is a moot point (anecdotal reports of deaths following attempts at resuscitation 'as shown on television' have appeared in newspapers).

9. This jars with the previously mentioned concern for medical authenticity. The *ER* production team constantly oscillated between the requirements of 'authenticity' and of 'drama' (Pourroy, 1996), although the medicine *per se* seems to have remained, on the whole, accurate (notwithstanding minor details).

10. Most UK medical dramas employ medical advisers, and early ones were overseen by medical associations (Karpf, 1988). Some topics are heavily censored on American networks (see Kingsley, 1990).

11. For other examples of pre-set groups collapsing at analysis, see Schlesinger et al. (1992), Dahlgren (1986), Corner, Richardson and Fenton (1990).

12. Machin and Carrithers (1996) and Liebes (1997), amongst others, show how different identity segments come into play according to the situation and contribute to different interpretations.

13. A large and fascinating body of work on the meanings of health and illness is available in the anthropology and sociology of medicine (see, for example, Calnan, 1987; Blaxter, 1990; Herzlich, 1973).

14. For other examples, see Smith, Flowers and Osborn (1997) on arthritis, Cain (1991) on alcoholism, BSC (1997) on disability.

15. Other identities are known to play a role in (interpretations of) health and illness: e.g. gender (Cornwell, 1984; Saltonstall, 1993), age (Quadrel et al., 1993), class (d'Houtaud and Field, 1984).

16. On the role of television in identity construction, see Buckingham (2000), Fisherkeller (1999), and Steele and Brown (1995).

REFERENCES

Adams, S., Pill, R. and Jones, A., 'Medication, Chronic Illness and Identity', *Social Science and Medicine*, 45:2 (1997), pp. 189–201.

Ang, I., *Watching Dallas* (London: Routledge, 1991).

Anger, D., *Other Worlds* (Toronto: Broadview, 1999).

BAC (Brooks Advisory Centre), 'When you meet someone you really like, you don't think of AIDS...' (London: BAC, 1999).

Barrère, I., Desgraupes, P. and Lalou, E., *En direct de la médecine* (Paris: Stock, 1976).

Barthes, R., *S/Z* (Paris: Éditions du Seuil, 1970).

Baudin, R., 'Le Phénomène de la série culte en contexte soviétique et post-soviétique', *Cahiers du monde russe*, 42:1 (2001), pp. 49–70.

Baudrillard, J., *Simulacres et simulation* (Paris: Gallimard, 1981).

Bausinger, H., 'Media Technology and Daily Life', *Media, Culture and Society*, 6 (1984), pp. 343–51.

Blaxter, M., *Health and Lifestyles* (London: Tavistock, 1990).

Brown, W. J. and Basil, M. D., 'Media Celebrities and Public Health', *Health Communication*, 7:4 (1995), pp. 345–70.

BSC (Broadcasting Standards Council), 'The Disabled Audience: a Television Survey', in A. Pointon and C. Davies (eds), *Framed – Interrogating Disability in the Media* (London: British Film Institute, 1997).

Buckingham, D., *Public Secrets* (London: British Film Institute, 1987).

Buckingham, D., *Moving Images* (Manchester: Manchester University Press, 1997).

Buckingham, D., *After the Death of Childhood* (Manchester: Manchester University Press, 2000).

Buckman, P., *All for Love* (London: Secker & Warburg, 1984).

Cain, C., 'Personal Stories: Identity Acquisition and Self-Understanding in Alcoholics Anonymous', *Ethos*, 19 (1991), pp. 210–50.

Calnan, M., *Health and Illness: The Lay Perspective* (London: Tavistock, 1987).

Cassata, M. B., 'The Soap Opera', in B. G. Rose (ed.), *Television Genres* (London: Greenwood Press, 1985).

Corner, J., Richardson, K. and Fenton, N., *Nuclear Reactions* (London: John Libbey, 1990).

Cornwell, J., *Hard-Earned Lives* (London: Tavistock, 1984).

Crawford, R., 'The Boundaries of the Self and the Unhealthy Other', *Social Science and Medicine*, 38:10 (1994), pp. 1347–65.

Crowther, B., 'Comedy, the Breast and the Knife', in N. Moody and J. Hallam (eds), *Medical Fictions* (Liverpool: John Moores University Press, 1998).

Cull, N. J., 'Bigger on the Inside…: Dr Who as British Cultural History', in G. Roberts and P. M. Taylor (eds), *The Historian, Television and Television History* (Luton: University of Luton Press, 2001).

Cumberbatch, G. and Negrine, R., *Images of Disability on Television* (London: Routledge, 1992).

Dahlgren, P., 'The Modes of Reception', in P. Drummond and R. Paterson (eds), *Television in Transition* (London: British Film Institute, 1986).

Davin, S., *Casualty: Reception Study of a Medical Drama* (London: Le Drac, 1999).

Davin, S., 'Medical Dramas as Health Promotion Resource – an Exploratory Study', *International Journal of Health Promotion and Education*, 38:3 (2000), pp. 109–12.

Davin, S., 'Healthy Viewing: the Reception of Three Medical Narratives', in C. Seale (ed.), *Media and Health: Ninth Monograph of the Sociology of Health and Illness Journal* (Oxford: Blackwell, 2003).

Davin, S., *Urgences: Les Spectateurs* (Paris: L'Harmattan, 2004).

Deacon, D., Pickering, M., Golding, P. and Murdock, G., *Researching Communications* (London: Edward Arnold, 1999).

d'Houtaud, A. and Field, M. G., 'The Image of Health', *Sociology of Health and Illness*, 6 (1984), pp. 30–53.

Duff, K., *The Alchemy of Illness* (London: Virago, 1994).

Elkamel, F., 'The Use of Television Series in Health Education', *Health Education Research*, 10:2 (1995), pp. 225–32.

Fisherkeller, J., 'Learning about Power and Success: Young Urban Adolescents Interpret Television Culture', *The Communication Review*, 3:3 (1999), pp. 187–212.

Fiske, J., *Media Matters* (Minneapolis: University of Minneapolis Press, 1995).

Gabbay, J., 'Asthma Attacked?' in P. Wright and A. Treacher (eds), *The Problem of Medical Knowledge* (Edinburgh: Edinburgh University Press, 1982).

Gerbner, G. and Gross, L., 'Living with Television: the Violence Profile', *Journal of Communication*, 26:2 (1976), pp. 173–99.

Gibbs, H. and Ross, A. D., *The Medicine of ER* (London: HarperCollins, 1996).

Gottlieb, V., 'Brookside', in G. W. Brandt (ed.), *British Television Drama in the 1980s* (Cambridge: Cambridge University Press, 1993).

Hagen, I., *News Viewing Ideals and Everyday Practices* (Bergen: University of Bergen, 1992).

Herzlich, C., *Health and Illness* (London: Academic Press, 1973).

Hill, A., *Shocking Entertainment* (Luton: University of Luton Press, 1999).

Hobson, D., *Crossroads* (London: Methuen, 1982).

Iser, W., 'Interaction between Text and Reader', in A. Bennett (ed.), *Readers and Reading* (London: Longman, 1995).

Karpf, A., *Doctoring the Media* (London: Routledge, 1988).

KFF (Kaiser Family Foundation), 'Documenting the Power of Television – a Survey of Regular *ER* Viewers', at www.kff.org/content/archive/1358/ers.html (1997).

Kingsley, H., *Soap Box* (London: Macmillan, 1988).

Kingsley, H., *Prisoner Cell Block H* (London: Boxtree, 1990).

Kingsley, H., *Casualty* (London: BBC/Penguin, 1995).

Kitzinger, J., 'Resisting the Message', in D. Miller, J. Kitzinger, K. Williams and P. Beharell (eds), *The Circuit of Mass Communication* (London: Sage, 1998).

Liebes, T., *Reporting the Arab–Israeli Conflict* (London: Routledge, 1997).

Liebes, T. and Katz, E., *The Export of Meaning* (London: Polity, 1993).

Lippman, W., *Public Opinion* (New York: Free Press, 1921–97).

Machin, D. and Carrithers, M., 'From "interpretive communities" to "communities of improvisation"', *Media, Culture and Society*, 18 (1996), pp. 343–52.

MacMahon, J., 'Imaginary Learners', in M. Meyer (ed.), *Educational Television* (Luton: John Libbey, 1997).

Meyer, M., 'Introduction', in M. Meyer (ed.), *Educational Television* (Luton: John Libbey, 1997).

Morley, D., *The Nationwide Audience* (London: British Film Institute, 1980).

O'Keefe, I., '"It's not like Frasier": Service Users' Experiences of NHS Therapy', *Journal of Contemporary Health*, 8 (1999), pp. 49–54.

Palmer, J., *Potboilers* (London: Routledge, 1995).

Pasquier, D., *La Culture des sentiments* (Paris: Maison des Sciences de l'Homme, 1999).

Philo, G., *Media and Mental Distress* (London: Routledge, 1996).

Poole-Hayward, J., *Consuming Pleasures* (Lexington: University Press of Kentucky, 1997).

Pourroy, J., *Behind the Scenes at ER* (London: Ebury Press, 1996).

Press, A. L., 'Class, Gender and the Female Viewer', in M. E. Brown (ed.), *Television and Women's Culture* (London: Sage, 1991).

Quadrel, M. J., Fischoff, B. and Davies, W., 'Adolescent (In)vulnerability', *American Psychologist*, 48:2 (1993), pp. 102–16.

Rapp, R., 'Chromosomes and Communication', *Medical Anthropology Quarterly*, 2:2 (1988), pp. 143–54.

Robinson, D., *The Process of Becoming Ill* (London: Routledge, 1971).

Rogers, D. D., 'Daze of Our Lives', in G. Dines and J. M. Hunez (eds), *Gender, Race and Class in the Media* (London: Sage, 1995).

Saltonstall, R., 'Healthy Bodies, Social Bodies: Men's and Women's Concepts and Practices of Health in Everyday Life', *Social Science and Medicine*, 36:1 (1993), pp. 7–14.

Schlesinger, P., Dobash, R. E., Dobash, R. P. and Weaver, C. K., *Women Viewing Violence* (London: British Film Institute, 1992).

Seiter, E., 'Making Distinctions in Television Audience Research', in H. Newcomb (ed.), *Television: The Critical View* (Oxford: Oxford University Press, 1994).

Singhal, A. and Rogers, E. M., *Entertainment-Education* (Mahwah, NJ: Erlbaum, 1999).

Smith, J. A., Flowers, P. and Osborn, M., 'Interpretative Phenomenology Analysis and the Psychology of Health and Illness', in L. Yardley (ed.), *Material Discourses of Health and Illness* (London: Routledge, 1997).

Steele, J. R. and Brown, J. D., 'Adolescent Room Culture', *Journal of Youth and Adolescence*, 24:5 (1995), pp. 551–76.

Strauss, A. L. and Corbin, J., *Basics of Qualitative Research* (London: Sage, 1990).

Tulloch, J., *Television Drama* (London: Routledge, 1990).

Turnock, R., *Interpreting Diana* (London: British Film Institute, 2000).

Wellcome Trust, 'A Review of Science Communication and Public Attitudes to Science in Britain', at www.wellcome.ac.uk/en/1/mismiscnepubpat.html (2000).

Woolley, B., *Virtual Worlds* (Oxford: Blackwell, 1993).

Health Promotion Campaigns for Ethnic Minority Groups: the Case of the Radio Campaign for Asian Populations in the UK

2

Yumiko Doi

Introduction

Britain is a multi-ethnic and multicultural society. According to the population census of England and Wales in 1991, the minority ethnic population[1] was almost 2.95 million; this represents 6 per cent of the total population (Balarajan and Raleigh, 1992). As many researchers have already highlighted, the original cultures, religions and lifestyles of these minorities differ, and this cultural difference is one of the major concerns for health service sectors (Arora et al., 2000; Henley and Schott, 1999; Nazroo, 1997). In a multicultural society, differences associated with culture affect different viewpoints with regard to the causes and treatments of ill health. Moreover, those cultural differences affect perceptions about the timing of seeking treatment, who to consult, and the appropriate treatment regimes to be undertaken (Henley and Schott, 1999).

Henley and Schott (1999, p. 23) note that 'health care is likely to be more effective when the beliefs, values and norms of both patient and professional are recognised and taken into account'.

There have been many considerations of ethnic minority health in Britain. However, research concerning this particular aspect is still limited. Nazroo (1997) points out that ethnic minority health study focuses on understanding the disease process rather than the cultural position of ethnic minority groups, and therefore, researchers of ethnic minority health are likely to focus on particular diseases which show a high prevalence among those groups, such as coronary heart disease. Here the emphasis is on enumerating pathologies rather than understanding the cultural, social and economic conditions which have an impact upon health. This can be contrasted with Kwan and Williams (1998, p. 188), who point out that:

cultural beliefs, together with perceptions of health, lifestyle, traditional health care practices and disease susceptibilities can have a profound effect on uptake of services among some minority ethnic populations and on the interactions with 'western' health professionals.

A comprehensive promotion strategy for ethnic minority health in Britain is confined and limited by the availability of resources, a situation that is reflected in the other fields of the health service sector. Bhopal and Donaldson (1988) assert that the priorities of health education/promotion programmes for ethnic minority groups are very narrow, attention being directed primarily to issues such as birth control, pregnancy and childcare. More than a decade later, one of the leading organisations in health promotion, the Health Development Agency (formerly Health Promotion England), focuses on health promotion for ethnic minority groups. However, the areas of concern are still narrowly selected, in this case being confined to issues such as alcohol, children and families, drugs, immunisation, and sexual health. These target areas do not make any allowance for cultural difference associated with ethnic minority groups, thus, there is no real differentiation made between these groups and the majority white population (Health Promotion England, 2002). In other words, in spite of the diversity of cultural, religious and social backgrounds prevalent among ethnic minority groups, and associated differences in health issue focus, the objectives of health promotion campaigns are still based on the established paradigm of the majority population. In addition, the numbers of such campaigns for ethnic minority groups are still relatively small, especially at the national level. As a consequence of these limitations, health promotion campaigns for ethnic minority groups are still likely to be designed and conducted without 'purpose-built' guidelines, the references used being drawn from existing health promotion methods, developed from experiences with majority populations.

For example, the use of the mass media is one of the most popular methods used in relation to conducting health campaigns for ethnic minority groups,[2] even though the effectiveness of this methodology is still controversial among health promoters (Gatherer et al., 1979; Klapper, 1960; Naidoo and Wills, 1999; Swinehart, 1997; Tones, 1993). One question to be addressed with regard to this usage is whether these health promotion methods – which have been used for recent health promotion campaigns (such as media health promotion) for ethnic minority groups – are suitable for the specific target populations. Do such methods act to encourage preventative actions (health-seeking behaviours) for better health within those populations?

The intention of this chapter is to discuss the above question through the lens of an actual ethnic health promotion campaign in the UK, the so-called *Malaria Radio Campaign*. An analysis of the methodologies used in this campaign, and the resultant outcomes, will act to highlight some of the advantages and disadvantages of adopting recent health promotion methods (majority population standards) in relation to those ethnic minority groups.

Case study: the Malaria Radio Campaign backgrounds

The Malaria Radio Campaign was based on the feasibility report for *The Malaria Awareness Project within Asian Populations in the UK*, a report that aimed to decrease the risks of imported malaria in the UK (Skidmore et al., 2001). The report identified that Pakistani populations, who are regular travellers between malarious countries and the UK, were generally knowledgeable about malaria transmission, but were not likely to take any precautions. The reasons for refusing to take precautions were reported as follows: (1) misunderstandings of the human immune system (such as being unaware that any immunity will be lost within a year's time); (2) no time to seek travel advice, due to frequent emergency travels; (3) the high cost of anti-malarials in the UK. Taking into consideration these findings, the Department of Health (DoH) planned to conduct a health promotion campaign in collaboration with Manchester Metropolitan University in order to encourage Asian populations to take precautions prior to their travel to Pakistan.

Content of the campaign

A private commercial advertising company, in consultation with the DoH, designed and made a radio advertisement as a major tool for this campaign. The radio advertisement contained the following information:

- In the UK, two thousand cases of malaria infection were reported in the year 2000;
- Any natural immunity will be lost within a few months if one continuously lives in the UK;
- A malaria-infected person has a high risk of transmitting malaria to other members in a community even within the UK;
- It is important to take anti-malaria medicine, and to use insect repellent whenever one goes to one's country of origin.

The information contained in the first three points was combined with ethnic music, and the last message was presented without musical accompaniment. This radio advertisement was translated into Hindu, Urdu and Bengali with the same structure (music and information).

The total length of the radio advertisement was approximately 30 seconds. The advertisement was broadcast via four ethnic radio stations in order to cover the major ethnic minority habituates, i.e. the Greater Manchester area, the Yorkshire area, and the Greater London and Midland areas. The advertisement was broadcast 3–4 times per day, morning and night, in December 2000, for four weeks; it appeared as an advertisement between scheduled radio programmes.

Evaluation of the campaign

The radio advertisement campaign was initially evaluated quarterly in the national anti-malarials prescriptions.[3] This data was used in order to examine the change in peoples' behaviour, which represented the overall aim of the campaign. In establishing an experimental design, the data examined trends before and after the radio campaigns, and between the same period in the years 2000 and 2001. There was no significant difference in the number of prescriptions before and after the radio advertisement campaign, in terms of the results of a chi-square test. Additionally, there was no significant trend in the prescription of anti-malaria medicine in the same quarter (Jan.–Mar.) in 2000 and 2001. This indicated that the radio advertisement did not affect peoples' behaviour in relation to seeking anti-malarials.

The second body of data was collected through questionnaires. The informants were recruited from Manchester (the Vice-Consulate of Pakistan and the Pakistan Community Centre), Sheffield (the Pakistan Advice Centre) and London (the Pakistan Community Centre, and the Asian Community Centre). A total of 127 completed questionnaires were used for this analysis.

In spite of the high audience figures for ethnic programming in general, and their listening consistency during the specific times when the malaria radio advertisement was broadcast, the recognition of the malaria advertisement was extremely low (only 2 out of 78 ethnic radio programme listeners). In addition to this result, 69.2 per cent of informants who travelled to Pakistan *after* the radio campaign failed to take anti-malaria medicine for preventive purposes.[4]

These results show that the radio advertisement was not broadly recognised, and thus the effect of the campaign upon changing the Asian population's behaviour was not significant. As a health promotion campaign project, the Malaria Radio Campaign did not achieve its aim.

Discussion: the reasons for the campaign's failure

Methodology

The most appropriate way to discover the reasons for the failure of this campaign is to re-examine its design process. In this section, I would like to rethink the Malaria Radio Campaign in terms of a critical analysis of its underlying theories and concepts, and of the empirical data obtained from qualitative research (in-depth interviews and group discussions) conducted among Pakistani populations in the period after the campaign.

The informants for the research were chosen from Sheffield (the Pakistan Advice Centre) and London (the Pakistan Community Centre, the Asian Community Centre). This qualitative research was conducted to identify the suitability of design, especially in the choice of channels, message-delivery styles and message design. The informants were asked to listen to the recorded radio advertisement in a quiet room, and were interviewed using pre-structured questions concerning the above points, in an informal environment. The structures for undertaking in-depth interviews and group discussion were similar. Ten Pakistani participants were recruited for in-depth interviews, and ten were recruited for each of the two group discussions. The interviews were recorded and transcribed for analysis using a quasi-statistical content-analysis method. The details of this analysis are available elsewhere (see Doi, 2002; 2003).[5]

Overall issues of the campaign: starting points for discussions

One major disadvantage of this radio campaign was the lack of a systematic design plan. Perhaps the first thing we should consider in examining this campaign in terms of health promotion methodology is to explore its theoretical/conceptual background. In order to do this, Atkin's guidelines for designing mass-media health promotion were used (Atkin, 2001). Taking into consideration these guidelines, Table 2.1 contains the author's summary of the Malaria Radio Campaign.

At a glance, the basic methodology uses a general health promotion paradigm. However, it is clear that there is still controversy over the effectiveness of some of the methods used. These are as follows:

1 the choice of channels (radio);
2 the delivery style of the message (one-sided content);
3 the entertainment method (using music for message delivery).

Other researchers have discussed the problems associated with these points, such as the effect of single media use (Atkin, 2001), and the entertainment–education

Table 2.1 Summary of the Malaria Radio Campaign

Points in the guideline discussion	The Malaria Radio Campaign plan
1 Target audiences	Asian populations in the UK as frequent travellers to malarious countries, e.g. India, Bangladesh, Pakistan
2 Target responses	To take precautions against malaria
3 Types of campaign messages	• **Awareness** of the risk of importing malaria and the importance of using precautions • **Persuasion** to use precautions
4 Channels	Radio (advertisement)
5 Quantitative dissemination factors	A few times per day between 6 a.m. and 9 p.m., for four weeks
6 Message design	• Incentive appeals with numerical evidence (providing the numbers of cases of imported malaria in the UK, the transmission process of malaria, and available types of precautions) • One-sided content • Entertainment method (using traditional music for message delivery in order to gain attention)

strategy (Singhal and Rogers, 2001). Interestingly, these same issues emerged from the qualitative research results for the Malaria Radio Campaign. They were:

1 the finding that radio is not an appropriate message tool;
2 criticism of the music used for the advertisement;
3 criticism of the 'spoon-fed' message-delivery style.

This consistency provides a hypothesis: that ethnic minority target populations would react similarly to a media health promotion campaign targeted at a major population. How did the minority ethnic groups describe these issues from their own perspectives? Did they, in fact, consider those issues from a perspective similar to that of the major population?

Point I   Choice of channels: Do media products influence everybody?

The first question is whether the choice of 'radio' was appropriate for this health campaign. Because of their powerful impact on society, the mass media have been recognised as among the most effective tools for health promotion for a long time (Backer et al., 1992; Flora and Cassady, 1990; Naidoo and Wills, 1999; Rendall and Jacobson, 1987). The use of mass media is also considered to be effective for health promotion directed at ethnic minority groups. There are two main reasons why health promoters have been attracted to mass media for ethnic minority health promotion: one is the 'penetration' of the health message to people who are relatively difficult to contact at health facilities; the second is associated with breaking through the communication barriers. Choosing radio for this malaria campaign was consistent with these two aims.

Ewles and Simnett (1999) note that the most significant advantage of the mass media for health promotion is the capacity to quickly establish channels of communication to large numbers of people who are often likely to be both ill defined demographically, and geographically scattered. In dealing with the situation of ethnic minority groups, this is a huge advantage. Nazroo (1997) notes that ethnic minority groups use less varied health services than white populations. This means that these groups are more likely to include a number of people who have not received direct health information from the health service sectors, and that even those who access health services receive limited information with regard to the specific service areas. In this sense, the choice of radio for the Malaria Radio Campaign seemed to be suitable for accessing hidden numbers of minority groups, not only those who were not taking anti-malarials, but also those who had no knowledge of the benefit of prophylactics, for example.

Another advantage of mass media for health promotion is their variety: visual/verbal communication, such as TV and radio, are especially important in communicating both with the general population and with specific communities which might have some difficulties in communication, the obvious example being illiteracy. This is why mass media have been commonly used for health promotion/education in developing countries where the illiteracy rate is normally very high. Withington and Samsujjoha (2000) give their reason for choosing mass media (in this case, radio) for their health promotion in Bangladesh: 'the use of the mass media is limited by access but does not require literacy and possibly increases the authenticity of the message received' (Withington and Samsujjoha, 2000, p. 83).

Illiteracy is not a major problem among Pakistanis, except among elderly people in the UK (Health Education Authority, 1994; Modood, 1997). Communication barriers associated with language differences among (mainly non-English speaking) ethnic minority groups are, however, often identified as one of the major concerns for health services provision (Ewles and Simnett, 1999; Health Education Authority, 1994; Henley and Schott, 1999; Kwan and Williams, 1998). This causes several problems among ethnic minorities in relation to accessing health services. The Health Education Authority (1994) revealed that ethnic minority groups, especially women, had a high requirement for formal/informal interpreters at their GP's practice. Kwan and Williams (1998) also reported that Chinese communities in the UK were anxious about health practitioners' (in this case, dentists') understanding of patient needs, arising from poor communication. This situation causes poor access to dental services. These communication barriers are an important issue for ethnic health management. According to King et al. (1999, p. 104): 'culturally appropriate and specifically targeted campaigns in community languages have been found to be effective in reaching their target groups'.

At the same time, some health promoters have revealed that non-English-speaking ethnic minority groups, in a multicultural society, are likely to use multicultural mass media as their major information sources – especially the terrestrial tools (Alcalay et al., 1993: King et al., 1999; Zúñiga de Nacio et al., 1999). This is because of difficulties in understanding information in English, but also because of 'straight' (immediate and clear) understanding of information both verbally and visually in their own languages. Alcalay and co-workers noted that multicultural messages provide ethnic groups with 'a crisper and more to-the-point feeling than the English translation' (Alcalay et al., 1993, p. 361). From this evidence, it is possible to say that ethnic minority groups, especially among the first generation, are more comfortable communicating in their own languages when it comes to health issues. For the above reasons, health promoters focus on mass media as a preferred tool to deal with communication barriers because of their easy adaptability to various languages. This was also the reason for choosing radio for the Malaria Radio Campaign.

The choice of radio is, however, associated with many communication difficulties with regard to the Malaria Radio Campaign. First, radio is a questionable communication tool among the target populations. Their attention to radio programming is generally very poor (Alcalay et al., 1993). Even though the target populations were, indeed, likely to listen to ethnic radio programmes (as outlined by the evaluation) – the result of the quantitative analysis showing that 61.9 per cent (78 out of 127) listened to Asian radio stations, the majority of them being categorised as regular Asian radio listeners – many informants in this study said that they watched TV more than they listened to the radio. Indeed, informants at the Pakistan Advice Centre in Sheffield *laughed* when they were asked the question: 'Do you listen to radio?' This is because, according to them, radio is a *primitive* information source compared with TV. Some of the informants also informed the interviewer that they had set up satellite channels on their TV, and that this was a much better information and entertainment source because it provided more news concerning Pakistan (with visual images) than either terrestrial TV channels or radio. Therefore, the number of potential radio listeners is in question, and thus, so is the effectiveness of radio as a campaign tool.

These perceptions of radio also influenced their listening habits. The Pakistani participants who listened to the radio used this information source for a relatively short time, e.g. while commuting to/from their work places. Additionally, they were less likely to concentrate on information from radio because of other activities going on at the same time (Singhal and Rogers, 2001). Under these circumstances, it is understandable that they did not remember the content of each radio advertisement. Indeed, a female informant at the Pakistan Advice Centre in Sheffield described her difficulties in understanding the content of the radio advertisement within such a brief time frame. She pointed out that it was almost impossible, within the 30 seconds of a radio advertisement, to deliver a quality message to break communication barriers.

From this discussion, we can identify what radio means for the target populations; it is perceived as merely a type of 'background music' and represents a non-attractive information tool. Because of these two negatives, radio does not fulfil the previously mentioned criteria as a mass media information tool. First, it is difficult for the message to penetrate to the ethnic minority group, and secondly, breaking down communication barriers is in vain without drawing attention to the message contained within the advertisement. These findings indicate that one of the important reasons for the failure of the Malaria Radio

Campaign is a misunderstanding of the reality of the target population's use of radio. It is, indeed, impossible to adapt people's perceived habits in Pakistan to the Pakistani populations in the UK. These findings suggest that health promoters who would like to use mass media for campaigns have to be more aware of the theories and concepts of mass media communication as well as theories of health promotion.

Health promoters dealing with ethnic minority issues are likely to refer to previous health promotion campaigns, campaigns that have normally been conducted in different multicultural communities – this may lead to the possibility of using misleading and inconsistent strategies. For example, Zúñiga de Nacio and co-workers (1999) noted that 99% of the Latino population in California listened to Spanish-language-format radio stations. However, this kind of access is not applicable to other ethnic minorities in other countries. For example, in the UK, Sreberny (1999) reports that more than 70% of the ethnic minority populations that she interviewed have, and use, more than two TV sets, and over 35% of her informants use cable or satellite channels. Sreberny's report is also consistent with the information from Pakistani informants in this study. The trend in the use of mass media is likely to differ from community to community, depending on a number of factors.

McLuhan (1964), for example, notes that technological innovation in the media is itself an important media 'message'. In other words, as more sophisticated technology for communication is invented, more people seek this technology – otherwise, people will miss the most up-to-date information (a kind of threat). This is a discussion concerning media and society in general, which is also applicable to ethnic minority groups. Ethnic minority groups are often cut off from their countries of origin and therefore have great enthusiasm in seeking up-to-date information, especially when it concerns their country.

Taking this into consideration, one can understand why ethnic minorities are likely to have up-to-date mass media tools (as long as they can afford them), and do not tend to use radio as a major information source. The comment, 'radio is a primitive tool', from a Pakistani informant in this study supports this tendency of media usage in the UK. This study was conducted after 11 September 2001, when Muslims, including Pakistanis, began to seek up-to-date information more enthusiastically than ever before, because of their home countries' possible involvement in international politics.

These findings indicate that strategies in the use of mass media for ethnic minority health campaigns is not only an important topic within health promotion methodology, but also an issue of debate in relation to mass media in general, being associated, as it is, with the users' lifestyles and social situation. Interestingly, the ethnic minority groups' enthusiasm for using mass media is not very different from that of the major population. This fact can only be understood in relation to detailed feasibility research into social trends and the lifestyles of mass media users. This means that health promoters need to pay attention to these aspects of ethnic minority society in order to conduct effective mass media health campaigns. This point will be discussed in more detail in the next section.

Point 2   Message delivery: Is a taste for the 'oriental' favoured by ethnic minorities?

The second issue to be considered is the delivery style of the message. One of the most important tasks for media health campaigns is to gain the target populations' attention. The delivery system for this campaign was designed as a combination of the message and traditional music that was seen as reflecting the target populations' cultural and social background. This is based on 'the entertainment–education strategy', which combines the use of entertainment (e.g. drama, songs etc.) and educational approaches in order to increase the audience's knowledge of a particular health issue, the desired effect being to create a favourable attitude and to change behaviour (Singhal and Rogers, 2001; Storey et al., 1999). This type of message-delivery system is popular for media health campaigns for ethnic minority groups. For example, Zúñiga de Nacio and fellow workers (1999) used two types of radio advertisement, using Spanish nursery lyrics combined with music in order to deliver immunisation information for children in the Latino population of California. As a result, the target population favoured the message-delivery style because of the advertisement's use of music, song and rhythm. As this example shows, using the target population's ethnic taste is one of the favoured message-delivery styles used by health promoters. However, the same type of message delivery for the Malaria Radio Campaign worked negatively, the informants being especially critical about the traditional music used.

The most important reaction from the target populations indicated that they were likely to be offended by this particular message-delivery method. Many informants noted the general popularity of the music used for this radio advertisement. However, their common opinion was that the music did not provide listeners with a serious image of health. As a consequence, listeners were not aware of the advertisement as a health warning. At the same time, many informants described their negative opinions concerning the radio advertisement (information with music) in terms of its being too 'childish'. During interviews, some informants sneered at the advertisement after the researcher played it, describing it as 'childish', 'too easy', or 'patronising'. In short, a combination of message and traditional music was not favoured; rather, it created feelings of offence among the target populations.

The reasons for the offended feelings created by the radio advertisement are intimately related to the social and cultural aspects of ethnic minority groups. One aspect is based on their social and cultural position in the UK and the second concerns their health-related behaviour. As Mirza (2000) discussed, ethnic minorities, including Asians, are struggling with long-standing western myths,[6] such as their intellectual inferiority to whites. In order to oppose such myths, Asian parents encourage their children to obtain higher educational degrees, with the result that the number of those who obtain British formal higher degrees matches the white population (Mirza, 2000; Modood, 1997; Skellington et al., 1992). However, overall, their social conditions are not as good as those of the white population: for example, ethnic minority groups have a higher unemployment rate (Modood, 1997). This history, and the issue of challenging social myths and images, seems to stimulate strong reaction against being treated in a childish way. The words used by informants concerning the advertisement ('childish', 'too easy', 'patronising') support this explanation. In addition, their attitude, such as in sneering at the advertisement, is evidence of the hidden resentment against this intellectual assault or implied reduction in their status as adults.

The informants' negative behaviour towards the radio advertisement accompanied by music also relates to their attitude towards health. Skidmore and his co-workers concluded that Pakistanis in the UK may give low priority to health as an issue (Skidmore et al., 2001). However, once they have a health problem, they are more likely to seek professional advice in health centres than any other ethnic groups (except Bangladeshis) in the UK (Health Education Authority, 1994; Nazroo, 1997). This tendency suggests that they do not give low priority to 'health issues', but they do give low priority to 'preventive medicine'. They perceive that health issues are a very serious matter.

To return to the process of designing this radio campaign, it is questionable whether health promoters thought about the deep social and cultural feelings of the target population and their ideas about health when adopting the 'entertainment–education strategy'. The applied message-delivery style reveals the different perspectives on 'ethnicity' held by health promoters and their target populations.

This 'gap' between the Authority's perceptions of ethnic minority groups and the ethnic minority's actual requirements reminds one of the famous debate in post-colonial theory between Edward Said and Gayatri Spivak (Moore-Gilbert, 1997). In this debate, Spivak highlights the difference in identity between ethnic minority groups who were forced slaves before 1850, and those who were voluntary migrants after the Second World War. The target populations who are the recent focus for health services in general in the UK are in exactly the same position as the latter black population. Their ideas concerning their ethnic backgrounds would tend not to be 'nostalgic' in relation to their country of origin. Their idea of 'ethnicity' is a more complicated matter, concerning their identity and social position in UK society, rather than nostalgia.

Importantly, the mass media contribute greatly towards the creation of this sensitivity 'gap' between the idea of 'ethnicity' among ethnic minorities and the major populations' 'stereotypical' images emanating from media products (e.g. soaps, advertisements). The media are likely to support stereotypical ideas adopted by the major populations in relation to minority groups (Dyer, 1993; Hall, 1997), such as that all owners of corner shops are Asians (Sreberny, 1999). Sreberny reports that ethnic minority viewers complain about ethnic minority actors' roles that seem to represent 'typical' ethnic identities and social situations, such as lower-class and unemployed black men in soap operas. The Broadcasting Standards Commission (2001) also reports the tendency towards stereotypical portrayals of ethnic minority groups – such as their involvement in criminal activities; the idea of using ethnic music in relation to ethnic minority groups establishes the same kind of 'stereotypical understanding' of ethnic groups. In short, no consideration is given to the complexities of social conflict within the minority group or, indeed, the minority ethnic population as a non-homogeneous group.

The findings of this case study suggest that health promoters should establish a wider perspective on ethnic minority groups, not only in the field of health, but when considering the concept of the 'ethnic community'. There needs to be a special awareness of the effects of mass media upon the creation of the 'social image' in relation to ethnic minorities. Mass media are not only a tool for message delivery, but also contribute towards social image and social structure (Dyer, 1993; Hall, 1997). If health promoters do not consider this complex inter-relationship between mass media and ethnic minority groups, the health message will not be accepted by these communities. Rather, it will contribute towards the creation of social offence and therefore rejection by the target populations.

Point 3   Overall design of the message: Is the content of the message appropriate for the target populations?

The last issue associated with this radio advertisement campaign is the content of the message. The message was designed to take account of the target populations' potential knowledge of malaria, i.e. they are highly knowledgeable regarding basic information about malaria, such as its transmission process. As a result, the message was created simply to provide information concerning numerical facts, such as the number of cases of imported malaria, and misunderstood facts, such as the immunity to malaria (Atkin, 2001). However, the message design was not consistent with the target populations' requirements regarding a health message given via radio.

First, the information given was 'too basic' to promote prophylactic use against malaria within a population of already experienced and frequent travellers. Indeed, many informants expressed their views about the advertisement using phrases such as, 'not enough', 'too simple', 'not new' or 'too general'. Their knowledge about malaria seems to be associated with information from their families and relatives, or their own experiences. Although there may be very limited knowedge about malaria in the UK,[7] people do have knowledge and experience of malaria in Pakistan. For example, some eradication campaigns have been conducted, such as the spraying campaign in Sheikhupura district (Rowland et al., 2000), and the pyrethroid-impregnated bednets (PIBs) project in North-West Frontier Province (Rowland et al., 1999). However, the national malaria eradication campaign has declined in the country[8] since the 1960s. Additionally, the Ministry of Health provides health services for malaria at a very local level[9] as well as conducting eradication programmes, e.g. insecticide spraying. This daily familiarity with malaria in Pakistan is highly likely to provide enough knowledge and experience to UK-born Pakistani travellers when they visit their relatives in Pakistan. The results of feasibility research concerning informed knowledge of malaria among Pakistanis in the UK can be explained by this situation. The advertisement, however, does not contain any new information that would induce them to take precautions. It is, therefore, a problem of the under-estimation of the potential traveller's experiential knowledge related to Pakistan combined with the health promoter's poor knowledge of this situation.

Health promoters also need to examine and analyse the reasons why people do not take medication. The following quotation is from one of the informants:

When we decide to go back to Pakistan, for two or three years you save the money (travel costs).... If you go there with other family, it costs like £2000. And now you have to pay airport tax, and have to pay security tax...People do not want pay any extra money. There is no money left. Why do people want to pay their money for injections?...We know it is a very important thing to take injections, but everything requires some money. (female, the Pakistan Centre in London)

This description reveals that the health message in the Malaria Radio Campaign did not consider this fundamental aspect of the target population's health-seeking behaviours.

The second issue is the 'one-sided' content of the message. An informant at the Pakistan Community Centre in London suggested a 'Q&A' (Question and

Answer) type of radio message, such as: 'Are you planning to go to Pakistan?' 'Have you taken anti-malarials?' This type of introduction would, in the informant's opinion, encourage listeners' curiosity, and also give more time to 'absorb' the risks of malaria. During this study, some informants suggested that a debate or discussion programme would be a much better method to raise people's awareness of the risks of malaria, as well as to encourage them to take precautions. According to such informants, radio listeners (Pakistanis) can thus share the core issues with the participants of a debate programme, and can think about the solutions along with those participants. The same positive opinion towards debate emerged from a focus group discussion. According to the informants, the focus group discussion provided a better opportunity to become aware of the risks of malaria, and the participants said that they were willing to take precautions after that session. This is an interesting finding.

These results, again, expose the 'gap' between the health promoter's perspective on target population's social and cultural behaviours and the population's actual requirements. The target population seemed to be more aware of some of the disadvantages of mass media communication, e.g. the ineffectiveness of one-sided content, in changing people's behaviour.

Conclusion

To summarise, a number of conclusions can be drawn from this study in relation to the use of the mass media in health education campaigns for ethnic minority communities.

First, the issue of the gap between health educators' perceptions of target audiences and their actual health needs and experiences needs to be addressed. The mass media are often used as a 'catch all' method and this is far too simplistic.

The question of which media to use is also important. In this case the target population seemed to have strong opinions about the 'primitive' nature of radio as a medium, and also its one-sided nature.

Care and attention also needs to be paid to the content of the message, and message designs – in this case message presentation was often seen as 'patronising' and containing references to stereotypical images of minority groups in the media, as well as ignoring the target population's prior experiences of and knowledge about malaria.

Finally, health education studies from the 1970s and 1980s (Davis, 1987; Koselka et al., 1976) have raised the question of the sole use of mass media in this type of campaign and advanced the argument that health education campaigns designed to change behaviour need additional components such as face-to-face intervention and possibilities for dialogue around the issue under discussion.

Others have pointed out the complexities of planning campaigns aimed at behaviour change, especially with minority communities (Bracht, 1990; Wallack, 1981, 1990; Werbner, 1990). These issues were also raised by the participants in this study, all of which adds weight to the argument that, when planning mass-media health education campaigns for ethnic minority groups, prior consultation with and knowledge of the target audience is essential.

NOTES

1. In this study, an ethnic minority group is defined as 'a social group with a distinctive language, values, religion, customs and attitudes' (Henley and Schott, 1999, p. xxi). In addition to this, the term 'major populations' is defined as 'the white British'.
2. The majority of health education/promotion resources for ethnic minority groups in the UK are media-related materials, such as audiocassettes and videos (Health Education Authority, 1999).
3. There were no ethnic categorisations in this data set.
4. The results of this evaluation are shown in Doi (2002).
5. The details of that qualitative research can be seen in Doi (2002).
6. Herrnstein and Murray (1994) discussed the intellectual inferiority of ethnic minorities on the basis of data from IQ tests. However, Mirza (2000) opposed the results because of the inaccuracy of the IQ test.
7. The NHS, of course, provides advice concerning malaria for travellers.
8. Herrel and co-workers (2001) reported that the decline of the national malaria control programme was 'due to economic constraints since the eradication efforts of the 1960s' (Herrel et al., 2001, pp. 236–7).
9. Government health services are basically free of charge, but the majority of the Pakistani population use private health services or self-treatments because they know that government facilities only provide primitive treatments for them (Donnelly et al., 1997). This is also a good example of their efficient knowledge of the current malaria situation.

REFERENCES

Alcalay, R., Ghee, A. and Scrimshaw, S., 'Designing Prenatal Care Messages for Low-income Mexican Women', *Public Health Reports*, 108:3 (1993), pp. 354–62.

Arora, S., Coker, N., Gillam, S. and Ismail, H., *Improving the Health of Black and Minority Ethnic Groups: A Guide for Primary Care Organisations* (London: King's Fund, 2000).

Atkin, C. K., 'Theory and Principles of Media Health Campaigns', in R. Rice and C. K. Atkin (eds), *Public Communication Campaigns*, 3rd edn (London: Sage, 2001), pp. 49–68.

Backer, T. E., Rogers, E. M. and Sopory, P., *Designing Health Communication Campaigns: What Works?* (Newbury Park, CA: Sage, 1992).

Balarajan, R. and Raleigh, V. S., 'The Ethnic Population of England and Wales: the 1991 Census', *Health Trends*, 24 (1992), pp. 113–16.

Bhopal, R. S. and Donaldson, L. J., 'Health Education for Ethnic Minorities – Current Provision and Future Directions', *Health Education Journal*, 47 (1988), pp. 137–40.

Bracht, N. (ed.), *Health Promotion at the Community Level* (London: Sage, 1990).

Broadcasting Standards Commission, *The Representation of Minorities on Television: A Content Analysis*, Briefing update, no. 9 (2001).

Davis, A. M., 'Heart Health Campaigns', *Health Education Journal*, 39 (1987), pp. 74–9.

Doi, Y., 'Health Risk Behaviour: an Evaluation Report on the Malaria Radio Jingle Campaigns for Asian Populations in the UK', unpublished report for the Department of Health Care Studies, Manchester Metropolitan University, Manchester (2002).

Doi, Y., 'The Uses of Mass Media and Health Promotion Campaigns for Ethnic Minority Groups: a Case', MSc dissertation, Manchester Metropolitan University, Manchester (2003).

Donnelly, M. J., Konraden, F. and Birley, M. H., 'Malaria-treatment-seeking Behaviour in the Southern Punjab, Pakistan', *Annals of Tropical Medicine and Parasitology*, 91:6 (1997), pp. 665–7.

Dyer, R., *A Matter of Images: Essays on Representations* (London: Routledge, 1993).

Ewles, L. and Simnett, I., *Promoting Health: A Practical Guide*, 4th edn (Edinburgh: Baillière Tindall, 1999).

Flora, J. A. and Cassady, D., 'Roles of Media in Community-based Health Promotion', in N. Bracht (ed.), *Health Promotion at the Community Level* (London: Sage, 1990), pp. 143–57.

Gatherer, A., Parfit, J., Porter, E. and Vessay, M., *Is Health Education Effective?* (London: Health Education Council, 1979).

Hall, S., *Representation: Cultural Representations and Signifying Practices* (London: Sage, 1997).

Health Education Authority, *Health and Lifestyle: Black and Minority Ethnic Groups in England* (London: Health Education Authority, 1994).

Health Education Authority, *Health-related Resources for Black and Minority Ethnic Groups*, 2nd edn (London: Health Education Authority, 1999).

Health Promotion England (2002), www.hpe.org.uk

Henley, A. and Schott, J., *Culture, Religion and Patient Care in a Multi-ethnic Society: A Handbook for Professionals* (London: Age Concern England, 1999).

Herrel, N., Amerasinghe, F. P., Ensink, J., Mukhtar, M., Van Der Hoek, W. and Konradsen, F., 'Breeding of *Anopheles* Mosquitoes in Irrigated Areas of South Punjab, Pakistan', *Medical and Veterinary Entomology*, 15 (2001), pp. 236–48.

Herrnstein, R. J. and Murray, C., *The Bell Curve: Intelligence and Class Structure in American Life* (New York: Free Press, 1994).

King, L., Thomas, M., Gatenby, K., Geogiou, A. and Hua, M., ' "First Aid for Scalds" Campaign: Reaching Sydney's Chinese, Vietnamese, and Arabic Speaking Communities', *Injury Prevention*, 5 (1999), pp. 104–8.

Klapper, J. T., *The Effects of Mass Media Communication* (Glencoe: Free Press, 1960).

Koselka, K., Pushka, P. and Tuomilheto, J., 'The North Karelia Project: a First Evaluation', *International Journal of Health Education*, 19 (1976), pp. 59–66.

Kwan, S. Y. and Williams, S. A., 'Attitudes of Chinese People toward Obtaining Dental Care in the UK', *British Dental Journal*, 185:4 (1998), pp. 188–91.

McLuhan, M., *Understanding Media* (London: Routledge, 1964).

Mirza, H. S., 'Race, Gender and IQ: the Social Consequence of a Pseudo-scientific Discourse', in K. Owusu, (ed.), *Black British Culture and Society* (London: Routledge, 2000), pp. 295–310.

Modood, T., 'Qualifications and English Language', in T. Modood, R. Berthoud et al., *Ethnic Minorities in Britain: Diversity and Disadvantage* (London: Policy Studies Institute, 1997), pp. 60–82.

Moore-Gilbert, B., *Postcolonial Theory: Contexts, Practices, Politics* (London: Verso, 1997).

Naidoo, J. and Wills, J., *Health Promotion: Foundations for Practice*, 2nd edn (London: Baillière Tindall, 1999).

Nazroo, J. Y., 'Health and Health Services', in T. Modood and R. Berthoud (eds), *Ethnic Minorities in Britain: Diversity and Disadvantage* (London: Policy Studies Institute, 1997), pp. 224–58.

Rendall, M. and Jacobson, B., 'Health Promotion in England, Wales and Northern Ireland: a State of the Art', in C. Robins (ed.), *Health Promotion in North America: Implications for the UK* (London: King's Fund, 1987), pp. 121–30.

Rowland, M., Hewitt, S., Durrani, N., Saleh, P., Bouma, M. and Sondorp, E., 'Sustainability of Pyrethroid-impregnated Bednets for Malaria Control in Afghan Communities', *Bulletin of the World Health Organisation*, 75 (1999), p. xx.

Rowland, M., Mahmood, P., Iqbal, J., Carneiro, I. and Chavasse, D., 'Indoor Residual Spraying with Alphacypermethrin Controls Malaria in Pakistan: a Community-Randomized Trial', *Tropical Medicine and International Health*, 5:7 (2000), pp. 472–81.

Singhal, A. and Rogers, E. M., 'The Entertainment – Education Strategy in Communication Campaigns', in R. Rice and C. Atkin (eds), *Public Communication Campaigns*, 3rd edn (London: Sage, 2001), pp. 343–56.

Skellington, R., Morris, P. and Gordon, P., *'Race' in Britain Today* (London: Sage, 1992).

Skidmore, D., Shah, M., Bhatti, H. and Chaudhry, A., *Health Risk Behaviour: Knowledge and Uptake of Travel Prophylactics within an Asian Population: A Close-up of Malaria*, a project report, Manchester Metropolitan University, Manchester (2001).

Sreberny, A., *Include Me In* (London: Broadcasting Standards Commission, 1999).

Storey, D., Boulay, M., Karki, Y., Heckert, K. and Karmacharya, D. M., 'Impact of the Integrated Radio Communication Project in Nepal, 1994–1997', *Journal of Health Communication*, 4 (1999), pp. 271–94.

Swinehart, J. W., 'Health Behavior Research and Communication Campaigns', in D. S. Gochman (ed.), *Handbook of Health Behaviour Research IV: Relevance for Professionals and Issues for the Future* (New York: Plenum, 1997), pp. 351–73.

Tones, K., 'Changing Theory and Practice: Trends in Methods, Strategies and Settings in Health Education', *Health Education Journal*, 52 (1993), pp. 126–39.

Wallack, L., 'Mass Media Campaigns: the Odds against Finding Behavior Change', *Health Education Quarterly*, 8:3 (1981), pp. 209–60.

Wallack, L., 'Improving Health Promotion: Media Advocacy and Social Marketing Approaches', in C. Atkin and L. Wallack (eds), *Mass Communication and Public Health: Complexities and Conflicts* (London: Sage, 1990), pp. 147–62.

Werbner, P., *The Migration Process: Capital, Gifts and Offerings among British Pakistanis* (Providence, RI: Berg, 1990).

Withington, S. and Samsujjoha, R., 'Radio as a Means to Enhance Early Case Finding in Leprosy', *Leprosy Review*, 71:1 (2000), pp. 83–4.

Zúñiga de Nacio, M. L., Price, S. A., Tjoa, T., Lashuay, N., Connell Jones, M. and Elder, J. P., 'Pretesting Spanish-language Educational Radio Messages to Promote Timely and Complete Infant Immunization in California', *Journal of Community Health*, 24:4 (1999), pp. 269–84.

Performing Disability: Impairment, Disability and Soap Opera Viewing

3

Alison Wilde

Introduction

Images of impairment and disability

> Does television have any influence; does it matter what people watch?
> (Silverstone, 1994, p. 132)

Although disability has seldom been a focus of cultural and media studies criticism, the disabled people's movement has campaigned for more 'positive' portrayals in the media since the late 1980s. Disabled peoples' campaigns have made a fundamental contribution to theory and practice within disability studies theory on this and other concerns. Building upon these foundations, theorists such as Barnes (1990) and Oliver (1990) have asserted a 'social model' of disability, which designates disability as the social oppression of people with accredited impairments (Barnes et al., 1999). This has provided a valuable corrective to the ideological strength of the 'medical model' of disability, whereby the body is constructed as disabled. This individualistic perspective of disability dominates social, political and professional approaches to peoples' lives in western societies, pervading most aspects of disabled peoples' lives and perpetuating exclusion (see, for example, Barnes, 1991; Oliver, 1990). Media images of disability, impairment and normality have been seen as an important facet in the construction and maintenance of these beliefs, perpetuating discriminatory attitudes towards impairment and providing few sources of identification for disabled people (Kent, 1987; Kitzinger, 1993; Longmore, 1987; Morris, 1991; Pointon and Davies, 1997; Rieser and Mason, 1992; Ross, 1997; Shakespeare, 1994).

However, disability studies on representation have focused primarily on the content of various media rather than on its 'effects'. Stereotypes of impairment, alongside the exclusion of disabled people at all levels of the production process, have been seen as central factors in the perpetuation of disabling images in these studies. One thing is clear from this body of work. Disabled people have been portrayed in an individualistic manner within a medical model, which emphasises personal rather than social pathology. That is, the basis of these representations tends to reflect impairment-specific archetypes, which are, thus, easily generalised to denote homogeneous characteristics of recognisable impairment 'groups', or the wider population of disabled people. As such, characters with impairments are usually portrayed in predictable, often temporary, roles and with narrative placements used to convey moral stories or as dramatic 'hooks' (Shakespeare, 1999). Moreover, they are regularly cast as: victims, deviant, bitter, foolish, and in contexts of violence (Barnes, 1992; Biklen and Bogdan, 1977; Cumberbatch and Negrine, 1992; Norden, 1994). Unsurprisingly, members or organisations within the disabled people's movement have complained that there are few 'accurate' images of the 'real world' of disability or impairment in the media (see, for example, Darke, 1995: Ross, 1997). Furthermore, disabled people are rarely seen as part of a network or community of disabled people (Klobas, 1988).

These studies have successfully identified a number of such problems which resonate with disabled peoples' concerns (Darke, 1995; Ross, 1997), highlighting those which have emerged from the disabled people's movement. However, it is unclear how these images are read by disabled and non-disabled people. The taxonomical approaches that have predominated in disability studies literature have usually pointed to the existence of negative and positive images, obscuring the complexity of representations and their reception, such as the interpellation of different viewing (subject) positions or situations. For instance, Fiske (1987) asserts that many popular texts, and television in particular, are polysemic.

This has been recognised in the growth of audience studies. In particular, a number of television studies have demonstrated that viewers approach and read television texts with a wide range of interpretations (see, for example, Curran, 1990; Silverstone, 1994). Solange Davin's chapter elsewhere in this book provides another such example.

None the less, however ambiguous these portrayals may be, it is likely, judging from the (limited number of) disability-specific audience studies (Cumberbatch and Negrine, 1992; Darke, 1995; Ross, 1997) that few, if any, viewers gain pleasure from current images of disabled people. However, it is also clear that significant numbers of disabled people watch soap operas, where some of the most exploitative images are to be found (Cumberbatch and Negrine, 1992; Shakespeare, 1997). Therefore, in undertaking 'audience' research I set out to examine issues of cultural identity and position through an exploration of the ways in which both disabled and non-disabled television viewers make sense of images and narratives of impairment, disability and 'normality' within soap operas. Before exploring these viewing performances, audience concerns need to be contextualised within previous academic concerns.

Audience and the soap opera text

Here and now we must be able to enjoy life – if only to survive.

(Ang, 1985, pp. 135–6)

Where pleasure is personal, discourse is social.

(Nightingale, 1996, p. 82)

It has been argued that the soap opera genre is an exemplar of polysemic popular texts (Modleski, 1997) and, in many ways, this is evident in the variety of meanings extrapolated from *Dallas* in a variety of audience research projects (see, for example, Ang, 1985; Liebes and Katz, 1993). Indeed the late 1980s saw a burgeoning body of work investigating soap operas, which coincided with the turn towards 'the cultural studies audience experiment' (Nightingale, 1996, p. 59) and its emphasis on the symbiotic analysis of textual production and response, utilising Stuart Hall's (1980) Encoding/Decoding model.

There seem to be a range of other reasons for the academic interest in soap operas. Alongside football coverage, soap operas are the most ubiquitous 'texts' within contemporary culture, occupying prominent sites within the 'mediascape' (Appadurai, 1993), particularly on television and in the print media. This is especially true in Britain, but soap operas and 'telenovas' also play an important role in other cultures. Not only are they popular viewing in the United States of America and western Europe, they have also had a considerable impact in the countries of the former Soviet Union and Latin America (O'Donnell, 1999). Indeed, Hugh O'Donnell has suggested that politics can have a direct effect upon the trajectories of telenovas, which can, in turn, exert significant influence in the political realm. He suggests that the narrative of political corruption in the Venezuelan *Por estas calles* was a significant contribution to the deposition of the former president Carlos Andrés Pérez (O'Donnell, 1999).

As the most popular genre on British television, soap operas have an important role to play. Not only do they achieve the highest viewing figures, but Nelson (1996) suggests that the soap opera format has become the dominant television mode, adopted by other dramatic forms and leaking into factual programming via the docu-soaps. Increasingly adopted to further political goals (e.g. by public figures such as Tony Blair, and Fernando Collor de Melo, in the Brazilian elections of 1989 [O'Donnell, 1999]), they are often expected to have a strong cultural verisimilitude (again, see Solange Davin's chapter for further discussion of viewers' expectations of realism within *ER*).

As such, they are expected to portray social and individual lives in an accurate and informative manner whilst simultaneously providing entertainment or 'escape'. Indeed, the goal of portraying accurate representations of 'real' social worlds is far from straightforward, given the differences that are likely to exist between viewing positions within such a large audience and the impossibility of defining reality (see the Introduction to this book). Furthermore, even though interest groups complain about inaccuracies, this is often at odds with their requests for 'better' representations of specific social groups, For example, 'positive representations' of successful people may obscure discriminatory social practices.

Additionally, the soap opera is usually perceived to have a low aesthetic and moral worth (Alasuutari, 1995; O'Donnell, 1999). This is often linked to its popularity (Seiter, 1999) and is likely to be linked to its reputation as a woman's genre (Ang, 1985; Hobson, 1982; Kuhn, 1997; Mattelart, 1986; Modleski, 1997; Seiter, 1999), with its association with and denigration of viewers who are confined to the house. Challenging views of low cultural worth, the feminist scholars (cited above) have suggested that the genre has been undervalued as a source of women's pleasure and identification and that it can be seen to have progressive, even Brechtian (Brunsdon et al., 1997) potential. For example, in terms of its form, it is seen to have a discontinuous mode and interruptive strategies, which allows viewers to adopt the, often adversarial, positions of different characters rather than privileging the voices of those occupying leading roles. Thus, it is suggested that it is a heteroglot (multi-voiced) text (Holquist, 2002). Arguing that it has an open narrative structure, Kuhn (1997) suggests that it avoids the ideological closure that typifies classic, realist, narrative forms, found in some other popular media texts, such as cinema that follows the enigma–retardation–resolution structure. Moreover, Fiske (1987) describes such television genres as *associative*, prioritising the 'laws of association' as organising principles, rather than imposing a structure of cause and effect.

Hence, as a relatively open, heterglot text, it can be seen as a genre which provides potential for multiple and resistive readings.

Indeed, some feminist scholars have suggested that soap operas challenge conventional patriarchal or masculinist modes of subjectivity, where the viewer is expected to identify with the leading character. Modleski (1997) argues that feminine subject positions are constructed, particularly that of the ideal mother, possessing multiple, limited identifications. Ang (1996) suggests that these different identifications pose a challenge to fixed identities. She argues that female viewers gain their pleasure through fantasising different subject positions. She contends that this is made possible by stimulating the viewer's *melodramatic imagination*, which is believed to interact with *the tragic structure of feeling* of the soap opera genre. Furthermore, Kuhn (1997) has suggested that there is a correspondence between women's experience of time and daily living and the soap opera's unending form and competing and intertwining plot-lines (Cantor and Pingree, 1983). Similar observations could be made for other people who spend significant amounts of time in domestic contexts, for example, disabled people and young people.

Moreover, the easy accessibility of soap operas seems to give them a significant role in bringing isolated audiences together within a symbolic community (Ang, 1985), introducing people to a more heterogeneous range of people and social concerns than they would otherwise expect to meet. Indeed, they have been recognised as a popular topic for debate within a range of social contexts, providing a basis of common ground for a wide range of people (Abercrombie and Longhurst, 1998). Arguably, then, the soap opera has potential to be a valuable site for the introduction of marginalised or counter-hegemonic perspectives to a large audience, a position which has been increasingly recognised by campaigning groups and television companies (Allen, 1995) over recent years in calls for and research into official realism (O'Donnell, 1999).

However, the majority of academic approaches towards soap opera audiences have emphasised the value of women's pleasure and identification with female characters, rather than their wider political potential. As such, they privilege particularist explanations of personal experience and consumerist identities (Stevenson, 1995) over analysis of the dissatisfactions underlying the melodramatic imagination (Nightingale, 1996, pp. 80–2). At a wider level there seems to be little opportunity for the introduction of alternative discourses, because, as O'Donnell argues (1999), the macro-narratives of soaps, as a collective, tend to create a national transnarrative of cultural values. He proposes, for instance, that ideals of solidarity and social democracy are pre-eminent in Norway just as sobriety and emotional restraint predominate in Dutch soap operas. Although it is clear that there are great variations between countries I am proposing that the 'normality' discourse pervades all levels of soap opera, across cultures. Indeed, it is insidiously present at every level of narrative, even within the diachronic, i.e. evolutionary, *hypernarrative* (O'Donnell, 1999, p. 24) dimension of each soap.

Hence, the participation of disabled people in such pleasures is of particular concern. It is unsurprising that the indications are that disabled people (despite their reputations as 'heavy viewers') would prefer to avoid images of people with impairments (Darke, 1995), particularly in soap operas (Cumberbatch and Negrine, 1992).

So, in investigating popular media images of disability and impairment, two of the central questions I sought to answer were:

■ Can a medium which is lauded for its ability to provide pleasure actually do so for disabled people?
■ Do images of impairment and disability give disabled or non-disabled viewers pleasure?

In order to investigate the political import of soap opera texts, and impairment/disability images, I wanted to explore their reception within everyday life, in the domains where meaning is continuously re-created (Nightingale, 1996; Silverstone, 1994). Hence, I foregrounded textual creativity (Nightingale, 1996) and discourse analysis. To these ends, relationships between texts and issues relating to the articulation of identities and meaning have been contextualised within the social concerns that lie at the heart of disability studies projects.

The project

Discussing the futility of gauging whether people are active or passive viewers, Silverstone (1994, pp. 169–70) argued:

> We are confronted with a different kind of empirical problem, which is not to discover presence or absence, activity or passivity, but on the contrary to understand engagement.

Understanding more about engagement with media texts bridges some of the gaps between political and identity concerns but it also necessitates approaches that navigate routes between individual interpretations and collective forms of meaning-making. Therefore, discussions were examined as specimens of interaction, emphasising the situatedness of the speech and writing acts as social/cultural phenomena, where media are utilised as a resource in performing and articulating identities.

In setting up the project, I intended to examine the ways in which people are attached or disaffected by media portrayals in a variety of contexts. This created a starting point for several endeavours: understanding, for example, the inter-actions between the reception of media images and the identity articulations of disabled people and non-disabled people; the dialectics of the moralities of soap opera texts and everyday life; the facilitation or obstruction of a sense of inclusion and belonging to society and/or the community of disabled people.

Strategies of *mutual aid* (Liebes and Katz, 1993) have been emphasised, i.e. processes of collective meaning-making and negotiation. Primarily, conversations took place within discussion groups made up of people who met with their peers in their everyday environments. There were seven discussion groups, four of whom met several times over a six-month period. Each group had between four and eight members. The sample was comprised of the following groups:

(a)   women;
(b)   men;
(c)   disabled adults, recruited at a day centre;
(d)   young women (aged 13–14 years);
(e)   young men (14–16);
(f)   disabled young people (of both sexes) who attended a segregated school;
(g)   disabled and non-disabled members of a youth club (of both sexes).

All these groups were recruited in the same town.

Twenty-one diarists were recruited from the focus groups and elsewhere. Eight were from young people (two were disabled) and the other seven were from local adults of both sexes (four of whom were disabled). Seven of the diarists came from other towns throughout England. The diarists were invited to write their entries in their own style, contextualising their comments within their daily lives.

Following Liebes and Katz (1993), a coding framework was adopted which identified six main topic areas: motivations for action; moral debates; gender norms; sexuality and relations; body performance; disability and impairment. Additionally, Liebes and Katz's classifications of referential and critical discussion were adopted, organising the data into two main categories of (a) experience, and (b) in the case of critical discussion, semantic, syntactic and pragmatic criticisms of soap opera texts and production processes.

However, most importantly, Liebes and Katz's study provided a methodological framework that has been useful in differentiating between levels and types of emotional attachments that can be found amongst viewers. That is, it has helped to highlight how the interpretations and levels of emotional pleasure of different groups tend to vary in ways that can be attributed to significant differences in 'involvement' according to cultural and socio-political values and influences. Furthermore, the use of diaries and focus groups has aided hermeneutic exploration by highlighting the crucial role of viewing and discussion contexts. Before evaluating these responses in terms of some of the themes identified above, I will turn to a brief examination of the storylines which were most frequently discussed.

The texts

Most of the characters that were discussed were male, reflecting the predominance of disabled men within dramatic genres (Shakespeare, 1997). This may be due to reliance on the Oedipal framework as the primary structuring factor for all 'narrative media' (Norden, 1994, p. 323). However, whereas the Oedipal scenario usually forms an over-arching structure within media such as cinema and novels (*Screen*, 1992), this is usually played out at the meta-narrative (topical) level in soap opera. This is invariably achieved through the use of temporary impairments, and resolution of the story by a rewarding or the re-establishment of non-disabled identities, i.e. a return to the moral authority of the normality macro-narrative. Predominantly, disabled male characters are used in this way to convey moral messages. These are resolved in a redemptive or punitive manner which strengthens the portrayal of disabled men as 'castrated' and invariably involves women as agents of moral reform or objects of 'diseased lusts' (Norden, 1994). The character Jim McDonald's (*Coronation Street*) impairment narrative was the clearest (and most frequently cited by research participants) of the first of these tendencies, whereby his personality was transformed from 'bad' to 'good' in the process of acquiring, coming to terms with, and eventually losing his impairment. On the other hand, the character Don Brennan's (*Coronation Street*) impairment (amputation) could not be restored through cure so impairment and masculinity became closely linked with sexual deviancy and the disruption of the 'normal' moral order, which left no (Oedipal) resolution other than death.

Many temporary impairment narratives follow similar sequences of 'natural justice': impairment as punishment – bitterness and personal decline – redemption – reform – cure; although this process is inherently gendered. For instance, in *Brookside*, the most explicitly political of British soaps, 'Jaqui Dixon' and 'Sinbad' both had temporary, sensory, impairments but this sequence took quite different trajectories. Jaqui became more of a *sweet innocent*, protecting her 'corporeal integrity' as an attractive woman whilst simultaneously denying her sexual subjectivity and weakening her personal autonomy, being literally unable to possess or to return 'the gaze' (*Screen*, 1992), whereas the close timing of Sinbad's impairment story, with allegations of paedophile behaviour, reiterated the themes of diseased lusts (Norden, 1994).

Textual performance

> Audiences create but, like Marx nearly said of history, not on the basis of texts of their own making.
>
> (Silverstone, 1994, p. 151)

Discussion group participants chose to spend far more time on specific storylines within the three most popular British soap operas: *Eastenders*, *Coronation Street*, and *Emmerdale*. The diarists reported watching a much wider range, including Australian soap operas such as *Neighbours* and American shows including *ER* and *Sunset Beach*.

Heterosexual relationship dramas were the main focus in all except the two male groups, both of whom asserted a preference for watching sports and programmes involving more 'action'. The preference for talking about relationships was particularly true where the male protagonist was deemed to be dangerous and good looking, in stereotypically aggressive masculine ways.

Otherwise, the groups and diarists tended to focus on storylines which were close to their own personal concerns: the women's group were keen on discussing portrayals of women they interpreted as strong and independent, such as 'Kerry Weaver' (*ER*), a confident and assertive doctor in an accident and emergency ward who is characterised by her propensity to make challenging medical decisions. In a similar vein the young women's group spent much time discussing teenage pregnancy storylines (see below) and other topics relevant to their age range and sexual identifications. Many of these came from programmes targeted at this age group, such as drugs-related storylines from *Hollyoaks*. Romantic relationship storylines involving 'gorgeous' young male characters were also a common topic of conversation, in particular, 'Beppe Di Marco' and 'Jamie Mitchell' (*Eastenders*). The disabled groups also chose to focus on relationships between core (non-disabled) characters, with a similar emphasis on age range and sexual predilection.

The diaries involve no observable interaction with other people, even though many of them were contextualised with everyday situations. Hence, there were marked differences between participants' diary entries and focus group interactions. This was particularly true among disabled people. Diary keeping is more likely to encourage disclosure of feelings that people would be less likely to risk demonstrating in a group context, for instance, disabled people may fear appearing to be 'defeated and angry' (see Klobas, 1988). Indeed, whereas the disabled adults acquiesced to stereotyped portrayals more readily than any other groups, one disabled diarist, Peter, wrote:

> Images of disabled people in soaps invariably make me feel worse about myself because they accentuate a negative sense of difference: – the disabled person/character exists by virtue of their disability or impairment – and seems to exist for that reason alone.

Non-disabled male participants, within the group, usually situated themselves as 'professional men' or 'providers' in relation to impairment and soap opera viewing. One member, for example, explained his viewing of a plane crash storyline (*Emmerdale*) in terms of his professional (medical) interest in information on post-traumatic stress disorder. Most of the time they went to considerable lengths to disassociate themselves from soap operas on gendered terms, despite the growing propensity for men to be soap opera viewers (Gauntlett and Hill, 1999):

> *Vince* Well one of the reasons I don't watch soaps is because I just think I've always categorised them as sort of kitchen sink stuff. You know I don't want to watch what is everyday and mundane, mediocre and monotonous. You know, I just want to, I'd rather watch erm, somebody scoring a spectacular goal or...
>
> *Harry* Yeah
>
> *Vince* ... climbing a mountain you know... and erm,

Conversely, the male diarists wrote more directly about how images of impairment made them *feel* (as shown above), with less shame attributed to soap operas, although disassociation seemed to increase with wider participation in the public sphere. Moreover, these clear differences in viewing performance, according to context, were demonstrated by several diarists who were also group members. For instance, the young women's group also spent much time in *referential* discussion (see Liebes and Katz, 1993) of teenage pregnancy storylines. During the fieldwork period *Coronation Street* and *Eastenders* were both running stories featuring a young teenage pregnant girl, 'Sarah Louise Platt' in the former and 'Sonia Jackson' in the latter. There was a considerably larger degree of identification with the character of Sarah Louise than with Sonia, by all members of the focus group. In the soap opera, related media and these discussions, Sarah Lou is depicted as pretty and quite passive in her relationships with boys, whereas Sonia is portrayed as a more aggressive and independent young woman, who is believed to be (comparatively) unattractive and less deserving of her boyfriend's affections. It seemed that, for members of the young girls' group, the 'sense of self as a performer under the constant scrutiny

of friends and strangers' (Lasch, 1980, p. 9) encouraged the collective performances of identification with a figure who is the best fit to the cultural ideal,
particularly in terms of body and gender performance.

Conversely, while Sarah Louise seemed to be the preferred character in the
younger people's focus group discussions, there was greater consideration given
to Sonia's portrayal within the diary entries of the same cohort, both in the
complexities of Sonia's situation as a school student with no parental support,
and particularly in terms of her body image:

> Sonia didn't think that Jamie really liked her because she thought that she wasn't skinny
> and pretty enough. It was nice to see a girl of 'normal' size go out with a nice bloke on
> TV. It always seems to be the beautiful, size 8 girls who get the best boyfriend so I
> thought it was good that Sonia and Jamie got together. It shows you that it's personality
> that counts.

Although these attitudes seem to contradict one another, it is understandable
that different identifications are made according to the imagined audience.
Within the focus group of peers it is probable that the viewed performance
would be judged on close identification with those who exhibited the best body
and gender performances within the soap opera. On the other hand, I was the
only audience for the diary entries, possibly shaping an image of 'the (disabled)
other' which elicited a different aspect of self-identification. This 'reflection on
the self in relation to others in imagination' (Abercrombie and Longhurst,
1998, p. 95) is, as Giddens (1991) suggests, re-ordered continuously and
according to different circumstances, even where the same text is being
addressed.

These enunciative differences raise a number of questions about body or
impairment performance, social context and the negotiation and articulation of
'disabled' and other identities. Moreover, they make the already fraught problems
of understanding relationships between media texts and questions of audience
more difficult. Added to the potential polyphony of the text and the complexity
of the mediascape, are the heterogeneity of audiences and their fluctuating
interpretive 'performances'.

In elaborating their idea of the 'diffused' audience, Abercrombie and Longhurst (1998) argue that being an audience is constitutive of everyday life, where
everyone becomes an audience and performer all the time. Thus, they contend
that the most salient feature of the diffused audience is its relationship with the
performative society (Kershaw, 1996). Whilst acknowledging that everyday life
has always been constituted by performance, Abercrombie and Longhurst
(1998) argue that contemporary society is *more* performative than previous

eras, a situation brought about in part by, and perpetuating the growth in, the resources provided by mass communications. They propose that this novel form of performativity results in the virtual elimination of cultural distance between performers and audience, whereby two simultaneous processes have occurred: the world has been constructed as 'spectacle' and individuals have become constructed as narcissistic.

These processes were evident in all the discussion groups and the diaries. For instance, each group demonstrated a range of over-evaluations of their own 'normalities' in their treatment of certain topics, for example, a disabled woman's exhibited homophobic attitudes towards lesbian and gay characters, reinforcing her 'normal' heterosexuality, within the focus group:

Betty   It's disgusting and I don't want to see it.
Alison Why?
Betty   Well, it's just not normal is it?

Therefore, in Betty's statement, her perception of lesbian sexuality simultaneously allows her to become an active, moral judge of 'others', whose 'minor differences' become amplified (Ignatieff, 1998), while locating herself as a self-constituting subject of 'normal' desire.

There was also a propensity for the younger groups to ridicule older characters and a tendency for the men to criticise female characters and genres as less exciting and dynamic. Furthermore, there is evidence from all groups and individual diarists that viewing practices are almost exclusively centred on what are perceived to be the 'normal' characters. This privileging of the 'normal' in its various forms usually focused upon narratives of heterosexual desire, involving characters who fit conventional standards of, usually white, attractiveness and stereotypical, if exaggerated, gender roles. As the participants in the disabled students' group, discussing 'alternative soaps', remarked:

Oliver You'd have to have a Grant.
Alison You'd still put Grant in?
Ruth   Yeah.
Daisy   Yeah. It'd be very boring without a Grant...especially when he's picking on everybody.

Indeed, this type of viewing practice is perhaps more marked in the disabled people's groups than in the others. This, and their dislike of impairment and disability images, suggests that soap operas have, at some level, created spectator positions which privilege (albeit exaggerated) forms of normality. The following statement demonstrates the propensity to adopt a 'non-disabled gaze', prioritising the imagined sensibilities of non-disabled viewers:

> *Andrew* I was just going to say. I suppose the soaps are really entertainments aren't they? And I suppose the people who do them don't want to see really bad cases. You know, people slavering all the time and . . . it would upset the ordinary people.

However, Darke (1995, p. 14) suggests that disabled people often reject portrayals of impairment and disability because they contribute to feelings of low self-esteem. He argues,

> a significant proportion of disabled people, tragically do not want to see themselves at all because they do indeed have so low an opinion of themselves that they feel worthless or in denial of their 'difference' or different treatment. For these people disablement refers to their bodies and not their social situation or discrimination.

These opinions are also likely to be linked to the negotiation of the complex relationship between constructed and material identities. None the less, although this group distanced themselves from representations which might reflect poor body and gender performances they also wanted soap operas to 'tell it as it is' in terms of 'impairment tragedy', suggesting a desire to communicate the experience of impairment and disability while minimising stigma. Hence, although they spent much time in referential discussion of their own impairments, a clear-cut distinction between individualist or social-orientated understandings of disability was not always discernible.

Despite the desire to see better images, many such discussions signify an acceptance of portrayals as normative 'reality', from which there is considerable potential for the disabled to judge themselves and other disabled people harshly, or at least, differently. As such, their discussions could not really be seen as examples of an active mediation between experience and text, which Barker (1999) proposes in his study of 'soap talk'. For instance, when asked to consider whether every disabled person is as nasty as 'Chris Tate', (*Emmerdale*), a core male character with a permanent impairment, who uses a wheelchair, they answered:

> *Jean* I suppose it's because he gone through certain things. That's why he's like that.
>
> *Andrew* I suppose if you are in a wheelchair permanently you can't upset people, can you? Because you need their help.
>
> *Geoff* No, you easily get frustrated.

While they were disassociating themselves from his angry and bitter persona, which continually re-enacts Oedipal crises (at the meta- and micro-narrative level) without full resolution, they were also accepting and identifying with experiences of impairment *and* disability (as social), even though they did not perceive their social situation as problematic or political. Once again the diary entries of disabled people demonstrated different attitudes to the same images. Peter believed Chris Tate to be a reiteration of traditional stereotypes or archetypes. He asserted:

> He is Richard III in a wheelchair – bitter, egotistical and bad.

Peter's diary entries became more critical over time as his life became fuller. Furthermore, he concluded the diary by stating that he no longer watched soap operas, and suggested that his prior viewing habits had occurred as a result of a relatively marginalised social position (as disabled and under-employed). Indeed, researchers such as Gauntlett and Hill (1999) and Smith (1994) have suggested that ill and disabled people tend to be over-represented in numbers of 'heavy' television viewers.

Unsurprisingly, the majority of disabled women diarists, who tended to spend more time at home, related to a wider range of soap operas with a different critical emphasis. Like the women's focus group, the female diarists had a much more critical approach to the programmes they were viewing, but they also expressed greater enjoyment and engagement with their content. Again, unlike the male preoccupation with issues of justice, they seemed to emphasise relationships and care. Talking of Jim McDonald (*Coronation Street*), a character with a (temporary) impairment, using a wheelchair, Molly wrote:

> Jim has mentioned his accident (which gained Gwen's sympathy, which was promptly lost again when he told her he had hit Liz).
> Interesting juxtaposition of victim and bully.

Generally, women expected soaps to be a resource for moral guidance as well as a source of entertainment. They tended to show a greater degree of emotional attachment to preferred storylines and characters. Overall, the men tended to have a more utilitarian attitude to representation. For example, they seemed to be more interested in accuracy and in how information is conveyed.

More than any other group, the women placed most of their critical emphasis upon semantic themes. For instance, the discussion of archetypes combined with debates about intentional production messages and discursive themes. They also talked about the prevalence of markers of 'sexual deviance' among

male characters with impairments and of the gendered character of stereotyping:

Sally   So it's the same thing that's still true, it seems, from the freak show circus, like,
that, you know, that was kind of added to the character for the sinisterness of
the character and . . .

Diane   Well, when we were thinking about what's portrayed, are the women portrayed
more tragically, then?

This type of discussion extended to a range of archetypical images and the ways
in which they are used to uphold a variety of normalities, e.g. the portrayal of
gay, lesbian or transsexual characters aspiring to heteronormative conventions.
In most other group discussions the ethical and moral debates emanating from
the soap opera narratives remained within the context of 'normality discourses'
rather than challenging the assumptions on which they are built. The only
exception to this was the young disabled people's (school) group, whose discussions occasionally explored ideas of 'normality reversals'.

Significantly, given the analysis of writers such as Modleski (1997), the
women's group were the only other group who extended their viewing identifications to include marginal characters. Furthermore they did not utilise evaluations
of 'abnormal' others in articulating their own identities or identifications with soap
opera characters. Indeed, despite expressing preferences and identifications
with certain characters and narratives, they often seemed to be occupying the
'feminine' subject positions of the *ideal mother*, posited by Modleski (1997),
whilst acknowledging and criticising many of the discursive strategies of particular representations, such as disabled men as sexually deviant or emasculated.
This seems to reflect a general female concern with 'ethics of care' (Gilligan,
1982) and private relationship issues, as Barker (1999) proposes. Although it is
clear that the 'articulation' of identities (Hall, 1996) cannot be correlated with
interpretations of discourse in an unproblematic fashion, there was a clear
gender division between ethical stances. That is, men's concerns tended to be
enunciated in relation to an ethics of social 'justice' and the public arena. The
men tended to focus primarily upon syntactic criticisms. However, these were biased
towards business, being geared towards economic or production interests and
viewing figures rather than soap opera formulae and the relationships depicted
within them. Indeed, on many occasions such concerns took precedence over
extended discussion of better images, which was generally believed to be a
futile exercise.

These gender divisions are apparent in non-disabled and disabled people's
groups, although the latter are usually anchored in an 'ethic of natural justice'

for older disabled people, whose lives are centred around the home or day centres. Talking of impairments, the following comments typify such responses:

Andrew   It is hard isn't it? When there's no apparent reason for it? Never thinking that you'd end up disabled yourself. It's a cruel world isn't it?

With the exception of the men's groups, the data gathered from the research participants in this project suggested a strong engagement at the micro-narrative level (O'Donnell, 1999), however contradictory these discussions may have been. O'Donnell explains that this level is concerned with relationships and who is doing what within them. In terms of body and gender performance these played a significant part in processes of identity articulation, for instance, when counterposed with referential discussions of their own lives.

When participants focused upon characters with impairments the discussions became more involved with what O'Donnell identifies as the meta-narrative, i.e. the topical themes, which often carry 'public service' content. At this level, soap operas are often judged to be progressive and could, ostensibly, promote the views of the disabled people's movement. However, there was a much weaker engagement with such issues. Moreover, several diarists questioned whether this content was commensurate with a genre designed for pleasure and 'escape'. Although the men's focus on justice involved the discussion of social concerns, these conversations did not stem from soap opera meta-narratives, but were largely derived from referential discussions about their working or public lives, and occasionally, the micro-narrative level of the soap opera.

O'Donnell argues that the macro-narrative level is the most crucial, carrying social and political values such as individualism and 'bestowing' moral protagonism. He argues that values of solidarity and cooperation are defended at all levels of the macro-narrative but this conclusion seems to be at odds with the individualistic discourses that soap operas carry, particularly that of normality. Furthermore, few participants questioned narratives at this level. However, in practice, one cannot separate these three levels so easily. As Barker's (1999) work demonstrates, much 'soap talk' is concerned with moral protagonism, particularly at the level of (micro-narrative) relationships. In this project, for instance, the women suggested that moral stories involving disabled men often helped in re-asserting 'normal' masculinities. Indeed, 'normality' seems to be the most crucial macro-narrative of the soap opera, structuring macro-narrative discourses of disability, gender and sexuality. In the light of the data, what seems most crucial about these normality macro-narratives is their virtual invisibility.

Indeed, Darke (1999) argues that impairment images are mythical, being founded on archetypes, thus accepted as 'universal' or 'timeless' truth, particularly as disability and abnormality usually are viewed as axiomatic. As such, the most explicit portrayals are those that are issue-based, invariably returning the viewer to normality (as Darke suggests of cinema [1998; 1999]). It is, therefore, unsurprising that viewers chose to discuss more obvious disability concerns at the meta-narrative levels, leaving micro- and macro-narrative discourses relatively unchallenged.

So, have soap operas provided pleasure for the disabled people in this project? Have impairment and disability images provided pleasure for any of the viewers? Are these viewing experiences compatible with disabled people's social and political goals?

A captive audience?

It was suggested that exercising the melodramatic imagination may be empowering for some women, even reflecting the 'melodramatic edge to feminism' (Ang, 1996, p. 165). However, the discussions of disabled people in this project suggest that characters with impairments do not evoke similar, albeit mixed, pleasures of identification. Moreover, it seems that the close relationship of melodrama to narratives of victimisation (Fiske, 1987) through the tragic structure of feeling (Ang, 1997) promotes or perpetuates the 'ethics of natural justice' identified in some disabled people's discussions. Given that Ang believed the melodramatic imagination to be 'a psychological strategy to overcome the material meaningless of everyday existence' (Ang, 1997, p. 79), which expressed a 'passive, fatalistic and individualistic reaction to a vague feeling of powerlessness and unease (Ang, 1996, p. 82), it is not surprising that less advantaged disabled viewers subscribed to the idea of natural justice. Ironically, given that soap operas are usually identified as a woman's genre, these ethics of tragedy and justice predominated in the narratives of disabled male characters and participants' discussions about them, whereas female characters such as Jaqui Dixon (*Brookside*) and 'Maud Grimes' (*Coronation Street*) tended to be viewed as ordinary. Arguably, in such cases, viewers are more likely to retain some emotional attachment.

Additionally, the predominance of referential discussions of impairment also suggested an over-identification with personal rather than collective issues. Indeed, the soap opera, as a melodramatic genre, seems likely to promote individualistic 'tragic victim' stereotypes (Barnes, 1992) rather than any other and is antithetical to the kind of images that the disabled people's movement have promoted.

In this and other respects, characteristics which have been attributed to the soap opera genre seem not to apply in similar ways to discourses of normality and disability. One of the most obvious of these is Fiske's (1987) claim that television genres are associative. Even in those groups who had weaker engagements with soap operas, it was widely recognised that characters with impairments invariably operated within structures of cause and effect, their stories being told and completed almost exclusively on the meta-narrative plane. It was a common observation that 'bad' male characters had accidents resulting in impairments (invariably involving the use of a wheelchair) until they underwent moral reform. Furthermore, these storylines rarely seemed to stimulate multiple or resistive readings but were seen by a few participants as a way of delivering a discriminatory and highly gendered moral discourse.

The women's and disabled adults' groups had a greater tendency to adopt different subject positions as Modleski (1997) has suggested. However, this 'ideal mother' position seems to encourage 'preferred' readings at the micro- and meta-narrative levels of discourse, leaving the macro-narratives intact, e.g. heteronormative and normality discourses. As such, the emotional attachments are likely to remain at the level of the tragic structure (Ang, 1997), quelling anger and stifling consciousness, which might otherwise emerge over a period of time (Crossley, 1998). The potential for reflection on these discourses is minimal, because of the fast pace of most storylines: rather than avoiding closure, narratives are frequently resolved over brief periods of time, most notably in the case of characters who acquire and are cured of impairments.

Whereas it is true that there are many voices speaking throughout the soap opera text, as theorists such as Brunsdon et al. (1997) and Kuhn (1997) suggest, the level of engagement with different characters demonstrates that these voices are far from equal. Issues such as prejudice against people with HIV, tackled at the meta-narrative level, seem to be superseded by attention given to the minutiae of the non-disabled characters' lives within the micro-narratives and undermined by the macro-narratives of normality, generating little interest for these viewers. Indeed, rather than pleasure being afforded through identification with characters in similar social situations, the discussions of these participants indicate far greater identifications with non-disabled characters. This is likely to have been exacerbated by the prevalence of impairment and disability issues addressed at meta-narrative levels and the 'feminising' or demonising of characters which occurs on this plane.

Thus, it seems that gaining pleasure from soap opera texts is incompatible with disability and impairment identifications. Just as Mulvey's (1992) theorising of feminine viewing positions with central female protagonists implied a contradictory and impossible 'phantasy of masculinisation' for female viewers, images of disabled characters return disabled viewers to an unachievable phantasy of normalisation.

This is a divisive factor in the creation of symbolic communities and is likely to perpetuate the viewing experience of isolation for disabled people. This is particularly true for under- or unemployed disabled people, whose viewing environment is too familiar and not the place of refuge or escape that so many television studies imagine it to be. Additionally, many disabled men may feel that their opportunities for masculine identifications are severely restricted by viewing disproportionately exploitative portrayals of men within the private sphere.

Furthermore, none of the non-disabled people in this project reported enjoying images of impairment or disability, and their engagement with such storylines was usually weak. Although the viewing contexts exert clear influence on reading practices, interpretations of impairment and disability were less ambiguous. Any pleasure gained from viewing these portrayals was not apparent. Moreover, several non-disabled diarists complained that portrayals of illness and impairment made them feel anxious. However, the latent discourse of normality is likely to be a more reassuring factor for non-disabled viewers (Darke, 1998, 1999), encouraging processes of normality over-evaluation, and leaving prejudices about disability intact.

It appears that British 'prime-time' soap operas have a captive, rather than 'model' (O'Donnell, 1999) audience, in many respects, particularly in households comprised of disabled people, parents and children. Socio-cultural positioning seems to be a key factor in explaining what people watch. Indeed, this has been recognised, in the original commercial appeal to 'housewives', and more recently, in the international growth of soap operas which target young people (O'Donnell, 1999).

Yet, disabled people, who are more reliant on domestic media owing to poor access to other cultural forms, have not been courted in the same way, although the softer approach to (rare) images of female characters with impairments may signify an acknowledgement that disabled women are an important constituency. None the less, it is possible to see the disproportionate degree of acquiescence to poor images of impairment and disability as a 'symptom of symbolic violence' (Seiter, 1999, p. 27). There is little evidence to demonstrate much multicultural variance, although O'Donnell's fleeting exploration of disability, or more accurately characters using wheelchairs, suggests that 'weakened' disabled female characters are much more frequent and that disabled male characters are relatively scarce but 'stronger' within other European soaps. With little opportunity to exercise choice it is understandable if disabled people as 'heavy viewers' become complicit with a form that naturalises disability pathologies, returns 'normality' to them in other forms and yet, supplies populist 'cultural capital'. As a previously ambiguous viewer, who now has the privilege of being part of a 'double access' (academic) audience (Gripsrud, 1995), I now have an unequivocally critical view of soap operas as a form of entertainment which, at best, delivers over-simplified, individualistic answers to serious social concerns and exploits the need for escape for those who can't.

REFERENCES

Abercrombie, N. and Longhurst, B., *Audiences* (London: Sage, 1998).

Alasuutari, P., '"I'm ashamed to admit it but I have watched Dallas": the Moral Hierarchy of Television Programmes', *Media, Culture and Society*, 14:1 (1995), pp. 651–82.

Allen, R. C., *To be Continued... Soap Operas Around the World* (New York: Routledge, 1995).

Ang, I., *Watching Dallas: Soap Operas and the Melodramatic Imagination* (London: Methuen, 1985).

Ang, I., *Living Room Wars: Rethinking Media Audiences for a Postmodern World* (London: Routledge, 1996).

Appadurai, A., 'Disjuncture and Difference in the Global Cultural Economy', in B. Robins (ed.), *The Phantom Public Sphere* (London: University of Minnesota Press, 1993).

Bakhtin, M. and Holquist, M. (ed.), *The Dialogic Imagination: Four Essays*, trans. C. Emerson and M. Holquist (Austin: University of Texas, 1993).

Barker, C., *Television, Globalization and Cultural Identities* (Buckingham: Open University Press, 1999).

Barnes, C., *Cabbage Syndrome: The Social Construction of Dependence* (London: Harvester, 1990).

Barnes, C., *Disabled People in Britain and Discrimination: A Case for Anti-discrimination Legislation* (London: Charles Hurst in association with the British Council of the Organization of Disabled People, 1991).

Barnes, C., *Disabling Imagery and the Media: An Exploration of the Principles of Media Representations of Disabled People* (Halifax: Ryburn, 1992).

Barnes, C., Mercer, G. and Shakespeare, T., *Exploring Disability: A Sociological Introduction* (Cambridge: Polity, 1999).

Biklen, D. and Bogdan, R., 'Media Portrayals of Disabled People: a Study of Stereotypes', *Interracial Books for Children Bulletin*, 8:6 and 7:4–7 (1977).

Brunsdon, C., D'Acci, J. and Spigel, L., *Feminist Television Criticism* (Oxford: Clarendon Press, 1997).

Cantor, M. G. and Pingree, S., *The Soap Opera* (Beverly Hills, CA: Sage, 1983).

Crossley, N., 'Emotion and Communicative Action', in G. Bendelow and S. J. Williams (eds), *Emotions in Social Life* (London: Routledge, 1998).

Cumberbatch, G. and Negrine, R., *Images of Disability on Television* (London: Routledge, 1992).

Curran, J., 'The "New Revisionism" in Mass Communications Research', *European Journal of Communication*, 5:2/3 (1990), pp. 135–64.

Darke, P., '"Link": an Evaluation', unpublished consultation paper for Yorkshire Television (1995).

Darke, P., 'Understanding Cinematic Representations of Disability', in T. Shakespeare (ed.), *The Disability Reader: Social Science Perspectives* (London: Cassell, 1998).

Darke, P., 'The Cinematic Construction of Physical Disability as Identified through the Application of the Social Model of Disability to Six Indicative Films made since 1970', PhD, University of Warwick (1999).

Fiske, J., *Television Culture* (London: Routledge, 1987).

Gauntlett, D. and Hill, A., *TV Living: Television, Culture and Everyday Life* (London: Routledge, 1999).

Giddens, A., *Modernity and Self-Identity* (Cambridge: Polity, 1991).

Gilligan, C., *In a Different Voice* (Cambridge, MA: Harvard University Press, 1982).

Gripsrud, J., *The Dynasty Years: Hollywood Television and Critical Media Studies* (London: Comedia/Routledge, 1995).

Hall, S., 'Encoding/Decoding', in S. Hall, D. Hobson, A. Lowe and P. Willis (eds), *Culture, Media, Language: Working Papers in Cultural Studies, 1972–79* (London: Hutchinson, 1980).

Hall, S., 'On Postmodernism and Articulation: an Interview with Stuart Hall', in L. Grossberg, in D. Morley and D. K. Chen (eds), *Stuart Hall* (London: Routledge, 1996).

Holquist, M., *Dialogism: Bakhtin and his World* (London: Routledge, 2002).

Hobson, D., *Crossroads: The Drama of a Soap Opera* (London: Methuen, 1982).

Ignatieff, M., *The Warrior's Honour: Ethnic War and the Modern Conscience* (London: Chatto & Windus, 1998).

Kent, D., 'Disabled Women: Portraits in Fiction and Drama', in A. Gartner and T. Joe (eds), *Images of the Disabled, Disabling Images* (New York: Praeger, 1987).

Kershaw, B., 'The Politics of Postmodern Performance', in P. Campell, *Analysing Performance: A Critical Reader* (Manchester: Manchester University Press, 1996).

Kitzinger, J., 'Media Message and What People Know about Acquired Immune Deficiency Syndrome', in Glasgow University Media Group, *Getting the Message* (London: Routledge, 1993).

Klobas, L. E., *Disability Drama in Television and Film* (Jefferson, NC: Macfarland, 1988).

Kuhn, A., 'Women's Genres: Melodrama, Soap Opera and Theory', in C. Brunsdon, J. D'Acci and L. Spigel (eds), *Feminist Television Criticism* (Oxford: Clarendon Press, 1997).

Lasch, C., *The Culture of Narcissism* (London: Sphere, 1980).

Liebes, T. and Katz, E., *The Export of Meaning: Cross-cultural Readings of Dallas* (Oxford: Oxford University Press, 1993).

Longmore, P., 'Screening Stereotypes: Images of Disabled People in Television and Motion Pictures', in A. Gartner and T. Joe (eds), *Images of the Disabled, Disabling Images* (New York: Praeger, 1987).

Mattelart, M., *Women, Media and Crisis: Femininity and Disorder* (London: Comedia, 1986).

Modleski, T., 'The Search for Tomorrow on Today's Soap Operas', in C. Brunsdon, J. D'Acci and L. Spigel (eds), *Feminist Television Criticism* (Oxford: Clarendon Press, 1997).

Morris, J., *Pride Against Prejudice: Transforming Attitudes to Disability* (London: Women's Press, 1991).

Mulvey, L., 'Visual Pleasure and Narrative Cinema', in *Screen, The Sexual Subject: A Screen Reader in Seuxality* (London: Routledge, 1992), pp. 22–34.

Nelson, R., *TV Drama in Transition – Forms, Values and Cultural Change* (London: Macmillan, 1996).

Nightingale, V., *Studying Audiences: The Shock of the Real* (London: Routledge, 1996).

Norden, M. E., *The Cinema of Isolation* (New Brunswick, NJ: Rutgers University Press, 1994).

O'Donnell, H., *Good Times, Bad Times: Soap Operas in Western Europe* (London: Leicester University Press, 1999).

Oliver, M., *The Politics of Disablement* (Basingstoke: Macmillan, 1990).

Pointon, A. and Davies, C., *Framed: A Disability Media Reader* (London: British Film Institute, 1997).

Rieser, R. and Mason, M., *Disability Equality in the Classroom* (London: Inner London Education Authority, 1992).

Ross, K., *Disability and Broadcasting: A View from the Margins* (Cheltenham: Cheltenham and Gloucester College of Higher Education, 1997).

Screen, The Sexual Subject: A Screen Reader in Sexuality (London: Routledge, 1992).

Seiter, E., *Television and New Audiences* (Oxford: Oxford University Press, 1999).

Shakespeare, T., 'Cultural Representation of Disabled People: Dustbins for Disavowal?' *Disability and Society*, 9:3 (1994), pp. 283–99.

Shakespeare, T., 'Soaps: the Story So Far', in A. Pointon and C. Davies, *Framed: A Disability Media Reader* (London: British Film Institute, 1997).

Shakespeare, T., 'Art and Lies? Representations of Disability on Film', in M. Corker and S. French (eds), *Disability Discourse* (Buckingham: Open University Press, 1999).

Silverstone, R., *Television and Everyday Life* (London: Routledge, 1994).

Smith, D. J., *The Sleep of Reason* (London: Century, 1994).

Stevenson, N., *Understanding Media Cultures: Social Theory and Mass Communication* (London: Sage, 1995).

Part II

Discourses of Health and Illness in the Print Media and the Internet

In this section the focus is on the print media and the internet. Here we pick up on some of the themes concerning representations, outlined in the Introduction. The chapters in this section address one of the central questions about the mass media – do they merely reflect reality or are they a key player in the construction of particular definitions of reality (Hall, 1997). A major theme of this section is representation and the construction of identity.

> The media contribute significantly to the definition of the world around us, and thereby also to the definition of ourselves.... They present parts and dimensions of the world that we ourselves have not experienced directly, and may never come to experience directly. As recipients of all this we simply have to form some sort of opinion about where we are located, so to speak, in the complex landscapes presented to us. (Gripsrud, 2002, p. 5)

Gripsrud (2002) argues that the media play a crucial role in the self-perception of the identity of individuals and groups. Building on the ideas of discourse offered by Foucault's (1973; 1977) work he argues that the media are crucial in creating (real or imagined) communities based on ideas of what it is to be British, Northern, black, male, etc. A study by Peter Hamilton (1997), for example, examines work done in France after the Second World War by French documentary photographers, producing a body of work which came to represent ideas about postwar 'France and Frenchness' as a national identity.

What is particularly interesting to us, here, is the way in which issues or groups are represented in the media – the ways in which discourses around particular groups or issues are constructed.

Gripsrud (2002, p. 11) states:

> Even if the media's offerings are plentiful and varied, this does not necessarily mean that they reflect and sustain all the identities and group formations that exist in society. That is why there may be political struggles over the rights to, and forms of representation in the media. . . . What is meant here is a depiction, description or account of fictive or real phenomena.

How, then, are particular groups 're-presented' through the media, or how do images of particular groups in the media represent or stand-for those groups in reality? Here, again, we address the question of reflection or construction in the media.

Dyer (1993, p. 1) argues strongly that there is a direct link between representation and reality, especially in relation to minority groups:

> how social groups are treated in cultural representation is part and parcel of how they are treated in life . . . that poverty, harassment, self-hate and discrimination (in housing, jobs, educational opportunity and so on) are shored up and instituted by representation. . . . How we are seen determines in part how we are treated.

Dyer is clear in his belief that the media's representation of groups in particular ways has an impact on public perception and social policy (Dyer, 1993).

Dyer's work is interesting because he engages with the issues outlined elsewhere in this book – power, discourse and the audience – a debate succinctly summed up by Berger and Luckmann (1967, p. 127): 'he who has the bigger stick has the better chance of imposing his definitions of reality'. Dyer, however, emphasises the complexities at work in this type of analysis. Much work has been done on the representation of women and other minority groups in the media (Brunsdon, 1997; Hooks, 1997; *Screen*, 1992). Dyer argues that the anger generated at negative representations in some of this work can be self-defeating. Gripsrud (2002), as we have seen, has identified the political and ideological struggles at work around representations, and Hall's (1997) work sets out the political framework in which these struggles occur. Dyer adds to this by pointing out that the whole concept of representation is a complex one and that the reality/ representation relationship is not straightforward.

The complex, shifting business of re-presenting, re-working, recombining representations is in tension with the reality to which representations refer and to which they affect. This is evident in three ways. Firstly, reality sets limits to what, barring idiosyncratic examples, humans can make it mean. . . . Secondly, reality is always more extensive and complicated than any system of representation can possibly comprehend and we always sense that this is so – representation never 'gets' reality, which is why human history has produced so many different and changing ways of trying to get it. Thirdly, representations here and now have real consequences for real people.   (Dyer, 1993, p. 3)

Dyer's (1993) own work on the film 'Victim' and on the complex representations of and about gay men and 'gay-ness' at work in this early 1960s work, is a good example of an attempt to come to terms with some of these complexities. Pollock's (1992) work on the role of ideology in visual representations of women is another good example, as is Kaplan's (1978) work on re-reading the representation of women in *film-noir*, in which she reinterprets and re-reads what were formerly seen as 'weak' and 'exploited' female characters in the *film-noir* genre as something quite different.

However, Dyer acknowledges that in producing 'typification' of certain groups the media use a short-hand coding system in order to represent these groups. For example, in producing representations of gay men he says:

typification is, as a mode of representation, immediate and economical. It dispenses with the need to establish a character's sexuality through dialogue and narrative by establishing it literally at first glance. Dialogue and narrative may themselves be stereotypical. There are conventional ways of indicating in dialogue that a character is gay.   (Dyer, 1993, p. 22)

As well as dealing with the media representation and construction of identity (and the opportunities for resistance to these dominant representations), the section also examines the role of the media in the making of health policy. There is a growing body of work which examines the ways in which the media, particularly the print media, influence policy through the representations of key health and social issues (Allen et al., 2000; Critcher, 2003; Miller et al., 1998).

Clive Seale's chapter explores through discourse and content analysis how newsprint media construct an idealised view of childhood subjectivity. Through his study of the representation of childhood cancer in the print media, Seale shows how the media offer cycles of value creation and subversion, and produce, maintain and rescue childhood in the face of the threat to the 'happy scenario' presented by cancer. In this process, he argues, there is also an erasure of subjectivity and a contrast and conflict between the representation of childhood cancer and the lived experiences of those with the disease.

Martin King and Clare Street provide a case study of print media coverage of the BSE crisis in the UK in the 1980s and 1990s. The study explores ideas advanced by Parsons (1995, p. 107):

> The mass media can shape the context within which policy responses take place and influence 'public opinion' by setting a public agenda in terms of an incident or event.

Using this work, and Gramsci's (1971) work on hegemony, the chapter draws conclusions about dominant and dissenting voices in the reporting of a public health crisis and about the role of the print media as a key player in the policy-making process. The print media's ability to present and represent the complexity of a public health issue such as BSE is questioned, as is the role of 'science' and 'scientific fact' in this process.

Michael Hardey looks at the internet as an important media site both in terms of providing health information and in offering resistance to dominant discourses around health and illness. He argues that news groups on the internet allow users to explore and form alliances concerning contested health and social problems, providing (potentially) a challenge to medical orthodoxy and a resistance to medical representations of personal troubles. He advances the notion of the possibility of multiple identities on the www: 'the home page, therefore provides a place where the author makes sense of life events and weaves together emotional and material transitions'. Following Giddens (1991), Hardey argues that therapy has replaced religion as a source of meaning, underlining yet again how important the study of discourses of health, illness, disease and the body, are in postmodern times.

REFERENCES

Allan, S., Adam, B. and Carter, C., *Environmental Risks and the Media* (London: Routledge, 2000).

Berger, P., and Luckmann, T., *The Social Construction of Reality* (London: Allen Lane/Penguin Press, 1967).

Brunsdon, C. (ed.), *Feminist Television Criticism: A Reader* (Oxford: Clarendon, 1997).

Critcher, C., *Moral Panics and the Media* (Buckingham: Open University Press, 2003).

Dyer, R., *The Matter of Images: Essays on Representation* (London: Routledge, 1993).

Foucault, M., *The Birth of the Clinic* (London: Tavistock, 1973).

Foucault, M., *Discipline and Punish* (London: Tavistock, 1977).

Giddens, A., *Modernity and Self-identity* (Cambridge: Polity Press, 1991).

Gramsci, A., *Selections from the Prison Notebooks* (London: Lawrence & Wishart, 1971).

Gripsrud, J., *Understanding the Media Culture* (London: Edward Arnold, 2002).

Hall, S. (ed.), *Representation: Cultural Representations and Signifying Practices* (London: Sage, 1997).

Hamilton, P., 'Representing the Social: France and Frenchness in Post-war Humanist Photography', in S. Hall (ed.), *Representation: Cultural Representation and Signifying Practices* (London: Sage, 1997), pp. 75–150.

Hooks, B., *Reel to Reel* (London: Routledge, 1997).

Kaplan, E. A. (ed.), *Women in Film Noir* (London: British Film Institute 1978).

Miller, D., Kitzinger, J., Williams K. and Behanel, P., *The Circuit of Mass Communication* (London: Sage, 1998).

Parsons, W., *Public Policy: An Introduction to the Theory and Practice of Policy Analysis* (Aldershot: Edward Elgar, 1995).

Pollock, G., 'What's Wrong with "Images of Women"?' in Screen, *The Sexual Subject: A Screen Reader in Sexuality* (London: Routledge, 1992), pp. 135–45.

Screen, *The Sexual Subject: A Screen Reader in Sexuality* (London: Routledge, 1992).

Threatened Children: Media Representations of Childhood Cancer

4

Clive Seale

Introduction

This chapter reports a sociological analysis of media accounts of childhood cancer, through an examination of news reports. Through portraying threatened children as innocently deserving of care, a potent symbol of need is constructed. Analysis focuses on the initial construction of childhood as a time of life in which children are entitled to certain activities that signify innocence and difference, with cancer being a threat to these entitlements. The task of helpers (family members, health care workers, the 'community') then becomes that of restoring these entitlements. In the process, a highly idealised view of childhood subjectivity is generated which contrasts markedly with studies of family experiences of childhood cancer. This has consequences for public debates about the funding of health services, as well as for families coping with childhood cancer.

More broadly, it is clear that images, mythologies and narratives about children abound in popular media, both reflecting and constructing contemporary ideals of childhood. Sociological analysis of these cultural representations has considerable potential for the general project of understanding the experience of childhood (and parenting) in a late modern context. Sociologists have argued that stories of threats to childhood, such as child abuse, child murder and missing or abducted children, are a fertile source for images of what is valued about children. Another such threat is childhood cancer, which is an important area of interest for news media. Several analyses of media portrayals of adult cancer experiences – particularly breast cancer – have been reported (reviewed in Seale, 2001a; 2001b; 2002), but there has been only one systematic study of media reporting of childhood cancer, done by Entwistle et al. (1996), focusing on coverage of a single case by British newspapers. The case of 'Child B' hit the headlines in March 1995, involving parents taking a Health Authority to court for refusing to fund experimental leukemia treatment for their daughter. Coverage, Entwistle reports, under-emphasised clinical considerations of the low likelihood of success and the potential for harmful side-effects, instead presenting it as a story about financial considerations denying a child a chance of life. One other relevant study (Manning and Schneiderman, 1996), this time in a US context, reports an analysis of children's hospital promotional literature. The authors note that ethical committees in US children's hospitals spend half of their time debating cases where parents of terminally ill children object to professionals' wishes to cease expensive treatments that the parents believe offer hope of a cure. They identify a cause of these unrealistic hopes as being an emphasis on medical miracles in the promotional literature of the hospitals themselves.

While there is a paucity of studies of childhood cancer in the media, there are a number of other analyses, by sociologists, of media stories about threats to children, which are therefore also accounts of the values that childhood represents. There is evidence to suggest that – at least in the US news media – there has been a general rise in recent years in the reporting of topics designed to evoke fear and anxiety, with reports about children being a particular focus (Altheide and Michalowski, 1999). Coverage of child abuse is a common vehicle for such themes (Atmore, 1996; Goddard, 1995; Gough, 1996; Jenks, 1994; 1995), allowing the archetypal division between child, as innocent victim, and abuser, as demonised monster, to be established and re-established. The false memory syndrome (FMS) story has then appeared as a challenge to the child abuse story (Kitzinger, 1998), which like many popular news themes had become 'old news', requiring the 'new' news of FMS to stimulate the jaded appetites of news editors and readers. The themes most obviously evident in reports of child abuse, though, have continued in more subtle form in other kinds of story.

For example, the construction of the 'missing children' issue in the US media in the 1980s has been analysed by close examination of rhetoric used to claim this as a social problem (Best, 1987; 1988) and through audience study to show how these claims are incorporated by media consumers into everyday knowledge about threats to children (Fritz and Altheide, 1987). The exaggeration of claims in these stories has been achieved by generalising from extreme cases, and selective presentation of fear-provoking statistics. This allows the rhetoric to then produce criticism of public authorities for inadequate responses to the magnitude of the perceived problem. Key premises of the reports (their 'warrants' as Best [1987] describes them) include the preciousness of children, their blamelessness (even in the case of 'runaway' children), and the invocation of associated known evils that threaten missing children, such as drug and sexual abuse, prostitution and child pornography.

Continuing the theme of abused childhood innocence, Giroux (1998) analyses coverage of US child beauty pageants in the wake of the murder of six-year-old JonBenet Ramsay (Figure 4.1). The media reflected widespread public disquiet at the displays of sexualised and commodified children encouraged in the

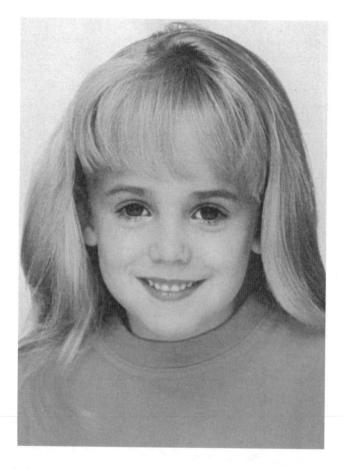

Figure 4.1   JonBenet Ramsey – a sexualised and commodified product of American culture

beauty pageant culture, prompting criticism of parents and organisers as engaging in a corruption of innocence analogous to child abuse. The contrast of innocence insufficiently protected against evil enables the production of a (sometimes romantic) opposition to institutions and bureaucratic law enforcement or welfare agencies. Media agencies position themselves and their reporters, on these occasions, as the voice of silenced majorities against the rule-governed impersonality of the state apparatus. Coverage of the 1996 Dutroux child murders in Belgium (Walgrave and Stouthuysen, 1996) prompted an international media debate about the deficiencies of Belgian public institutions, centred on their failure to defend vulnerable children or to detain and punish their abusers. The Bulger child killing case in Britain (James and Jenks, 1996) generated a rather similar soul searching, although in this case the surprising indifference of the 'general public' (here constructed as the faceless mass of a crowd, rather than as a majority oppressed by faceless bureaucracy) to the scenes of child abduction that had happened before their very eyes was the focus of media-orchestrated criticism.

However, the Bulger case also allowed new themes to emerge, demonstrating the capacity of the media to provoke interest through challenging the categories which media agencies themselves help create. The Bulger case, through contemplation of the young child killers themselves, allowed the category of childhood innocence to be questioned very deeply (Figure 4.2). While stories of transgressive teenage behaviour have long been part of the common stock of news accounts (Lumley, 1998), the Bulger case enabled more fundamental questions about the inherent nature of children as innocent or evil to emerge into public discourse, due to the age of the killers. In such ways, the media can offer a continual provocation and excitement for consumers, in a cycle of value creation and subversion that satisfies the requirement for 'news'. As James and Jenks (1996) point out, however, careful exploration of the subjective experience of childhood is largely missing from news accounts, as the stories involve adult fantasies of the inner worlds of children. This lack of exploration of subjectivity contributes to an image of children as largely passive victims of events, rather than active agents, a portrayal that acquires a starkly political edge in portrayals of children in famines (Burman, 1994a; 1994b), allowing western aid agencies and charities to maintain a self-image as powerful benefactors on behalf of helpless dependants.

Paradoxically, a similar lack of careful regard for subjectivity may characterise portrayals of highly successful, active children in media stories. This may particularly be the case where illness and disability are concerned, where inspirational stories of children heroically overcoming obstacles are often told. Rolland (1997) has argued that these idealised portrayals of successful coping strategies

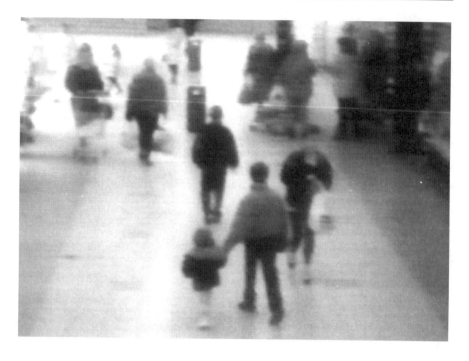

Figure 4.2   The Jamie Bulger case – a question mark over childhood innocence
(reproduced from CCTV footage)

represent adult fantasies that may be experienced as oppressive by disabled children and families who find themselves unable to cope in this way. Romanticised images of the family life of children with cancer, with parents positioned as endlessly self-sacrificing, children as invariably optimistic and brave, can involve serious distortions (Moller, 1996). Family discipline, for example, can break down in the face of the immense pressure to treat one child as possessing special rights to parental attention; sibling rivalry may become intense under these conditions, especially if the painful procedure of bone marrow donation becomes the sibling's obligation. Young et al. (2002) have shown that parents' descriptions of what it is like to have a child with cancer bear little resemblance to media portrayals. Children can be unhappy, distressed and hard to influence, especially where frightening and painful medical procedures are proposed (see also Dixon-Woods et al., 2003).

Media accounts of childhood cancer, then, can be analysed sociologically in so far as they relate to themes of childhood innocence in the face of threat, the degree to which children are portrayed as active agents, the extent to which a full variety of subjective experience is allowed to emerge, and for images of appropriate behaviour by parents and other adults – including expectations of health care. Such analysis assists in understanding the cultural component of illness experience and health care in late modernity (Lupton, 1994a), an aspect which has been somewhat under-explored in medical sociology. As part of a larger study of news reporting of cancer experiences, the present account will show that the manner in which childhood cancer is reported has implications at several levels: for sociologists concerned with the issue of the social construction of childhood, for health policy makers and practitioners, and for children and their parents facing life-threatening disease.

The study

Details of the study are published in fuller detail elsewhere (Seale, 2001b), so a brief summary is provided. A commercially available on-line database (NEXIS) of newspaper articles worldwide was used to retrieve 2,419 articles appearing in the English-language press during the first week of October 1999 that contained the words 'cancer', 'leukaemia' or 'leukemia'. From this, I chose a sub-sample of 358 articles in which there was significant coverage of the life or death of a person with cancer (hereafter PWC). There was a predominance of North American (72%) and UK (26%) papers in the sample. Because PWC stories often occurred across a number of articles, as well as some articles containing several PWCs, it was decided to make the unit of analysis the PWC rather than the article. There were 382 PWCs in all.

There were 42 child PWCs in the sample, of whom 22 were male. Their stories appeared in 26 US newspapers, 7 UK papers and 3 Canadian papers. The emphasis on children with cancer (most frequently leukaemia) is, numerically, disproportionately high if compared with the age distribution of cancer in relevant populations. In fact, there was also a disproportionately high focus on younger adults with cancer, reflecting news values that prioritise the reporting of tragic events and 'bad' news (Entwistle et al., 1996; Galtung and Ruge, 1973). Thus the deaths of elderly people from disease is rarely considered newsworthy.

Analysis of the language of PWC stories involved, first, using NVIVO software to code every section of text in which a PWC was depicted. Selecting only this text, a word concordance was then done and linguistic terms associated with a variety of themes were identified. This was used as a sensitising device in a further NVIVO coding exercise, in which sections of text concerning themes of interest were identified and retrieved. These sub-selections were then run through further word concordances. This systematic and iterative procedure enables both a quantitative and qualitative report that seeks to draw on the strengths of interpretive sociological methods such as discourse analysis (Potter and Wetherell, 1987; Fowler, 1991) and objectivist methods such as content analysis (Weber, 1990), a mixed methodological approach whose rationale has been outlined elsewhere (Seale, 1999).

Representing childhood cancer

Maintaining childhood

The childishness of the children in the stories was intensively signalled by the frequent demonstration of their entitlement to the category-bound activities (CBAs) of childhood. This is a concept taken from Harvey Sacks (Silverman, 1998), who uses it in his broader project of analysing membership categorisation devices in talk. CBAs are the activities taken to be appropriate, in a given society, for particular groupings of persons. Children are thus expected to enjoy childlike things, and if they do not there may be a threat to established assumptions about normal behaviour. The activities and things of childhood are nowadays subject to quite careful age-gradations, which themselves have a scientific foundation in the disciplines of child development, and a commercial aspect in the provision of age-graded products such as toys (Buckingham, 1997; Burman, 1994a; Luke, 1994). The experience of adolescence can, in part, be understood as a negotiation of identity through complex manipulations of category-bound entitlements, so that the 15-year-old who 'still plays with toys' can be understood in certain contexts as one who is inappropriately 'childish'. In the news reports the entitlement of children to childlike activities was used to produce the subjects of the reports as children, to show that illness threatened this production, and to engage in rescue dramas in which communal activity (of which the journalistic report is itself a part) repaired this damage.

Producing childhood

A commonly cited activity of children with cancer in the news reports was that of sport. Sixteen-year-old Michael Penon, for example, 'loved basketball' (*News Tribune*); 8-year-old Steven Newkirk 'liked sports so much that he began reading the newspaper when he was 4, to learn about his favourite Chicago teams, the Cubs and the Bulls...."he loved baseball and basketball" [said his father]' (*Chicago Tribune*). Otto Tang, who died aged 17, 'swam in the Class 4A state championships' (*Seattle Times*). Other sports activities of children with cancer included watching car racing and playing golf.

The possession, enjoyment and grateful reception of toys and other kinds of present was the next most common indicator of childish category-bound activity.

At a charity event, 3-year-old Hunter Elizabeth Jones was presented with 'a stuffed animal dog...she gratefully named him "Atlas"' (*Press Journal*). The cancer clinic where 11-year-old David Stewart was treated contained 'Mickey Mouse toys and bright tropical fish stickers' and he spent much of his time there 'playing charades, exploring an aeronautics museum, and riding a toy bike around the pediatric ward' (*Boston Globe*). Eight-year-old Sarah Dowson 'can ride a bicycle and roller skate with help' in spite of her leg amputation (*Daily Press*). Ashley Suian's 'love of dogs keeps her in good spirits most of the time' (*Edmonton Sun*).

Another common device was to cite educational and other achievements as evidence of future potential, which is of course an entitlement of children in particular. ' "He completed 2nd grade at Pritchett last year and would've entered 3rd grade this year" [said his mother]' (*Chicago Tribune*); Kelly Freeman, who died aged 17, was a 'school athlete and an author of childrens' books on "dogs, school and other subjects" ' (*Cincinnati Inquirer*). In Michael Penon's case, educational achievements combined with his sporting interests: 'Michael Penon loved swimming and scuba diving, basketball and math. He was a junior historian and knew the Bible backward and forward' (*News Tribune*).

Appearance also indicated childishness: 'little Louis Dwyer, 5...[is a] cute, blond-haired, chirpy rascal' (*The Mirror*); 'Zachary Collins's chubby 2-year-old face smiled' (*Providence Journal-Bulletin*); 6-year-old Jason Stephenson is described as a 'bubbly youngster' (*Birmingham Evening Mail*). David Stewart's appeal for those who raised money for his experimental treatment lay in his appearance as well as his other category-bound activities:

> hundreds of Massachusetts residents weren't about to extinguish hope. Not for an 11-year-old boy in cargo pants and basketball sneakers, who smiled and waved at the door of the plane taking him to his uncertain medical future.... His father says, 'Here's a boy out riding his bike and doing magic tricks, and I'm not ready to see this end.' (*Boston Globe*)

Additionally, childhood was depicted as a time of entitlement to parental love and support, friends and playmates. Michael Rutter's mother took leave of absence from her job to care for her son (*St Petersburg Times*); Ulises Magana's mother is pictured as she 'hugs her son', another picture shows 'hugs from his sister' and yet another poses Ulises with his father (*Ventura County Star*). Five-year-old Autumn Jensen, who is partially paralysed and unable to swallow because of radiation treatment, 'rested her head on her mother's shoulder' (*Milwaukee Journal Sentinel*). Eleven-year-old David Gaetke 'got a hug from his mother' (*San Diego Union-Tribune*). Louis Dwyer's adoption as a charitable cause for 'Superstar Daniel O'Donnell' involves the said superstar being described as 'a new playmate' in a picture caption (*The Mirror*); David Stewart's 'playmates keep in touch' during his hospital treatment in another city (*Patriot Ledger*).

Thus childhood is routinely produced as a time of life in which certain stereotyped activities, entitlements and relationships are considered normal, healthy and desirable. As was shown earlier, sociologists have pointed out the socially constructed nature of this idealised image in recent years. The analysis of threats to the image is therefore a potentially fertile source of insight into its constructed character.

Threatening childhood

With normal childhood signalled by these means, sickness could then be brought in as the destroyer of such innocently enjoyed entitlements and activities. Thus the mother of 14-year-old Bradley Rutter found that

> It was a rare day this summer when Dora Rutter could keep 14-year-old Bradley inside. Her son's inline skates, dirt bike and fishing pole were his constant companions. But that changed in August when Bradley was diagnosed with Burkitt's lymphoma, a rare form of cancer. Since then, Bradley's days have passed either in a hospital or at home in bed. 'Before all of this, he lived outside,' Rutter said. 'It's hard on a kid, especially in the summer.' (*St Petersburg Times*)

The effect of cancer in threatening normal childlike or teenage appearance was emphasised: 'chemotherapy has claimed his blond hair' (*St Petersburg Times*); Jason Stephenson's determination to 'live life to the full' is achieved 'despite losing his hair' (*Birmingham Evening Mail*). Natalie Willis, 14, underwent treatment 'which caused her long hair to fall out' (*Houston Chronicle*).

The tragedy of the death of Steven Newkirk is given emphasis by the stress on how this disrupted his future, whose especial brightness is emphasised by his teachers:

> 'He was a very bright child. He was one of those kids you could see a bright future for,' said Jane Kier, principal of Pritchett Elementary School in Buffalo Grove, which Steven attended. 'He was charismatic. He was interested in things.' Steven went through kindergarten, first grade and second grade at Pritchett. His illness prevented him from starting the third grade this year. 'Our whole staff, we've all known him. We're all grieving together,' Kier said. 'You hate to lose a kid, any kid, and Steven was a very special one.' (*Chicago Daily Herald*)

Similarly, the promising school careers of two teenagers 'both from the school's gifted and talented classes...classmates who compete with each other for the highest grades at Westfield Middle School' have been blighted by diagnoses of brain tumours (*Indianapolis News*). Because of his illness, Eric Gilliland had to take courses at home last year rather than attending junior high school: ' "He was so sick at times, but he never really complained" [his mother] said. "He got four A's and two B's that year" ' (*Ventura County Star*). David Stewart's ambition to be a pilot is produced poignantly by his father, who waits to see whether his son will respond to last-ditch experimental treatments after conventional therapy has failed (*Boston Globe*).

Contrast between the innocent enjoyment of childish activities and the looming threat of illness is clearly, then, a key device for journalists wishing to increase the human interest value of their stories. This contrast between innocence and evil was particularly marked in the *Toronto Sun* story of Tina Beauvais who, having died from a malignant melanoma aged 13, was laid to rest next to the grave of Dennis Melvyn Howe, a suspected 'sex killer', 'career criminal and child killer' in whose apartment was found a bag of 'a little girl's underwear... [perhaps] some kind of macabre trophy'. The reporting of his death from cancer made much of the fact that this man (who, we learn, smelled, abused alcohol, was covered with nicotine stains and had no friends) had not told anyone of the existence of his pet dog, so that it starved to death in his apartment as he lay dying a 'painful death' in hospital. The Tina Beauvais story focuses on her mother's response to the news that her daughter's grave may be disturbed by plans to exhume Howe's body, but its chief appeal lies simply in the (literal) juxtaposition of the two bodies, representing opposite poles of good and evil: 'The suspected career criminal and child killer is surrounded by Christian crosses and headstones carefully tended by surviving loved ones.' In this story, then, we see a conflation of two threats to childhood innocence – cancer and sex abuse – providing a powerful journalistic opportunity.

More usually, cancer alone is used to represent evil, and the fact that much childhood cancer is now curable has allowed journalists to engage readers in the kind of tense speculation about the outcome that is a familiar ploy in the reporting of sports events. Here, we may note the close connection between the reporting of sports and of cancer that has been established in other media analyses (Clarke and Robinson, 1999; Seale, 2001b), since both genres can be understood, either metaphorically or literally, to invoke a struggle for survival. The underlying drama in the childhood cancer stories reported here is the issue of which force will win: the evil cancer or the innocent child; the more immediate news interest being the way the contest was fought. The drama of searches to find bone marrow donors before a child died was a particularly exciting way to present this tension: ' "We've been to hell and back countless times, hoping and praying the right donor would come along before it was too late" said grandmother Teresa Dwyer' (*Belfast Newsletter*). Seven-year-old Coby Howard failed to make it to the finishing line: 'Howard's family mounted a desperate fund-raising effort [to pay for a bone marrow transplant] but could not raise the money in time to save Coby' (*Boston Globe*). Stephen Lumsden, on the other hand, learned some good news about the bone marrow he had donated, suggesting a successful contest: 'It was amazing to hear about the little girl, and that she was doing well' (*Aberdeen Press and Journal*).

As in all good fairy tales (Langer, 1998; Propp, 1968), heroes must over-come obstacles in spite of villains and with the help of friends. The villains of these stories were commonly obstructive health care bureaucrats, denying children last-hope treatments for reasons kept deliberately obscure by journalists. Thus the David Stewart story hinges on the decision 'last month when the state Medicaid program refused to pay hospitalization costs associated with the disease and its treatment' (*Patriot Ledger*), prompting a surge of community fund-raising activity that resulted in David being flown to Seattle for 'experimental' treatment. His parents 'remain angry at Massachusetts officials who they say cost David precious weeks in his fight for life.... "They cost us some time" [his father] said of the state officials. He said David's condition had worsened considerably' (*Boston Globe*). In another report we learn that 'The Relland foundation is named for a cancer survivor whose parents had to raise money themselves after Alberta Health rejected their plea for coverage of his treatment in the US' (*Edmonton Sun*). A British report, by contrast, focuses on the bungling efforts of Derby City Council, who took two years to fit a specially adapted shower for 16-year-old Zoe Woods, whose operation for cancer had resulted in a leg ' "so delicate they say that if I fall and damage it they will not be able to save it" '. Once fitted, the shower seat fell off the wall: ' "I couldn't believe it..." [said her father] "If that had been Zoe she would have been in serious trouble" ' (*Derby Evening Telegraph*). Health and social service bureaucrats, then, are aligned with the cancer itself in conspiring to destroy children's health.

In view of Manning and Schneiderman's (1996) analysis of the promotion of hopes for miracle cures in children's hospital promotional literature, it is of interest to note the reported words of David Stewart's doctor who, while commenting on the slim chances the experimental treatment offers, is quoted saying: ' "I feel that this is valuable for the family because, obviously, if he has a successful response, that's wonderful.... If he has not, that really clarifies for the family that they have not left a stone unturned" ' (*Patriot Ledger*). As was shown earlier, commentators on medical soap operas (Gerbner, 1981; Signorielli 1993; Turow, 1989) have long been concerned about the effects of portraying medical care as an apparently unlimited resource. Reports of children's cancer appear to reinforce this tendency by generating a readiness to stigmatise bureaucrats. They also fail to dampen hopes for miracle cures since, unlike bureaucrats, doctors (who provide these extremely expensive treatments) are nowhere criticised in the news reports, being aligned with the family and community in leading efforts to rescue children.

Rescuing childhood

Parental love, community support and friendship are not shown as threatened, but instead are shown as enhanced by the cancer experience. Indeed, much of the newsworthiness of the stories is derived from events that depict almost super-human efforts on the part of parents and others to protect and in some cases restore the threatened entitlements of childhood. Identification of heartless bureaucrats, for example, enables the family, friends and 'community' to demonstrate their own heroism in opposing such figures. In US news reports this tension could be made particularly poignant where parents were under-insured for the massive expenses of treatment, so that much of the immediate news interest sparking the stories was in charity fundraising events for the treatment of particular children.

The contrast between the world of childhood and the world of sickness could be made especially poignant if the child could be designated as innocently unaware of a danger that only an adult mind could properly perceive:

> Even at the most difficult moments, his family says, David [Stewart's] mind lingers on typically boyish thoughts. [His mother] recalls seeing David look glum and introspective after a Friday bone marrow test. When she sat down to console the boy, David revealed his thoughts: he prefers Monopoly to war games. 'He's doing better than I expected' [his father] said. (*Boston Globe*)

Here, the continuation of childish activity helps the journalist imaginatively 'rescue' David from the looming threat of illness by emphasising his immersion in the category-bound activity of game playing. David's interest in a variety of childlike activities was, as has been shown earlier, repeatedly emphasised in the reports of his bike riding and museum visiting in Seattle. Rescue efforts were more usually reported as literal, concrete community activities, which often surrounded the children with (newsworthy) special events and ceremonies whose effects were predictably positive and resulted in the continuation or restoration of category entitlements threatened by illness.

The focus of a benefit for 8-year-old Jason Perch, for example, was on a drag race and car show, enabling the journalist to write about Jason's 'passion for cars' and to quote his father saying 'Jason is a car buff' (*Allentown Morning Call*). Teenager Eric Gilliland's passion for golf was such that it inspired the

Orange County chapter of the Make-a-Wish Foundation to get him a member-ship of a local golf club: 'the day got better when Gilliland was presented with bag after bag of golf shirts, balls, hats and tees. He even received a golf bag.... "This is better than Christmas" said Gilliland' (*Ventura County Star*).

Perhaps the most elaborate arrangement for restoring the category-bound entitlements of childhood was in a report from the *Houston Chronicle* describing 'Camp Periwinkle', a holiday camp for children treated at the Texas Children's Cancer Center. The report initially focuses on the story of 14-year-old Kayla Cooper who, 'confined to a wheelchair' because of cancer that had affected her spinal column, was visiting the camp for the first time. Her feelings of anxiety about leaving home, and an initial loneliness, are contrasted with the state she was in soon after her arrival:

> Within a few days, Kayla realized she should never have worried so much – she was having the time of her life. At Camp Periwinkle she was experiencing a lot of 'firsts.' She swam, played volleyball, met Monica Lamb when the Houston Comets center visited the camp, and boogied at two big dances. 'I've been to dances at school, but I never danced. At this dance I did,' she says excitedly. She also took part in an Olympics-style team com-petition, in which she navigated an obstacle course while dodging water balloons, and she scooted in a relay race while balancing a jug of water atop her head. 'I'm really shy. I usually don't cheer, clap or get loud. But I did. Wow, it all came out,' she says. 'Here, I'm a different person.' ... [o]ne of the best things about the camp experience was just hanging around and talking with friends.'

Kayla is thus restored to normal teenage life by the communal repair of her category-bound entitlements. The emphasis on the camp as a special place for rescuing childhood is emphasised in another part of the *Houston Chronicle* report, pointing out the inadequacy of the child's usual home environment for this purpose, recounted by one of the volunteer helpers remembering his sister's experiences: '[My sister] was really fond of this place. My mom was very protective of my sister. Swimming or climbing the wall would never happen at our house. They encourage that here. This is a place she could be herself.'

Idealised subjectivity

Thus far we have seen that newspaper accounts produce or construct childhood as a stage of life involving particular entitlements and activities, so that cancer, by threatening these, may then be understood as an assault on childhood itself. Attempts to rescue childhood by others can then be cast as attempts to restore entitlements. Where does this leave the thoughts, feelings and personal accounts of the children themselves? Analysis suggests that these are commonly reported by people other than the children, resulting in a highly selective presentation.

The subjective moods or perceptions of 21 of the 42 children with cancer were reported, in three cases by direct quotations from the children themselves, but in all other cases by adults associated with the child. Parents were the most common spokespeople (for 14 children), but sometimes other relatives spoke (4 children), other adults (5 children) or journalists themselves wrote about the child's subjective experiences (7 children). This is a marked contrast to the reporting of adult cancer experiences, where people with cancer are more usually quoted directly, or at times author their own reports for newspapers. This is particularly the case for breast cancer 'confessional' accounts, where women appear keen to bear witness in public to their inner experience (Seale, 2002).

The three reports where children 'spoke for themselves' (although clearly we must recognise the hand of journalists in selecting and arranging quotations) included Kayla Cooper at Camp Periwinkle, another child in that location who spoke of her renewal of confidence brought about by the camp experience, and Eric Gilliland, the grateful recipient of golfing presents. Clearly these are all 'upbeat' stories of success and gratitude that demonstrate the benefits of community rescue efforts. The Kayla Cooper story is particularly marked by its realism and emotional impact in charting the transition from frightened child to blossoming teenager.

In other reports of children's subjectivity there was a distinct tendency towards idealisation of the child's character, perhaps made particularly poignant by the fact that five of these involved children who had died, thus introducing a eulogistic element to the report. Thus Michael Penon's qualities were remembered by his parents, whose reminiscences are introduced sympathetically by the journalist:

> Throughout his illness, Penon never lost his propensity for caring. When interviewed on national television shows, he repeatedly called upon potential marrow donors to help the many people in need. 'He didn't just say "Help me,"' Angela Tucker said. 'He was looking out for other people. Most kids would say "Help me."' (*News Tribune*)

Steven Newkirk was remembered fondly by his teacher and his parents: ' "Steven was a child who could light up the room," said Jane Kier, principal of Buffalo Grove's Pritchett Elementary School, where Steven was a pupil' (*Chicago Tribune*). Kelly Freeman was remembered by her mother: ' "As sick as she was, she would go and comfort all the other kids in the hospital," her mother said. "She was amazing. She never questioned why this had happened to her"' (*Cincinnati Inquirer*).

Children still living with cancer, however, could also attract such eulogising discourse. Kelly Tatum's mother was quoted saying: 'She's showing us how to deal with this. . . . She's very brave and has been an inspiration to us both' (*Indianapolis News*). Sarah Nelson's mother said 'Sarah gets up with a smile every day. She has always been a cheerful fighter. She really loves life and it shows' (*Dayton Daily News*). Nine-year-old Ulises Magana attracted a number of comments from members of the community engaged in supporting him and his family:

> 'He just draws you to him,' she said, choking back tears. 'Now you're going to make me cry. He's just very sweet and special and, what can I say, he's just a great kid.' Ulises is 'one of God's jewels,' said Martha Brunner, a school worker who is close with the Magana family. 'He's just a wonderful, wonderful person,' Vlahakis said. 'I don't know what it is.' (*Ventura County Star*)

Thus, qualities of special insight, bravery, cheerfulness and altruism were commonly reported qualities of children with cancer. With the exception of the anxiety felt by Kayla Cooper on entering Camp Periwinkle, the only negative emotions said to have been expressed by children with cancer concerned two children who were reported to have cried before their deaths. These are searing, if brief, images and stand in stark contrast to depiction of the moment of death as akin to a peaceful sleep, which might have been expected of this journalistic genre: ' "During this entire ordeal, he [Michael Penon] never complained," Andre Penon said. "It wasn't until the very end that he cried a little" ' (*News Tribune*). ' "We tried to make him [Otto Tang] as comfortable as we could," Mattson said. "He was crying" ' (*Seattle Times*). Perhaps these (albeit brief) references to terminal distress are introduced to reinforce the tragic element of the stories, already tragic through their focus on a life cut short.

Conclusion

This analysis has shown that news reports of children with cancer participate in the construction of childhood as a time of life where children are entitled to childish activities. Sporting endeavours and the possession and use of toys are presented as obvious markers of childhood, along with an appropriately childlike appearance and the assumption that childhood is a preparation for future potential through educational activity and progress. Additionally, an entitlement (and perhaps incitement) to parental love and affection, and the company of friends and playmates is asserted. Threatening to break up this happy scenario, childhood cancer initially begins by disrupting the most obvious signs of childhood:

children can no longer play with their toys, maintain their appearance, pursue their educational careers under such threat. Cancer, in fact, is an evil, equated to other evils that threaten childhood identified by media sociologists, such as the spectre of child abuse, abduction and the more distant evils that seem to happen to children in poorer countries (Burman, 1994a; 1994b).

Help, though, is at hand. Medical professionals, who of course benefit from this unquestioning valorisation of their expensive efforts, are conceived as allies and helpers in the childhood cancer story. Primarily, though, help at the most heroic level emanates from 'the community', conceived as gathering round equally heroic but nevertheless overwhelmed sets of parents, who are portrayed as confronting the limits of an almost endless supply of parental love. Thus parents both represent the best and most intensive aspects of community endeavour, and are at the same time in need of community support against the combined forces of disease and occasionally obstructive bureaucracy. Hence the opportunity for the journalistic report, which both records and orchestrates community effort.

Through the heroic efforts of these individuals, children are sometimes rescued, this primarily being symbolised by the continuation or restoration of the category-bound entitlements and activities of childhood. It appears, as in the case of Camp Periwinkle, that this can at times involve the removal of the child from the parent and into the arms of quasi-professionalised communities who may possess specialist expertise in the restoration of children – the resumption of childlike activities heralding a return to childhood for grateful participants. At other times, children's charities gather around to 'make a wish come true' by providing presents, award ceremonies and celebrations for the stricken individual, again portrayed in grateful receipt of this attention. Whether children with cancer live or die, however, it seems that they are all special characters, with unusual levels of insight, cheerfulness, courage or altruism. Rarely do children with cancer speak for themselves, or express distress at any length. This absence allows generous scope for idealised depictions of child heroism.

Lupton (1994b), in a study of Australian news reports of women with breast cancer, found (in contrast to other studies of cancer reports, see, for example, Seale, 2002) that these involved the 'exclusion of the needs, wants, and feelings of women in the general population' (Lupton, 1994b, p. 83). If applied to the reports of children with cancer analysed here, rather than to women, the comment is accurate, in so far as children rarely speak for themselves. The adults who speak for them introduce a powerful element of idealisation, often involving triumphant or awestruck accounts of the child's special qualities that apparently enable the children to make light of the illness, or to retain their childlike interests in spite of it. Only occasionally is this idealised picture broken up by reminders of the intensity of suffering endured by these children, perhaps introduced by journalists concerned to heighten the interest in human tragedy represented by stories of dying children. The rare moments where children speak for themselves are notably more realistic about the ups and downs of feelings involved in serious illness and disability, but nevertheless focus on upbeat accounts, reminding us that in the last analysis journalists (and editors) select the stories they are going to tell.

Unlike the news reporting of adult cancer experience – and of breast cancer in particular, where an activist movement has been strikingly successful in gaining a voice in press reports – children with cancer are largely denied the opportunity to voice their experiences on their own terms. In this respect, representations of sick children are similar to those of disabled people some years ago, before the critique of 'Telethon mentality' led to new thinking about such stigmatising images (Elliott and Byrd, 1982; Rolland, 1997). A very simple range of emotions is allowed them, with negative feelings, distress, aggression and pain receiving either no attention or only fleeting mention, and then only to rhetorically heighten tragic effects, rather than to allow readers to enter sympathetically into the complex subjective world of illness experience. Thus the knowledgeability of children about cancer (Oakley et al., 1995) is also denied by this style of reporting. The erasure of subjectivity in reports of children has been noted by sociologists who have analysed other areas of the media, such as charitable aid campaigns (Burman, 1999) and sex abuse coverage (Goddard, 1995). There is, then, in these news reports, no discussion of the wisdom of expensive and traumatising medical treatments for which parents are said to lobby so anxiously. Parents' and 'community' wishes for rescue at all costs seem to be paramount. Children are denied an active role in treatment decisions, or in expressing their own views of the meaning of disease, in deference to images of childhood that render children largely passive and grateful recipients of the busy efforts made by adults on their behalf. The idealised newspaper portrayal of family life is also significantly at odds with studies that have directly investigated families where a child has cancer (Dixon-Woods et al., 2003; Young et al., 2002).

The dramatic emphasis on life-or-death situations in media portrayals is clearly enhanced if potential victims of disease can be portrayed as innocently deserving of care and compassion. Thus the disruption of childhood by the threat of cancer offers journalists a perfect opportunity to identify villains and helpers and so add to calls for increased funding of health services. This rhetorical exploitation of characters standing in opposition to each other is a somewhat standardised feature of news reports designed to evoke sentiment and identification in human dramas (Langer, 1998; Seale, 2003). A ready supply of villains who, at least in imagination, are conceived as the allies of cancer itself, are the heartless and bungling bureaucrats who run health care systems without prioritising the unique demands of sick children, who are depicted as deserving limitless resources of care. Bureaucrats, then, are stigmatised in a way that is analogous to the stigmatisation of the social work profession in child abuse stories (Gough, 1996). There are also parallels to be drawn with the criticism made of 'authorities' by parents lobbying for the recognition of ADHD as a widespread social problem deserving drug treatment (Lloyd and Norris, 1999).

The view that health care ought to be an unlimited resource is in fact promoted in a variety of other media representations of health, illness and health care. The portrayal of health care in television soaps, for example, analysed by Joseph Turow in his book *Playing Doctor* (1989), has consistently involved the stigmatisation of health care administrators, who are shown variously obstructing, impeding or attempting to cut back on the health care that doctors (usually heroically) attempt to provide. Drs Kildare and Casey possessed apparently limitless resources for patient care. The harassed medics in later soaps, such as those working in 'St Elsewhere', were perhaps less heroic, but were nevertheless depicted as oppressed by a hospital bureaucracy that obstructed the implied ideal of endlessly available health care. The economic context of health care receives little serious attention in such fictional portrayals and probably contributes to a generally low level of public understanding of political debates about health care (Gerbner, 1981; Signorielli, 1993). It appears from the present analysis that stories about childhood cancer share this characteristic with soap opera.

REFERENCES

Altheide, D. L. and Michalowski, R. S., 'Fear in the News: a Discourse of Control', *Sociological Quarterly*, 40:3 (1999), pp. 475–503.

Atmore, C., 'Cross-cultural Media-tions: Media Coverage of Two Child Sexual Abuse Controversies in New Zealand/Aotearoa', *Child Abuse Review*, 5 (1996), pp. 334–45.

Best, J., 'Rhetoric in Claims-making: Constructing the Missing Children Problem', *Social Problems*, 34:2 (1987), pp. 101–21.

Best, J., 'Missing Children, Misleading Statistics', *Public Interest*, 92 (1988), pp. 84–92.

Buckingham, D., 'Dissin' Disney: Critical Perspectives on Children's Media Culture', *Media, Culture and Society*, 19 (1997), pp. 285–93.

Burman, E., 'Poor Children: Charity Appeals and Ideologies of Childhood', *Changes*, 12:1 (1994a), pp. 29–36.

Burman, E., 'Innocents Abroad: Western Fantasies of Childhood and the Iconography of Emergencies', *Disasters*, 18:3 (1994b), pp. 238–53.

Burman, E., 'Appealing and Appalling Children', *Psychoanalytic Studies*, 1:3 (1999), pp. 285–301.

Clarke, J. and Robinson, J., 'Testicular Cancer: Medicine and Machismo in the Media 1980–94', *Health*, 3:3 (1999), pp. 263–82.

Dixon-Woods, M., Seale, C., Young, B., Findlay, M. and Heney, D., 'Representing Childhood Cancer: Accounts from Newspapers and Parents', *Sociology of Health and Illness* (2003).

Elliott, T. R. and Byrd, E. K., 'Media and Disability', *Rehabilitation Literature*, 43: 11/12 (1982), pp. 348–55.

Entwistle, V., Watt, I. S., Bradbury, R. and Pehl, L., 'Media Coverage of the Child B Case', *British Medical Journal*, 312 (1996), pp. 1587–91.

Fowler, R., *Language in the News: Discourse and Ideology in the Press* (London: Routledge, 1991).

Fritz, N. J. and Altheide, D. L., 'The Mass Media and the Social Construction of the Missing Children Problem', *Sociological Quarterly*, 28:4 (1987), pp. 473–92.

Galtung, J. and Ruge, M., 'Structuring and Selecting News', in S. Cohen and J. Young (eds), *The Manufacture of News: Social Problems, Deviance and the Mass Media* (London: Constable, 1973).

Gerbner, G., 'Health and Medicine on Television', *The New England Journal of Medicine*, 305:15 (1981), pp. 901–4.

Giroux, H. A., 'Nymphet Fantasies: Child Beauty Pageants and the Politics of Inno-cence', *Social Text*, 16:4 (1998), pp. 31–53.

Goddard, C., 'Read All About It! The News about Child Abuse', *Child Abuse Review*, 5 (1995), pp. 301–9.

Gough, D., 'The Literature on Child Abuse and the Media', *Child Abuse Review*, 5 (1996), pp. 363–76.

James, A. and Jenks, C., 'Perceptions of Childhood Criminality', *British Journal of Sociol-ogy*, 47:2 (1996), pp. 315–31.

Jenks, C., 'Child Abuse in the Postmodern Context: an Issue of Social Identity', *Childhood*, 2 (1994), pp. 111–21.

Jenks, C., 'Constituting Child Abuse: a Problem of Late Modernity?' *Sociological Studies of Children*, 7 (1995), pp. 155–75.

Kitzinger, J., 'The Gender-politics of News Production: Silenced Voices and False Memories', in C. Carter, G. Branston and G. Allan (eds), *News, Gender and Power* (London: Routledge, 1998), pp. 186–203.

Langer, J., *Tabloid Television: Popular Journalism and the 'Other News'* (London and New York: Routledge, 1998).

Lloyd, G. and Norris, C., 'Including ADHD?' *Disability and Society*, 14:4 (1999) pp. 505–17.

Luke, C., 'Childhood and Parenting in Popular Culture', *Australian and New Zealand Journal of Sociology*, 30:3 (1994), pp. 289–302.

Lumley, K., '"Teeny Thugs in Blair's Sights": Media Portrayals of Children in Education and their Policy Implications', *Youth and Policy*, 61 (1998), pp. 1–11.

Lupton, D., *Medicine as Culture: Illness, Disease and the Body in Western Societies* (London: Sage, 1994a).

Lupton, D., 'Femininity, Responsibility, and the Technological Imperative: Discourses on Breast Cancer in the Australian Press', *International Journal of Health Services*, 24:1 (1994b), pp. 73–89.

Manning, S. and Schneiderman, L. J., 'Miracles or Limits: What Message from the Medical Marketplace?' *HEC Forum*, 8:2 (1996), pp. 103–8.

Moller, D. W., *Confronting Death: Values, Institutions and Human Mortality* (Oxford: Oxford University Press, 1996).

Oakley, A., Bendelow, G., Barnes, J., Buchanan, M. and Husain, O. A. Naseem, 'Health and Cancer Prevention – Knowledge and Beliefs of Children and Young People', *British Medical Journal*, 310:6986 (1995), pp. 1029–33.

Potter, J. and Wetherell, M., *Discourse and Social Psychology: Beyond Attitudes and Behaviour* (London: Sage, 1987).

Propp, V. I., *Morphology of the Folk Tale* (Austen: University of Texas Press, 1968).

Rolland, J. S., 'The Meaning of Disability and Suffering: Sociopolitical and Ethical Concerns', *Family Process*, 36:4 (1997), pp. 437–40.

Seale, C. F., *The Quality of Qualitative Research* (London: Sage, 1999).

Seale, C. F., 'Cancer in the News: Religious Themes in News Stories about People with Cancer', *Health*, 5:4 (2001a), pp. 445–60.

Seale, C. F., 'Sporting Cancer: Struggle Language in News Reports of People with Cancer', *Sociology of Health and Illness*. 23:3 (2001b), pp. 308–29.

Seale, C. F., 'Cancer Heroics: a Study of News Reports with Particular Reference to Gender', *Sociology*, 36:1 (2002), pp. 107–26.

Seale, C. F., *Media and Health* (London: Sage, 2003).

Signorielli, N., *Mass Media Images and Impact on Health* (Westport, CT: Greenwood Press, 1993).

Silverman, D., *Harvey Sacks: Social Science and Conversation Analysis* (Cambridge: Polity Press, 1998).

Turow, J., *Playing Doctor: Television, Storytelling, and Medical Power* (New York: Oxford University Press, 1989).

Walgrave, S. and Stouthuysen, P., 'From Tears to Clenched Fists, about the Politicization of Private Emotions: the Dutroux Case', *Tijdschrift voor Sociologie*, 19:3 (1996), pp. 347–76.

Weber, R. P., *Basic Content Analysis* (Newbury Park, CA: Sage, 1990).

Young, B., Dixon-Woods, M., Findlay, M. and Heney, D., 'Parenting in a Crisis: Conceptualising Mothers of Children with Cancer', *Social Science and Medicine*, 55 (2002), pp. 1835–47.

Mad Cows and Mad Scientists: What Happened to Public Health in the Battle for the Hearts and Minds of the Great British Beef Consumer?

5

Martin King and Clare Street

Introduction

The BSE (Bovine Spongiform Encephalopathy) crisis of the 1980s and 1990s raised a number of questions about the mass media's role in the protection of public health in the UK. In this chapter we focus on the role of the mass media as messenger in a crisis of confidence in the food supply chain. We also examine the role of the media in the policy making process and its relationship to other key players – in this case the UK government, other European governments, the farmers, supermarket chains, consumers and public health 'experts'.

It is our intention to focus on the UK print media and, using the BSE crisis as a case study, examine some of the complexities of the media's role in relation to public health issues.

The chapter will examine the value of using media and cultural studies techniques in relation to specific public health 'problems' or 'crises' and look at what this can tell us about these 'problems' and 'crises'. It will also examine the role of the media in relation to public health issues, exploring some of the debates about the role of the media in reflecting and constructing 'problems'.

It will then raise questions about the role of Government in protecting the public health and look at some of the conflicts of interest which seemed to emerge in the BSE crisis in the UK (Figure 5.1).

The major 'panic' about BSE – the 'discovery' that turned it into a major public health issue – was the link made between BSE in cattle and variant CJD (Creutzfelt-Jakob Disease) in humans, in 1996 (Maxwell, 1999). However,

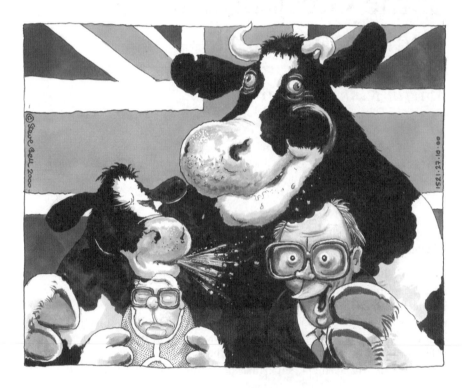

Figure 5.1   BSE: The *Guardian* cartoonist Steve Bell portrays politicians in the grip of 'mad cow disease' still waving the flag (*Guardian*, 27 October 2000)

this link has been disputed more recently (Mills, 2000). Maxwell (1999) offers a chronology of key events from 1986 to 1995, which is reproduced here (Table 5.1), and this provides useful background to this case study.

The use of media and cultural studies techniques in a public health context

The development of interdisciplinary work which recognises the value of using the techniques of media and cultural studies to investigate health 'texts' is a relatively recent development (Bunton, 1997; King and Watson, 2001; Seale, 2003).

> If we view cultural studies as an 'intellectual strategy' that is 'mobile and adaptive' (Bennett, 1998) then its application to the field of 'health studies' seems self-evident. Rather than viewing cultural studies as a discrete discipline with fixed boundaries, we would advocate the use of the 'strategies' associated with cultural studies to interrogate 'health' issues. (King and Watson, 2001, p. 405)

In the field of public health a number of authors have done this with interesting results (Lupton, 1993; Bunton, 1997; Southwell, 2000).

As King and Watson (2001, p. 406) state:

> there has been a recent recognition in the sphere of public health that the study of media representations of 'health' and the audience catered for by such representations is centrally important to that discipline.

Southwell (2000) emphasises the central importance of looking at media representations of public health issues when he states:

> in so far as such realisations are worthwhile, analysis in this vein is not idle perusal of arcane documents but rather vital work for public health researchers. (Southwell, 2000, p. 317)

We would argue that the techniques of documentary research (May, 1993; Plummer, 2001), discourse analysis (Chouliaraki and Fairclough, 1999; Torfing, 2002) as well as Foucault's (1989) work on power and Hall's (1980) work at the Centre for Contemporary Cultural Studies in Birmingham in the 1970s and 80s, provide excellent analytical tools to examine public health issues and the way that they are reflected and constructed in the mass media. Later in this

Table 5.1   Chronology of events

Date	Event
November 1986	BSE first identified by Central Veterinary Laboratory.
5 June 1987	Chief Veterinary Officer (CVO) informs Minister of Agriculture about new disease.
15 December 1987	Initial epidemiological studies completed, which conclude that ruminant-derived meat and bone meal (MBM) was the only viable hypothesis for the cause of BSE.
3 March 1988	Department of Health informed. Expert Advisory Committee recommended.
21 April 1988	Southwood Working Party established. As a result, government indicated it would legislate to make BSE notifiable and to ban ruminant-derived MBM.
21 June 1988	BSE Order 1988 made BSE notifiable.
July 1988	Following advice from Southwood, decision announced to introduce slaughter of all affected cattle, and ban on ruminant-derived MBM comes into force.
8 August 1988	Compensation Order introduced. Compensation set at 50% of value for confirmed cases, 100% for negative; both subject to ceiling.
February 1989	Southwood Report received and published, with government's response. Establishment of Tyrrell Committee on research announced (as recommended by Southwood).
10 June 1989	Tyrrell Report received by government.
13 June 1989	Decision to introduce offals ban announced – not a Southwood recommendation but a government initiative.
28 July 1989	EC ban on export of cattle born before 18 July 1988 and offspring of affected or suspect animals.
13 November 1989	Ban on specified bovine offals (SBO) comes into force.
9 January 1990	Tyrrell Report on research, and government response to it, published.
14 February 1990	Compensation figures changed (see 8 August 1988). Full compensation would be paid, up to a ceiling.
1 March 1990	EC restricts exports of cattle to animals under six months.
1 April 1990	Disease made notifiable to European Commission.
3 April 1990	Spongiform Encephalopathy Advisory Committee (SEAC) established under chairmanship of Dr David Tyrrell.
9 April 1990	EC decision to ban export of SBO and other tissues.

11 April 1990	Humberside County Council withdraws British beef from school meals.
24 July 1990	Dr Tyrrell writes publicly to the Chief Medical Office to say 'any risk as a result of eating beef or feed products is minute. Thus we believe that there is no scientific reason for not eating British beef and that it can be eaten by everyone.'
25 September 1990	Ban on the use of SBO extended to its inclusion in any animal feed. Export of such feed to other EU member states also banned. (Exports outside the EU banned 10 July 1991.)
15 October 1990	Farmers required to maintain breeding and movement records.
27 June 1994	Prohibition on the feeding of mammalian protein to ruminants throughout the EU, other than Denmark.
1 April 1995	Compulsory blue staining of SBO.
15 August 1995	The Specified Bovine Offal Order 1995 consolidated and tightened the existing rules for processing SBO.

chapter we will be applying these techniques to newspaper coverage of the BSE crisis in the UK.

Science, public health and food scares

Williams and Miller (1998) outline the increase in the British Press of health coverage throughout the 1980s, leading to the establishing of 'health' reporters or 'health' teams on all major newspapers. A major feature of this type of reporting has always been the reporting of the views of the scientist or expert, which, Allan (2002) argues, creates a tension between the superficiality of journalism and the serious expertise of the 'boffin' in the white coat:

> journalists, struggling to report on a scientific development . . . will more often than not succumb to the forces of sensationalism to make their news account attract the public's wandering eye.   (Allan, 2002, p. 2)

He goes on to argue that it is the discourse between science and the media that creates the 'reality' of any given public health issue, such as the BSE crisis, and that the public draws on these discourses and the media's representation of 'science' and 'scientific fact' to make sense of such issues.

Food scares, throughout the 1980s and 1990s, have provided good copy for journalists. In addition, Allan (2002) argues, the associated media interest in campaigning consumer journalism, celebrity chefs and cooking shows, and an increase in food advertising, have placed food at the centre of the national consciousness.

The mass media and the construction of public health 'problems'

There are a wide variety of views regarding the role and influence of the media in society (Boyd-Barrett and Newbold, 1995; Gripsrud, 2002; McLuhan, 1964; Silverstone, 1999). These range from those who, like Gramsci (1971), believe that institutions such as the mass media operate in the interests of the ruling elite and powerful interests in society, to those with a more pluralistic vision (Parsons, 1995) who see those in the media as players in a process which brings issues into the political arena and shapes policy.

Beardsworth and Keil (1997, p. 171) state:

> once issues of food safety have escaped the control of a closed, oligarchical policy community and entered into the public domain, the official voice becomes only one voice among many, each presenting its competing account.

Adam (2000) argues that journalists are constantly trying to re-frame public health debates within an economic discourse and we will look at this later in the chapter when examining the health vs wealth debate around BSE. In order to make the debate 'fit' into something more manageable, he argues, the economic discourse tends to predominate. However, with a food scare or panic like the BSE crisis, this is not always successful and the debate cannot always be contained. What is interesting when looking at the reporting of the BSE crisis is that evidence can be found to support these differing perspectives and viewpoints.

To illustrate this we can pull out a couple of examples of different 'voices' speaking through the media. There are numerous examples of the voice of the political elite, or the official government line on the link between BSE and variant CJD. An article in *The Times* from the early 1990s (Hornsby, 1993) with the headline 'Cow disease does not affect humans' includes a number of statements from the Chief Medical Officer (CMO) and farmers' leaders emphasising the safety of eating beef. Dr Calman, the CMO, is quoted as saying: 'I wish to emphasise that there is no scientific evidence of a causal link between BSE in cattle and CJD in humans' (Hornsby, 1993, p. 1).

However, dissenting, sceptical 'voices' are also in evidence. An article from the *Financial Times*, published three years earlier (Bloom, 1990) with the headline 'Mad Cows and Englishmen', reports the fear and uncertainty felt by the public in the wake of the Southwood Report of 1989, which, Bloom states, is 'full of reservations and its conclusions are tentative' (Bloom, 1990, p. 7). Coming early in the debate about BSE in the print media this article is interesting in beginning to report (or is it construct?) a 'panic'.

> There are largely unspoken and deep-seated fears behind today's most emotional British debate, centring on the so-called mad cow disease. . . . BSE is alarming, not least because so little is known about it.   (Bloom, 1990, p. 7)

This is what Wilkins (1964) means when he states that the media 'sensitises' and 'amplifies' problems. This is, we would argue, especially true of the print media, our main focus in this chapter. The tabloid media in particular have a tendency to sensationalise what are sometimes minor events into a major social problem.

Perhaps the classic study which illustrates this is Cohen's (1972) *Folk Devils and Moral Panics – the Creation of the Mods and Rockers*, in which he describes how a few minor skirmishes between rival groups on Brighton beach in 1964 became a 'moral panic' about the state of youth and its deviant behaviour in modern society, through its reporting and amplification in the tabloid media.

Cohen states:

> The student of moral enterprise cannot but pay particular attention to the role of the mass media in defining and shaping social problems. The media have long operated as agents of moral indignation in their own right: even if they are not self-consciously engaged in crusading or muck racking, their very reporting of certain 'facts' can be sufficient to generate concern, anxiety, indignation or panic.   (Cohen, 1972, p. 16)

This study observes that the print media has a pivotal role in the creation of 'panic' around particular issues and there have been a number of public health 'panics' and 'scares' in the media over the past twenty years to support this thesis – HIV, salmonella, the contraceptive pill, the MMR vaccine and, of course, BSE – to name just a few. It is interesting, to illustrate these points, to look at the reporting of a particular event in the crisis by a broadsheet (the *Financial Times*) and a tabloid (the *Daily Mail*). The event in question is the death of a farmer from variant CJD, which therefore provided the media with its first real 'case' to link BSE and CJD.

The reporting in the *Daily Mail* (Henderson and Oldfield, 1993), under the headline 'The First Victim of Mad Cow Disease', is much more personalised, with its tabloid 'human interest' angle and very emotive language. The use of the term 'mad cow disease', and the description of the farmer in question as being 'transformed from a healthy extrovert into a slurring unsteady hospital patient requiring constant care' and suffering a 'dramatic decline' (Henderson and Oldfield, 1993, p. 1), are woven together into a tale of human tragedy.

Characterised as 'the life and soul of the party ... a lovely fellow ... a typically healthy outdoor type' (Henderson and Oldfield, 1993, p. 5), the farmer is contrasted with faceless 'Government scientists' who 'reported anonymously' his death, commissioning 'further scientific studies' (Henderson and Oldfield, 1993, p. 1). The structure of the report uses these binary oppositions (Lévi-Strauss, 1968) to create a sensational story, creating its own certainty about the link between BSE and variant CJD in the midst of uncertain and contradictory evidence.

The official denial of a causal link between BSC and variant CJD, which features in the *Daily Mail* article, is given prominence in the *Financial Times* report of the same incident (Cookson, 1993). Under the headline 'Government seeks to allay fear of "Mad Cow" disease', the report gives voice to 'Government veterinary and health experts' (Cookson, 1993, p. 6) and prominence to the Government Chief Medical Officer's statement: 'there is no scientific evidence of a causal link between BSE in cattle and CJD in humans' (Cookson, 1993, p. 6).

In a much shorter, less emotive and personal report than that of the *Daily Mail*, the emphasis is on science and statistical analysis, with a disclaimer from the doctor who published the report of the death in the *Lancet*.

> Dr Robert Will of Western General Hospital, Edinburgh who is monitoring all CJD cases in the UK for the Department of Health, drew attention to Mr Warhurst's case without naming him in the *Lancet*, a medical journal. He says he now regrets writing to the *Lancet* because of the unnecessary alarm caused.   (Cookson, 1993, p. 6).

The policy making agenda

Parsons (1995) explores the role of the media as a player in the policy making process. He states:

> The mass media can shape the context within which policy responses take place and influence 'public opinion' by setting a public agenda in terms of an incident or event. (Parsons, 1995, p. 107)

The contrasting previous examples provide a good illustration of this point. This view of the mass media – and, especially, we would argue, the print media – as a key player in the policy making process is supported by Newby (1993, p. 320), who says:

Twenty years ago social science would have made the arrogant claim that it alone could produce solutions to social and economic problems according to some rational model of social engineering. However, as we now know all too well, social science does not provide solutions for policy makers in this way. . . . Policy 'problems' are highly contextual and contingent; they are defined and framed by certain historical circumstances and configurations. Any 'solution' has, therefore, to take into account this contingency, which includes the way in which 'problems' are perceived, interpreted and also manipulated by actors in the policy process.

Miller et al. (1998), in their work on the reporting of HIV and AIDS in the media, argue that news organizations play an active role in defining social problems and shaping solutions. These views challenge the notion that the media merely reports or reflects on social issues. Instead they advance the view that the media are part of a process which constructs them. Parsons (1995) puts forward a framework which illustrates the way in which the media feed into the public policy making process. As he states:

the media . . . by being in the business of 'manufacturing' news are also involved in the production of problems. The media select what is 'newsworthy' and in so selecting include and exclude issues, events and ideas.   (Parsons, 1995, p. 107)

The process he outlines is as follows:

- An incident
  - Media take up story
    - Incident portrayed as illustrating a wider/bigger social problem
      - Stereotypes emerge
        - Distortion of issues
          - 'Out of proportion' coverage
            - Public panic
              - Demands for policy makers to do something.

This argument incorporates Hall et al.'s (1978) ideas on the media as secondary definers of important social issues in the news – an institution which translates the messages and discourses of the primary definers, such as government, into a product for public consumption.

We have already looked at an example of 'an incident' ('The first victim of mad cow disease'), which, using Parsons' (1995) framework, triggered the need for a policy response. The turning point or 'public panic' in the BSE crisis occurred in 1995 as evidence of links between BSE and variant CJD seemed to grow.

One example, from the *Independent* (Castle et al., 1996), under the headline 'Now Ministers have to eat their words', illustrates how TV news, in particular, plays a key role in establishing the parameters of debate around key social issues and is active in deciding what is included and excluded (Fiske, 1987). This article links two key themes which emerge throughout the reporting of the crisis – the threat to public health and the economic threat.

> Ministers are in no doubt of the scale of the calamity now unfolding. On the one hand, there is the possibility, identified by the Chairman of the Scientific Committee on BSE, that thousands or even hundreds of thousands of people could fall victim to a fatal disease. On the other, there is the prospect that an entire industry, the flower of our agricultural system, could be devastated at a cost of billions of pounds and thousands of jobs. (Castle et al., 1996, p. 16)

Prior to this point the print media had reflected the elite/dissenting voices' debate. After 1996 what we see is the move on Parsons' (1995) framework to 'a demand for policy makers to do something' coupled with venomous attacks on the previous 'official' or 'elite' line. This is well reflected in an article from the *Daily Mirror* (Wilson, 1996) under the headline '10 year battle against scourge: the denials: 10 year history of mad cow disease'. This article charts events in the crisis:

> At every turn, at every new crisis, the Government has reacted with smug complacency... today the *Daily Mirror* looks back on the shameful story of BSE in Britain.   (Wilson, 1996, p. 4)

This type of reporting then becomes the norm, and numerous examples can be found (Allison, 1998; Anon., 1998; Martin, 1996).

This provides evidence that the intervention of the journalists (and their role in creating a 'panic' in such a crisis) establishes them firmly as key players in the policy making process.

In addition McQuail and Windahl (1993) would assert that agenda setting can be initiated by the media or policy makers and that this can be a complex and interactive process. Downs' (1972) work adds to this by stating that the media has a limited issue-attention span – public health concerns such as BSE and its links to CJD are eventually displaced from the front pages by the infidelities of politicians, the threat of evil foreign dictators or the break-up of the latest manufactured singing sensation.

Downs' issue-attention cycle (1972) asserts that policy issues and concerns go from a pre-problem stage, to alarmed discovery/euphoric enthusiasm, to realising the costs of significant progress. Then a gradual decline of public interest eventually leads to the post-problem stage, with some kind of policy solution in place.

This can be seen in the reporting of BSE, when fresh interest in the issue was generated by the government's official inquiry into the crisis in 2000. Under the headline 'Named and Blamed . . . the decision makers' (Anon., 2000, p. 17), the *Daily Mail* reports on the results of the inquiry, apportioning blame and taking on the voice of 'the public'.

Health vs wealth

The question of who are the key players in a public health crisis is particularly pertinent to our case study on BSE, where a number of key stakeholders – the UK government, public health professionals, scientific 'experts', farmers, super-market chains, consumers and foreign importers of British beef – seem to have been vying for influence in the policy making process. The way in which the media reported the views of these stakeholders, how the messages given by different stakeholders over the period of the crisis changed, whose views became the dominant discourse (Foucault, 1989) and whose were filtered out, are important questions for those interested in public health in the UK.

We have already mentioned two key themes – the concern over public health, and the threat to economic wealth posed by the crisis. There is an obvious tension between these two issues – conspiracy theorists would obviously see early (pre-1996) reporting of the 'cow disease does not affect humans' (Hornsby, 1993) and 'Government seeks to delay fear of "mad cow" disease' (Cookson, 1993) type as being intentionally misleading, putting concerns about wealth before health. Partisan views are certainly reflected in the reporting of the crisis – we have discussed how these shifted in 1996. This is also obvious in the reporting of another key theme in the crisis – the ban by the EU on British beef products – which led to, perhaps predictable, tabloid jingoism. Even the Press Association provides us with the headline 'Beef Ban humiliation for Britain' (Meade, 1996), describing a 'humiliating defeat', and 'Draconian Ban' (Meade, 1996, p. 1), while at the same time politicians of all persuasions refused to be daunted by potentially dangerous British Beef – 'I'll keep eating beef, says Blair' (McCarthy, 1996, p. 1).

This resulted in the production of obviously contradictory messages from the print media – at a time when outrage was being expressed about the withhold-ing of information and a possible threat to public health, anger was also being expressed at 'foreigners' (the old enemy) refusing to eat 'our' beef. Thus an 'it may be dangerous but its ours' mentality emerges in much of the reporting at

this time. It is important to recognise that the print media are capable of sending out such mixed messages and developing often conflicting themes through
selectivity in reporting. Fiske's (1987) work examines the notion of selectivity
in news reporting and draws on a body of work in the field of media and cultural studies which debates the notion of power.

> The news tells the story of the key events of the last twenty-four hours. This simple defi-
> nition introduces the contradictions. . . . For events seem to be part of nature, whereas
> the telling of stories and the selection of the key events are clearly cultural activities. The
> first struggle of news is to impose the order of culture upon the polymorphous nature of
> 'the real'. The news text is engaged in a constant struggle to contain the multifarious
> events and their polysemic potential within its own conventions.   (Fiske, 1987, p. 783)

Of particular interest to us here is the relationship between government and
media during the BSE crisis, and the whole notion of conflicting interests. The
role of information was obviously a vital factor. Lang (1996, p. 40) states:

> a key factor was government misunderstanding of the role of information in the market
> place of ideas. It failed to realise that the British public, in crucial senses, was and is rela-
> tively BSE literate. It has experienced years of media coverage.

Here he highlights the seeming contradictions between the Government's assertion that 'British Beef is safe to eat' in the early part of the crisis, with information
being reported in the same period which suggested a link between infected meat
and variant CJD, and a failure of government policy at that point to prevent
infected beef getting into the food supply (Baggott, 2000; Maxwell, 1999).

Science and the role of the 'expert'

This is where the role of the scientific 'expert' and the use of and reporting of
'scientific fact' become extremely important. Lang (1996, p. 39) asks:

> what is the role of the state in such a crisis? More precisely, how is a balance to be struck
> between the state, the public, science and scientific interests and evidence?

The use of 'science' and 'expert' opinion by the government to support its
often changing messages in public health issues is a contentious area for public
policy analysts (Adam, 2000). The print media often provide a forum for such
messages. However, in the reporting of the Phillips Inquiry into BSE and variant
CJD in the *Lancet* (Anon, 2001) this approach was criticised.

The Inquiry report highlights the way that the UK Government wrongly put expert scientific committees into the policy making limelight, especially by **manipulating** [our emphasis added] its Spongiform Encephalopathy Advisory Committee (SEAC). On December 7th 1995, ministers and officials from the Ministry of Agriculture, Fisheries and Food (MAFF) 'decided to use SEAC to try to get the message across that beef was safe'. (Anon., 2002, p. 1535)

The uncertainty created by conflicting scientific 'fact' and 'expert' opinion was one of the dominant features of the BSE crisis. The media provided a forum for exchange of these opinions but what we see in this report is an assertion that the government used this forum in a manipulative way. As Lang (1996, p. 41) states: 'science has been on trial, yet ministers hid behind science'.

This brings us back to questions about the government's role in protecting public health, the conflicting interests of stakeholders in the crisis, and the media's role in helping or hindering the uncovering of 'the truth' or in presenting a number of different versions of 'the truth' in a balanced way. We have already seen examples of the media's ability to present contradictory 'truths' concurrently. We can certainly see examples of the use of 'science' and 'scientific fact' to support the status quo:

> Government veterinary and health experts were yesterday putting out reassuring messages about bovine spongiform encephalopathy (BSE) or 'mad cow' disease in the face of growing public anxiety. (Cookson, 1993, p. 6)

We can also see examples of conflict between ministers and scientific opinion and evidence of suppression of 'scientific fact' when it does not support the 'official Government line'.

> Richard Southwood, the University of Oxford Zoologist who was the Government's Chief Adviser on BSE in 1998 and 1990 ... told *New Scientist* 'I bridled when I heard ministers saying they were doing everything they'd been asked. The signals I got from Senior Civil Servants at the time were very different.' (Pearce, 1996, p. 4)

Evidence to support outright conspiracy theory also exists. Under the headline 'Top BSE Scientist "duped" to retire' (Leonard, 1998, p. 9), *Scotland on Sunday* reports on Professor Richard Lacey, a microbiologist who had voiced concerns about links between BSE and variant CJD early in the crisis:

> the maverick scientist who first warned that BSE in cattle would eventually be passed to humans, believes he was duped into early retirement by civil servants. (Leonard, 1998, p. 9)

Underlying these different uses of 'science' to support different positions is the media's (and also government's) tendency to manipulate what is actually meant by 'scientific fact'. The scientific 'fact' of a proven link between BSE and variant CJD, which lies at the heart of the BSE crisis as a public health issue, although, interestingly, not necessarily at the heart of the BSE crisis as an economic crisis, remains open to debate and challenge. This is partly due to the fact that BSE does not provide a classic case of 'risk' in public health terms (Adam, 2000). Unlike more certain established public health risks, such as smoking, food scares such as BSE provide an element of uncertainty and lack of probability.

We have seen examples in this chapter of the ways in which the print media attempt to contain this uncertainty and translate it into more certain and understandable discourses. This, argues, Leach (1998, p. 128) is really an impossible task: 'the BSE event offers no narrative closure, no ending by which the truth is recovered, boundaries stabilized, or uncertainties made certain'. Beck (1992) looks at this type of risk in the context of the relationship between capitalism, the media and science and argues that society can no longer contain and handle the risks engendered by modern-day capitalist production. The BSE crisis would certainly seem to provide such an example. Leach (1998) argues that, within this changed environment, the discourse of science within the media is actually shifting, and that being uncertain is 'the mark of the respected scientist' while being certain is the mark of the 'quack or snake-oil salesman' (Leach, 1998, p. 124).

As we have seen in the examples given, it is often the media that step in to provide a certainty and a set of solutions through their representation or interpretation of scientific fact. However, this process has become problematic for the print media and brings its own uncertainties, especially in the relationship between the short-term news priorities of the print media and the long-term nature of public health issues. Adam (2000, p. 22) states:

> Environmental 'news' . . . is almost a contradiction in terms. In the case of BSE and the BSE v CJD link, the long-term continuous pertinence of possible danger constitutes a major challenge to news work: news as the delimited here and now of events has to be rethought in the context of the long-term. . . . The complexity of the issues and the substantial level of uncertainty involved frustrate the journalist's need to be fast and succinct under deadline pressure.

Conclusion

The first conclusion that we would draw is that the application of media and cultural studies techniques to the examination of public health issues is something which can further our understanding of the ways in which public health issues are communicated to the public. Linked to this is the debate about which 'voices' predominate. In using the BSE crisis as a case study we have found examples which support both Gramsci's (1971) notion of the media as mouth-piece for a ruling elite and Parsons' (1995) more pluralistic approach. Parsons (1995) provides a useful model through which the media's role in the policy making process can be examined. This draws on Wilkins' (1964) ideas about 'amplification' of problems and Cohen's (1972) concept of the creation of a 'moral panic' by the print media.

Certainly there seems to be strong evidence that we need to regard the media as key players in making health policy rather than as an institution which merely reflects and reports on health issues. Clive Seale's chapter elsewhere in this book provides further evidence of this process.

The 'health vs wealth' tension revealed through the reporting of the BSE crisis is a recurring theme in the public health context in the UK, and it is useful to focus on the way in which this theme emerges at key points throughout the 1990s in this particular case study. The print media's ability to present conflicting opinions within its own editorial policy as well as representing conflicting 'voices' is something well worth noting. The implications for the public's understanding of public health issues need thinking through, especially if we accept that the print media are a vital source of information on health issues for many people. Concerns and debate about public health issues often seem to have been subsumed under more sensationalist approaches to the reporting of the crisis.

The use and role of 'science' is another key theme for public health practi-tioners. In this case study it is interesting to note the way in which important players in the crisis were willing to use or ignore 'scientific fact', depending on their own aims and ends. Adam's (2000) work on the difficulties generated for the print media by the uncertainties and long-term nature of a public health crisis of this type, and Beck's (1992) work on the changing nature of risk in modern-day capitalist societies, are useful contributions to this debate.

Finally, we are led to conclude that the populist print media products (but also publications which would characterise themselves as more 'serious') do not seem to have the will or the ability to provide a balanced educational argument around health and risk, nor are they suited to the task of providing a forum for a 'grown-up' debate about public health in the UK. However, their power and influence on the policy making process means that those concerned with public policy must regard the print media as a 'key player' in this process and recognise that the ways in which public health issues are represented in print have far-reaching consequences.

REFERENCES

Adam, B., 'The Media Timescope of BSE News', in S. Allen, B. Adam and C. Carter (eds), *Environmental Risks and the Media* (London: Routledge, 2000), pp. 117–29.

Allan, S., *Media, Risk and Science* (Buckingham: Open University Press, 2002).

Allison, S., '"I won't be gagged" says BSE scientist', *Newcastle Evening Chronicle*, 10 June (1998), p. 19.

Anon., 'BSE: Was Enough Done?' *Leicester Mercury*, 19 October (1998), p. 1.

Anon., 'Named and Blamed...the decision makers', *Daily Mail*, 27 October (2000), p. 17.

Anon., 'The Phillips Report on BSE and v CJD', *Lancet*, 356: 241 (2002), pp. 1535–6.

Baggott, R., *Public Health, Policy and Politics* (London: Macmillan, 2000).

Beardsworth, A. and Keil, T., *Sociology on the Menu* (London: Routledge, 1997).

Beck, U., *Risk Society: Towards a New Modernity* (London: Sage, 1992).

Bennett, T., 'Cultural Studies: A Reluctant Discipline?' *Cultural Critique*, 12:4 October (1998), pp. 528–45.

Bloom, B., 'Mad Cows and Englishmen', *Financial Times*, 27 January (1990), p. 7.

Boyd-Barrett, O. and Newbold, C., *Approaches to Media: A Reader* (London: Edward Arnold, 1995).

Bunton, R., 'Popular Health, Advanced Liberalism and Good Housekeeping Magazine', in S. Peterson and R. Bunton (eds), *Foucault, Health and Medicine* (London: Routledge, 1997), pp. 223–48.

Castle, S., Watts, M., Cohen, N., Routledge, P. and Cathcart, B., 'How Ministers had to Eat their Words', *Independent*, 24 March (1996), p. 16.

Chouliaraki, L. and Fairclough, N., *Discourse in Late Modernity: Rethinking Critical Discourse Analysis* (Edinburgh: Edinburgh University Press, 1999).

Cohen, S., *Folk Devils and Moral Panics – the Creation of the Mods and Rockers* (Oxford: Basil Blackwell, 1972).

Cookson, C., 'Government Seeks to Alley Fear of 'Mad Cow' Disease', *Financial Times*, 13 March (1993), p. 6.

Downs, A., 'Up and Down with Ecology: the Issue Attention Cycle', *Public Interest*, 28:1 (1972), pp. 38–50.

Fiske, J., *Television Culture* (London: Routledge, 1987).

Foucault, M., *Birth of the Clinic: An Archaeology of Medical Perception* (London: Routledge, 1989).

Gramsci, A., *Selections from the Prison Notebooks* (London: Lawrence & Wishart, 1971).

Gripsrud, J., *Understanding Media Culture* (London: Edward Arnold, 2002).

Hall, S., Critcher, C., Jefferson, T., Clarke, J. and Roberts, B., *Policing the Crisis: Mugging, the State and Law and Order* (London: Macmillan, 1978).

Hall, S., 'Encoding/Decoding', in S. Hall, D. Hobson, A. Lowe and P. Willis, *Culture, Media, Language: Working Papers in Cultural Studies, 1972–79* (London: Hutchinson, 1980), pp. 128–38.

Henderson P. and Oldfield, S., 'The First Victim of Mad Cow Disease?' *Daily Mail*, 12 March (1993), pp. 1, 5.

Hornsby, M., 'Cow Disease "does not affect humans"', *The Times*, 12 March (1993), p. 1.

King, M. and Watson, K., 'Transgressing Venues: Health Studies, Cultural Studies and the Media', *Health Care Analysis*, 9 (2001), pp. 401–16.

Lang, T., 'The Food Policy Lessons: How Not to Approach Consumers', in K. Torque and M. Bellis (eds), *BSE and Public Health: Perspectives from Agriculture, Food Policy and Epidemiology*, I, October, North West Public Health Association (1996).

Leach, J., 'Madness, Metaphors and Mis-communication: the Rhetorical Life of Mad Cow Disease', in S. C. Ratzen (ed.), *The Mad Cow Crisis: Health and the Public Good* (London: UCC Press, 1998).

Leonard, S., 'Top BSE Scientist "Duped to retire"', *Scotland on Sunday*, 1 March (1998), p. 9.

Lévi Strauss, C., *Structural Anthropology* (London: Penguin, 1968).

Lupton, D., 'AIDS, Risk and Heterosexuality in the Australian Press', *Discourse and Society*, 4:3 (1993), pp. 13–19.

McCarthy, R., '"I'll keep eating beef" says Blair', *Press Association*, 21 March (1996), p. 1.

McLuhan, M., 'Understanding Media', *The Extensions of Man* (Boston, MA: MIT Press, 1964).

McQuail, D. and Windahl, S., *Communication Models for the Study of Mass Communications* (London: Longman, 1993).

Martin, P., 'The Mad Cow Deceit', *Night and Day – The Mail on Sunday Review*, 12 May (1996), p. 7.

Maxwell, R., 'The British Government's Handling of Risk: some Reflections on the BSE/CJD Crisis', in P. Bennett and K. Calman, *Risk Communication and Public Health* (Buckingham: Open University Press, 1999).

May, T., *Social Research* (Buckingham: Open University Press, 1993).

Meade, G., 'Beef Ban Humiliation for Britain', *Press Association*, 20 May (1996), p. 1.

Miller, D., Kitzinger, J., Williams, K. and Beharrell, P. (eds), *The Circuit of Mass Communication* (London: Sage, 1998).

Mills, J., 'Scientists Fail to Find any Link between CJD and Beef', *Daily Mail*, 4 November (2000), p. 4.

Newby, H., 'Social Science and Public Policy: the Frank Foster Lecture', *RSA Journal*, May (1993), p. 365–77.

Parsons, W., *Public Policy: An Introduction to the Theory and Practice of Policy Analysis* (Aldershot: Edward Elgar, 1995).

Pearce, F., 'Ministers Hostile to Advice on BSE', *New Scientist*, 30 March (1996), p. 4.

Plummer, K., *Documents of Life*, vol. 2 (London: Sage, 2001).

Seale, C., *Media and Health* (London: Sage, 2003).

Silverstone, R., *Why Study the Media?* (London: Sage, 1999).

Southwell, B., 'Audience Constructions and AIDS Education Efforts: Exploring Communication Assumptions of Public Health Interventions', *Critical Public Health*, 10:3 (2000), pp. 314–19.

Torfing, J., *New Theories of Discourse: Laclau, Mouffe and Žižek* (Oxford: Blackwell, 2002).

Wilkins, L.T., *Social Deviance, Social Policy Action and Research* (London: Tavistock, 1964).

Williams, K. and Miller, D., 'Producing AIDS News', in P. Miller, J. Kitzinger, K. Williams and P. Beharrell (eds), *The Circuit of Mass Communication* (London: Sage, 1998), pp. 147–66.

Wilson, E., '10-Year Battle against Scourge, the Denials: 10-Year History of Mad Cow Disease', *Daily Mirror*, 21 March (1996), p. 4.

Writing Digital Selves: Narratives of Health and Illness on the Internet

6

Michael Hardey

Introduction

In the 1930s, when radio was the new medium, Bertolt Brecht noted that it

> would be the finest possible communication apparatus in public life . . . if it knew how to receive as well as transmit, how to let the listener speak as well as hear, how to bring him into a relationship instead of isolating him. (Brecht, 1964, p. 52)

The internet has overcome these deficits and, like radio, the use of the internet has grown rapidly. In 1993 there were just 130 computer servers that underpinned the internet, yet by 1999 this figure had increased to an estimated 9.5 million servers. A survey undertaken in July 2000 found that 43 per cent of all adults in Britain had accessed the internet (Office for National Statistics, 2001). Such generic figures, however, disguise inequalities of access. For example, men are more likely to use the internet than women and while nearly all people under the age of 24 years have used the internet, it has been used by only 6 per cent of those aged 75 and over. Ownership of a computer and home access to the internet are less common in poorer communities; however, this is rapidly changing.

For the growing population of internet users, it is information related to health that is one of the most important resources it has to offer (Miller, 2001).

In Britain, the Departments for Health and Social Services have included in proposals the suggestion that all government services should be available through the internet by 2005, so that 'patients will be helped to navigate the maze of health information through the development of NHS Direct online, Digital TV and NHS Direct information points in key public spaces' (Department of Health, 2000, para. 10.2). In North America the potential market in drugs and other health-related products and services that can be delivered through the internet has been valued at an estimated $1.7 billion (CyberAtlas, 2000). Consumer use of the internet is also growing rapidly, with one survey reporting that 98 million Americans, who represent 86 per cent of adult internet users, had sought health information on the internet (Harris Interactive, 2000). However, such surveys should be approached with caution given the difficulties associated with defining and measuring such a highly dynamic population.

This chapter focuses on the new digital media of the internet. The first section of the chapter reviews some of the key features of the 'electronic' spaces fashioned by the internet. In particular, it looks at the social spaces represented by newsgroups and the World Wide Web and relates them to broader commentaries about the internet and social and economic change. The second section examines how users represent themselves and interact with others. Here I explore the possibilities of intimacy and trust in a space that is essentially anonymous and where identity is uncertain. The third section develops the idea that users are able to publish their own stories and challenge the interventions made into their lives by doctors, social workers and other authorities. Here we see how the home page of a person I call David can be read in various ways and can give the author access to a global audience. The final section speculates on how use of the internet may shape our notions of expertise, knowledge and lay/professional relationships.

The internet and new social spaces

Writing about the computer, McLuhan (1960, p. 567) noted that the 'advent of a new medium often reveals the lineaments and assumptions, as it were, of an old medium'. If the print and broadcast media represent the old and the internet the new media, it throws into relief assumptions about the production and consumption of information. In soap operas, film and print media, considered elsewhere in this book, there is commonly a clear distinction between those who consume and those involved in the production of the media. For McLuhan (1964) it is what he refers to as 'hypermedia' that promise to revolutionise writing by overturning author-centred text and its attendant apparatus of publishers and distribution systems. As we shall see later, the embedding of hypertext linkages within a web page transforms reading into a process that involves the construction of a narrative so that the author/reader dichotomy is challenged. Moreover, the same technology that enables users to identify and view information also makes it possible for users to create and publish their own material. Before we examine this challenge to established assumptions about knowledge, power and consumption it is necessary to outline briefly the development of the internet and describe two significant social spaces within it.

The global communications network brought together through the internet includes email, newsgroups and the World Wide Web. Its origins are rooted in the cold war and the United States military's need to provide a diversified communications system that lacked centres vulnerable to attack. However, subsequent development was undertaken largely by academics, students and hobbyists who shared a disdain for commercial and government attempts to control the emerging system (Rheingold, 1994). One of the original aims behind linking computers in different localities was to enable people to send messages to each other quickly and easily. Established technology like the telephone had been doing this for over a hundred years but scientists and others needed to rapidly transmit, view and revise complex diagrams, pictures and other material. Moreover, they needed to retain the interactivity possible though the telephone in order to create a virtual co-presence interaction. The key technological development behind Computer Mediated Communication (CMC) was packet-switching, which, briefly, allowed digital information to be broken down into blocks that could be transmitted between computers. This enabled the same 'piece of wire' or channel to carry a number of simultaneous transmissions with a high degree of reliability. It made possible applications, including electronic mail, that came into use in the 1970s and captured the imagination, to become a ubiquitous part of the internet. This development alone could have promoted new forms of collaborative working within and across organisations. However, people have been exchanging letters for hundreds of years and although email can be instantaneous, the content and form of the messages transmitted may not be that different.

The first space within the internet we need to select for consideration consists of newsgroups. These are related to email and are focused on particular subjects, and allow members to read and post messages. They range from closed discussion groups that are carefully moderated and where membership is by invitation only, to groups open to anyone. There are similarities to email-based mailing lists. However, newsgroups are more diverse, versatile, and easier for those outside professional or otherwise defined groups of users to identify and join. Newsgroups share a common message hierarchy so it is possible to read previous exchanges and follow specific discussion 'threads'. This contrasts with chat rooms, where exchanges are essentially 'typed conversations' and are not retained. There are advantages here for researchers, who are able to examine the history of individual newsgroups, participate within them and even create their own groups (Mann and Stewart, 2000).

In North America, newsgroups rapidly developed to replicate many of the themes around which self-help groups were organised (Finn, 1999; Pleace et al., 2000). Indeed, an early impact of newsgroups and bulletin boards was as part of the campaign to gain recognition and funding for HIV/AIDS research and therapy. A similar pattern of newsgroups as places for self-help is discernible in Britain and elsewhere in Europe. Such 'wired self-help' groups (Burrows et al., 2000; Muncer et al., 2000) are global but because of differences in health and social care, as well as in therapeutic approaches and language, there is a strong association with national locality. Prescription drugs, for example, may be identical in all but name in Europe and the United States. This means users may subvert national regulations or controls over particular drugs or therapies by exchanging information about sources beyond national boundaries (Hardey, 2002a). One of the driving forces behind the emergence of these groups is the way they allow users to explore and form alliances around contested health and social problems. By 'contested', I mean to indicate problems that have no generally agreed causality, symptoms or therapy amongst health and social care practitioners. Moreover, the information exchanged in these newsgroups is based on bodily and emotional experiences that often present lived experience as a social truth. There are, for example, many newsgroups clustered around complementary and alternative approaches to health. Exchanges within these groups draw on individual experiences and often include a questioning of medical treatment. As with off-line self-help groups, participation, it is suggested, can be empowering and provide a serious individual and collective challenge to medical orthodoxy (Vincent, 1992).

The second space we need to examine is the most complex and diverse. The World Wide Web was developed in Europe in the late 1980s, in part, as a reaction against the hierarchical structures found in, for example, newsgroups. The idea of the 'Web' was of a 'flat' system within which users could access and create material centred on their individual requirements. A hypertext language was developed that allowed links to be embedded into material so that 'web pages' could be associated. Viewing it by means of a graphically based browser, users could now move from one page to another by simply clicking a hypertext link or graphic. Moreover, the physical locality of the computer that stores any particular web page is frequently not known, or indeed relevant, to users. This invisibility of sources is congruent with the original ideal behind the design of a CMC system and, as we shall see, poses particular challenges to the control of information. In effect, while browsing across the Web, users are constructing their own material or assembling their own sets of information. With a few technical skills, any users can now create their own 'home pages', which can include text, graphics, photographs and video.

Email, newsgroups and the Web have been increasingly drawn together as browsers such as Internet Explorer have integrated access through one piece of software. Indeed, it is the networked nature of interconnected computers that makes information technology so powerful and which commentators such as Castells (1996) have argued is behind a 'technological revolution' and a conse-quent 'new mode of development, informationalism' (Castells, 1996, p. 14). Castells's three-volume exploration of society, economy and culture has been compared to earlier and now classic texts like Weber's *Economy and Society* (Giddens, 1996) and Marx's *Das Kapital* (McGuigan, 1999). Whatever the merits of such comparisons they draw attention to how Castell and other theorists regard information technology as essentially social in its development, use and impact on economies and cultures. This is important because analysis of this kind tends to foreground technology as the key driver of social change rather than as a feature of it. McLuhan's (1964) vision of a 'global village', for example, assumed that television broadcasting technology would create a homogeneous world culture. The story of the emergence of the internet, like other technologies, is one of unforeseen and unintended consequences that flowed from the work of many individuals and organisations (see Winston, 1998).

Representing digital selves and the possibility of intimacy

The internet has been celebrated as a medium which allows individuals to avoid the constraints of the 'real world' and to take on new and often multiple identities. There is a desire to 'leave the "meat" behind and to become distilled in a clean, pure, uncontaminated relationship with the computer technology' (Lupton, 1995, p. 100). In commentaries about the internet there is a thread that coun-terpoises the 'purity' of technological space with the 'dirt' and 'decay' of the off-line world. This apparent escape from the corporeal body promises to 'free up' or liberate those who feel locked into damaged bodies or spoilt identities (Goffman, 1967). A paraplegic confined to the home, for example, can explore the internet and be an active participant in newsgroups, and other virtual communities and places. The disembodied self or selves that interact with others are essentially anonymous and may have little resemblance to the off-line indi-vidual who creates them. At a simple level this may be done by creating a name to be know by, for example, within a newsgroup. Internet identities therefore lack many of the constraints, including a sense of responsibility for interactions, that are associated with face-to-face encounters (cf. Goffman, 1967). This may enable users to become who they wish to be without hindrance but it also makes it possible to manipulate and mislead others. An unusual example can be found in the increasingly odd postings from a member of a newsgroup which was focused on feminist issues, and which were eventually revealed to be coming from a completely computer-generated persona (Ogan, 1993).

Despite the increasing use of photographs, video and other imaging technology, identities on the internet are predominantly written in text. Interactions in newsgroups, email and elsewhere are conducted through the text. This renders invisible the outward signs of bodily form, dress, posture, movement, facial decorations and emotional expressions that are usually so important in determining how individuals perceive themselves and how others respond. The loss of 'vocabularies of bodily idiom' (Goffman, 1967) represents an opportunity for those who feel disadvantaged in the co-present 'presentation of self' (Goffman, 1969). While lacking such cues and rituals associated with face-to-face interactions, there are established 'netiquette' conventions that shape interactions in many internet places. For example, it is commonly regarded as 'good manners' for newcomers to a newsgroup to make sure they understand its purpose and the broad form of exchanges that take place. The incident we noted earlier of the computer-generated identity being planted in a feminist newsgroup became visible because it did not adhere to the expected netiquette. Some interactions can appear strange to outsiders because they follow a netiquette that may include the use of acronyms (e.g. BTW: 'by the way'). In addition, commonly used 'emoticons' (;-] to denote a wink) act as shorthand for bodily signs used in off-line encounters. Such abbreviations distinguish CMC and, as early users of email noted, enable 'one to write tersely and type imperfectly, even to an older person one did not know very well, and the recipient took no offence' (Licklider and Vezza, 1978, p. 1330). There is, therefore, a freeing up of formalities and constraints commonly observed in letter writing or other communications.

Research into CMC sociability has highlighted the impersonal, anonymous and often hostile communication (e.g. 'flaming' – sending insulting messages via email) within newsgroups and argued that it is difficult for users to develop trusting and close on-line relationships. This suggests that those who are seeking a sense of belonging and an escape from what they experience as a hostile or uncomfortable off-line world may be disappointed. However, others have argued that internet selves have new opportunities for sociability and personal relationships that may develop into internet communities unhindered by locality or time (e.g., Plant, 1998; Rheingold, 1994; Shields, 1996). Whatever the merits of such arguments, environments, especially MUDs (multi-user dimensions), provide unique opportunities for taking on identities unhindered by bodily constraints, including gender (Roberts and Parks, 2001).

Internet dating sites are designed to enable strangers to develop an on-line relationship in order to arrange co-present meetings that may lead to close relationships (Hardey, 2002b). This contrasts sharply with other environments such as MUDs and multi-user interactive games, where fantasy selves interact in a virtual landscape. However, the possibilities of such virtual relationships have been highlighted in the media, and have contributed to the opening up of lifestyles that are a 'prime connecting point between body, self-identity and social norms' (Giddens, 1991, p. 15). The search for intimacy 'is at the heart of modern forms of friendship and established sexual relationships' (Giddens, 1991, p. 95). The emphasis on growing individualisation, the decline of public authority, and other social and economic anchors, is a common theme in theories about the nature of societies where ICTs have a significant role. While Giddens argues that such conditions allow individuals to make choices and build self-reflexive identities in open societies others have a darker analysis. They emphasise anxieties, uncertainties, frustrations and fears of solitude (Bauman, 2001; Beck and Beck-Gernsheim, 2001). Intimacy and love are always uncertain, fragile and achieved in spite of an increasingly rationalised and impersonal world (Beck and Beck-Gernsheim, 1995, p. 178). Purely virtual encounters between disembodied users of cyberspace echo this vision of 'second modernity' (Beck and Beck-Gernsheim, 2001). Indeed, cybersex may be an ultimate expression of disembodied risk-free engagement with others (Wiley, 1995).

While the media have helped open up choices they have also created new barriers and disadvantages by privileging images of the 'fit body' and desirable lifestyle (Falk, 1994; Featherstone, 1981; Shilling, 1993). Internet dating sites do not escape such influences but provide a place where there is an emphasis on communication. The predominantly text-based environment provides a place where users can 'get to know' others and negotiate their differences, similarities and desires. However, these interactions remain anchored in off-line bodies and lives because on-line relationships are only a prelude to meeting and possibly forming a relationship off-line. Giddens (1991) has argued that negotiation and communication are central to what he has identified as 'pure relationships'. With the falling away of traditional constraints, he argues, such 'confluent love' is based on the maintenance of 'clear personal boundaries' and consequent interdependence. It is 'above all a matter of emotional communication, with others and with the self, in a context of interpersonal equality' (Giddens, 1992, p. 130). As Shilling (1997) points out, this may be an unrealistic ideal rather than a valid ideal type but the 'pure relationship' does suggest a discursive, disembodied vision of late modern intimacy. Representations of the self, constructed, maintained and negotiated on and through the internet, therefore contain the possibility for intimacy that some strive to achieve in off-line lives.

Narratives of the self as challenges to authority

The personal home page represents a space in the internet where users can write their own stories and publish them to a global audience. Simple to construct, such pages are 'hosted' by an Internet Service Provider (ISP) where they can be identified through search engines and linked to other areas of the Web. It has been argued that, as reflected in the label 'home', these pages contain symbolic material that has meaning to an individual in the same way that, for example, a picture has when displayed on a living room or bedroom wall (Chandler, 1999). As Selvin (2000) notes, how home pages are presented to visitors and the links made to other parts of the internet constitute a means of self-expression. The personal home page is, therefore, a distinctive space within the internet with some of the attributes commonly associated with broadcast media. In effect, users can design, create and broadcast material about issues that concern them. While lacking the immediate interactivity of, for example, newsgroups or chat rooms, the home pages often contain an email address so that visitors can contact the author.

Web pages are often said to be 'under construction' and may be unstable as they appear and disappear on the internet. Such disappearing acts may reflect individuals moving to different ISPs in the search for better service or as a strategy to enable contentious and potentially litigious material to remain available. As elsewhere on the internet, the pervasive substitution for the 'real' by the simulated poses questions about authenticity. The readers of this chapter cannot, for example, conduct their own analysis of the 'data' on which it is based. However, this is true of most narratives that are rendered into data in academic books and journals. Such issues are not confined to the internet and are reflected in broader and long-established debates within ethnographic and other research (Plummer, 1999; 2000). Ethics are uncertain in internet-based research (Hakken, 1999) and it is too easy for researchers to view the contents and activities in virtual space as a vast collection of data just waiting for analysis. The personal home page, like an autobiography or a work of art displayed in a gallery, is in the public domain. Indeed, most authors are keen for their site to be visited and read and they often encourage comments through email.

These are the circumstances of a person I shall call 'David' as he described them on his personal home page, which is hosted by a UK ISP. The web page was identified during a study of home pages that contained accounts of illness, which is described elsewhere (Hardey, 2001, 2002c). David is in his 40s and has worked, between periods of unemployment, in the computer industry since leaving college. David's parents moved from Jamaica and he has lived in Brixton all his life. He describes how he gained access to the internet at public libraries to:

find out stuff that they don't want you to know. I got to know what I was addicted to and got off that. The Net is powerful. I used it to get out from doctors who wanted to control me and take away what I was. Not all were bad but they would only listen because I had the knowledge I got from Net stuff and friends I have on there.

The following text is taken from the opening sentences of his home page. The bracketed text has been used to indicate hyperlinks:

Welcome to my cyber home. I started two years ago as I traced my family history [hyperlink to a detailed family tree complete with many photographs, and links to other sites about black history]. It has grown into the story of my troubles and how I got back my life from the social workers and psychiatrist by finding Jesus. It might help you not to fall under their power and find ways of dealing with issues that life throws at you. I don't pretend to have the answer but you won't hear my story from the professionals.

What follows is a detailed account of his family, his childhood in London and how he was diagnosed as suffering from depression. It is sometimes difficult to follow, occasionally contradictory and embedded with hyperlinks to documents and other material that has been scanned and pasted into the home page. This allows David to comment on, for example, letters sent to him by a hospital and reports provided by social workers. He rejects medical language displayed in the documents that refer to his 'case' and frames his experiences within a professional and managerial structure. He also expresses some vitriolic views about doctors and warns readers about what he sees as the prejudices and biases of the largely white practitioners he has come into contact with:

I'm not saying that there are not some doctors that don't try their best but you must remember that you are a case not a person and they don't have much time or interest in you. The best solution for them is drugs as they are quick, control you (especially big black men) and giving out pills is what doctors do. White doctors don't understand black experience. Some of them thought 'Give the man the drugs, he won't bother me and I've done what's expected'. No therapy. No reality. No hope.

Such encounters mark sequential transitions in his identity as an 'outsider' who has depression. As the narrative moves on there is an increasing sense of being seen as 'trouble', 'difficult' and 'black'. Such experiences are not unique and a disproportionate number of African Caribbeans are diagnosed as having some form of mental illness (Littlewood, 1993). Indeed, the use of popular conceptualisations of blackness by psychiatry can lead to racialised forms of identity being relatively open to various psychiatric diagnoses (Parker et al., 1995).

David uses his experiences and knowledge of medicine and its organisation to challenge the assumptions and judgements that are made about him:

> Doctors see a black man, read the case notes and give him the pills. It is the church [hyperlink to picture of a church] that made my life. It is with black people I found my way. Blackness is part of me and it is a black therapist at the church helps me.

Antagonism and resolution through religion represent the grand narrative that enables David to interpret and work through his experiences. It also shapes his development of a new life after a period in hospital and living on the street. Indeed his home page is part of the way he seeks to do this, by re-framing his identity around his conceptualisation of 'blackness' (Knowles, 1999). The writing and re-writing of the home page, therefore, provides a place where the author makes sense of life events and weaves together emotional and material transitions. It also enables individuals to share their experiences with others. If writers of biographies have in mind a reader (Elbaz, 1987), the authors of personal home pages construct them with visitors in mind. David notes early on that he hopes to 'reach people who are in situations like mine' and indeed uses key words, including 'depression' and 'social work', in header information that can be picked up by search engines.

Giddens (1991, p. 53) argues that, in the contemporary era, the self is 'reflexively understood by the person in terms of her or his biography'. This is developed through an engagement in relationships and activities that can enhance this narrative, which is a mode of cognition rather than a literary construction. Such 'autobiographical thinking' in a 'broad sense of an interpretive self-history produced by the individual concerned ... whether written down or not ... is actually the core of self-identity' (Giddens, 1991, p. 53). There is an affinity here with the narratives that are always 'under construction' and mapped out by home page authors. The self is, therefore, essentially cognitive and may be written on the internet together with digitised images of places and people. The self that is written about may only exist as a narrative and what is told about the self may change according to circumstances.

The writing of the narrative and the reproduction of documents and images of places and others who figure in David's life reflect the self-formation of identity that shapes and is shaped by relationships and events. As Polkinghorne (1988, p. 11) suggests, narratives are 'the primary scheme by means of which human existence is rendered meaning-ful'. Freeman (1993) argues that, in oral narratives, questions about the coherence and plausibility of accounts can be assessed by applying what he refers to as the 'narrative order of experience'. This questions whether the story utilises the experiences and information available in a plausible manner. David's home page does this and provides many documents and other material to support the narrative he constructs. Therefore, it is unlikely to be a complete fabrication and the documentation and family/community history anchor the narrative in an off-line life and community. Unlike the majority of narratives reported by academics, David has not created a story in collaboration with an interviewer who has a particular research agenda (Erban, 1993; 1998). His is a different global audience.

Meanings and relationships through the internet

The personal home page explored here reflects a disembodied identity that is cased in the off-line self rather than a virtual escape from the self (cf. Stone, 1996). It also marks a resistance to, and redefinition of, medical and other representations of personal troubles. However, people who visit a personal home page do so as readers who construct their own text and images. Unlike print media, a web page contains text and often pictures that are nonlinear, because hypertext links can take the reader to different parts of the home page or into other areas of the internet. Such pages are not created in a linear sequence but constructed out of images, text and other information as they occur to the author, who may include material from other parts of the internet or import it from other sources via a scanner or other technology. One reading of David's page is as a family/community history that contains only a hint of his engagement with the medical profession. This interactivity challenges the privileged position of the author as the distinction between author and readers becomes blurred, with the latter 'making up' a narrative as they read. Boller (1992, p. 20) argues that 'an electronic text only exists in the act of reading – in the interaction between the reader and textual structure'. For hypertext enthusiasts this liberates users from the hierarchies and inequalities between producers and consumers that exist in other media, and as such is inherently democratic (Poster, 1995).

Caution is needed here, in that the apparent escape from the ascendancy of the author and the power of copyright envisaged by some should be placed in the context of a number of successful corporate and state initiatives to define and control various aspects of the internet. For example, the use of internet software to make music freely available on-line, despite copyright restrictions, has resulted in the successful removal of the software resources.

The asymmetrical nature of the professional/lay relationships is central to Parsons' (1951) formulation of the 'sick role' where the technical expertise of the doctor casts patients into a situation of 'helplessness' and 'technical incompetence' (Parsons, 1951, p. 440). The ill person is 'generally not in a position to do what needs to be done' and 'does not "know" what needs to be done' (Parsons, 1951, pp. 441–5). The significance of information and expertise is highlighted by Parsons' use of cybernetic theory (the science of systems). Public access to medical information was therefore mediated by doctors through the consultation, where their authority and status was rarely challenged. As we have seen, the internet and other media enable anyone to seek out health information and evaluate competing therapies. This is congruent with the expectation that the internet, amongst other developments, is facilitating partial or full-blown re-skillng of the users of health and social services (Giddens, 1991). However, a disengagement or disenchantment with practitioners and the health care system may provoke a misplaced apprehension of medical therapies and advice. Other developments in information technology have created opportunities for the surveillance and evaluation of the work of doctors and other professionals in order to make them 'accountable' to consumers and the state.

Taken together these developments are transforming professional/lay relationships as the former are removed from the insulation of 'observability' they have enjoyed in the past (Coser, 1961). It is psychiatrists' and other practitioners' access to, and command of, information and expertise that generates their position of dominance over clients. This is depicted on David's home page by the inclusion of official letters and his sometimes detailed notes of interviews with practitioners. While interpretations of identify *vis-à-vis* psychiatry frame medical and social-work discourses as authoritative, other interpretations expose lay agency as a viable resistance. Poster (1997, p. 211) notes that:

> The 'magic' of the internet is that it . . . puts cultural acts, symbolizations in all forms, in the hands of all participants; it radically decentralizes the positions of speech, publishing, film-making, radio and television broadcasting, in short the apparatuses of cultural production.

The absence of the authoritative voice in newsgroups, chat rooms and home pages allows issues to be discussed and advice to be given by those 'who experience or "are" the problem', in contrast to relatively constrained and 'expert'-led discourses that are the foundations of talk shows and reality television (Shattuc, 1997, p. 194).

For Giddens (1991), religion has been replaced by therapy as a source of meaning and a resource to navigate the complexities of high modern life. The diversity of therapies and lifestyle advice available to consumers constitutes an expert system that resonates with the reflexive project of the self as a way of promoting autonomy and self-knowledge. As we have seen, newsgroups and home pages contain a vast amount of information, including western medicine, New Age therapies, Ayurvedic healing, and so forth. Moreover, in facilitating the globalising tendencies of late modernity the internet has increased awareness of 'manufactured' risks and uncertainties in health and other aspects of life (Beck, 1992; Giddens, 1991, 1994). Medicine has a heritage of state registration, with attendant codes of practice, so that it is able to lay claims to act in the public interest (Crompton, 1990; Saks, 1995). Telemedicine and other projects point to how ICTs have been used and incorporated into the expert system represented by medicine. However, they also expose knowledge previously closed to non-practitioners to the public gaze (Hardey, 1999).

In response to this and the increasing questioning of medical practice (Slater, 2001), the problem of the 'quality' of information available to users has become a significant discourse within the medical domain and one that is frequently couched in terms of clinicians' duty to protect the public. The price of 'protection', however, is often the consolidation of expert knowledge and the relegation of other forms of expertise. For example, there is a proliferation of organisations that evaluate and rate health-related internet resources (e.g. the HON Code, American Medical Association, Internet HealthCare Coalition, MedCertain). Indeed, there has been an unsuccessful attempt to establish an internet domain, identified by the suffix '.med', that would only contain material grounded in medical science. However, national standards and clinical guidelines vary and so what is good practice in one country may be not accepted in another. Moreover, the use of the internet to purchase prescription drugs that are not available in the user's country poses important questions related to trade, national regulation and law as well as health care systems.

Conclusion

In Giddens's vision of a fluid and reflexive world (Mellor and Shilling, 2001), anything is possible. The internet helps to open these new possibilities and enables users to make new connections, both virtual and off-line, with others. However, care needs to be taken not to follow the course of the internet utopian commentators who offer a vision of democratised global communities. Despite the increasing number of people who have access to the internet the digital divide remains a significant barrier to the promotion of social equality through ICTs (Social Exclusion Policy Action Team, 2001). The predominance of English usage on the internet also disadvantages those who have no knowledge of it (Berland et al., 2001). Notwithstanding such qualifications, the internet is a new medium that is shaping the understanding and consumption of health. Featherstone and Lash (1999, p. 5) argue that, 'In cyberspace we move beyond the old realist divisions of space/time, sender/receiver, medium/message.' We may want to add to this list of modernist dualities those of author/reader and expert/lay. The blurring of such categories reflects the newness of the space provided by the internet and the opportunities it offers for representing health in new ways that will increasingly shape individual and global health and well-being.

NOTE

The author of the home pages cited here was contacted through email and gave permission for extracts to be used for research purposes. At the time of writing he has taken his page off the internet while he re-designs it.

REFERENCES

Bauman, Z., *The Individualized Society* (Oxford: Polity Press, 2001).

Beck, U., *Risk Society: Towards a New Modernity* (London: Sage, 1992).

Beck, U. and Beck-Gernsheim, E., *The Normal Chaos of Love* (Cambridge: Polity Press, 1995).

Beck, U. and Beck-Gernsheim, E., *Individualization* (London: Sage, 2001).

Berland, G. K., Elliot, M. N., Morales, C. S. and McGlynn, E. A., 'Quality of Health Information on the Internet' – Reply, *Journal of the American Medical Association*, 286:17 (2001), pp. 2094–5.

Boller, D., 'Literature in the Electronic Writing Space', in M. Tuman (ed.), *Literacy OnLine* (Pittsburgh: University of Pittsburgh Press, 1992).

Brecht, B., 'The Radio as an Apparatus of Communication', in J. Willett (ed. and trans.), *Brecht on Theatre: The Development of an Aesthetic* (London: Methuen, 1964).

Burrows, R., Nettleton, S., Pleace, N., Loader, B. and Muncer, S., 'Virtual Community Care? Social Policy and the Emergence of Computer Mediated Social Support', *Information Communication and Society*, 3:1 (2000), pp. 23–31.

Castells, M., *The Rise of Networked Society* (Oxford: Blackwell, 1996).

Chandler, D., 'Personal home pages and the construction of identities on the web', www.aber.ac.uk/~dgc/webindent.html; accessed 06 /11/01 (1999).

Coser, R. L., 'Insulation from Observability and Types of Social Conformity', *American Sociological Review*, 25 (Feburary) (1961), pp. 28–39.

Crompton, R., 'Professions in the Current Context', *Work, Employment and Society*, Special Issue (1990), pp. 34–68.

CyberAtlas, 'OnLine healthcare market looks energized', www.Cyberatlas.internet. com/markets/retailing/article/0.1323.6061_153701.00html; accessed 12/05/02 (2000).

Department of Health, *Information for Social Care* (London: HMSO, 2000).

Elbaz, R., *The Changing Nature of Self: A Critical Study of the Autobiographical Discourse* (Iowa City: University of Iowa Press, 1987).

Erban, M., 'The Problem of Other Lives: Social Perspectives on Written Biography', *Sociology*, 27:1 (1993), pp. 15–26.

Erban, M., 'Biography and Research Method', in M. Erban (ed.), *Biography and Education: A Reader* (London: Flamer Press, 1998).

Falk, P., *The Consuming Body* (London: Sage, 1994).

Featherstone, M., 'The Body and Consumer Culture', *Theory, Culture and Society* 1(2) (1981), pp. 18–33.

Featherstone, M. and Lash, S., Introduction, in M. Featherstone and S. Lash (eds), *Spaces of Culture* (London: Sage, 1999).

Finn, J., 'An Exploration of Helping Processes in an Online Self-help Group Focusing on Issues of Disability', *Health and Social Work*, 24:3 (1999), pp. 220–31.

Freeman, M., *Rewriting the Self* (London: Routledge, 1993).

Giddens, A., *Modernity and Self-Identity* (Cambridge: Polity Press, 1991).

Giddens, A., *The Transformation of Intimacy, Sexuality, Love and Eroticism in Modern Societies* (Cambridge: Polity Press, 1992).

Giddens, A., *The Constitution of Society* (Cambridge: Polity Press, 1994).

Giddens, A., 'Out of Place', *Education Supplement Higher*, 13 December (1996).

Goffman, E., *Interaction Ritual* (Harmondsworth: Penguin Books, 1967).

Goffman, E., *The Presentation of Self in Everyday Life* (Harmondsworth: Penguin Books, 1969).

Hakken, D., *Cyborgs@Cyberspace? An Ethnographer Looks to the Future* (London: Routledge, 1999).

Hardey, M., 'Doctor in the House', *Sociology of Health and Illness*, 12:6 (1999), pp. 820–35.

Hardey, M., 'E-health: the Internet and Transformation of Patients into Consumers and the Producers of Health Knowledge', *Information, Communication and Society*, 4:3 (2001), pp. 388–405.

Hardey, M., 'Health for Sale: Quackery, Consumerism and the Internet', in W. Ernst (ed.), *Plural Medicine*, Routledge Society of the Social History of Medicine (London: Routledge, 2002a).

Hardey, M., 'Life Beyond the Screen: Embodiment and Identity through the Internet', *Sociological Review*, 24:3 (2002b), pp. 570–85.

Hardey, M., '"The Story of my Illness": Personal Accounts of Illness on the Internet', *Health: An Interdisciplinary Journal*, 6:1 (2002c), pp. 31–46.

Harris Interactive, 'Explosive Growth of "Cyberchondriacs" Continues New York', Harris Interactive, 11 August, available at: www.harrisinteractive.com/news/index.asp; accessed 12 May 2002 (2000).

Knowles, C., 'Race, Identities and Lives', *Sociological Review*, 110–35 (1999).

Licklider, P. E. and Vezza, A., 'Applications of Information Technology', *Proceedings of IEEE*, 66:11 (1978).

Littlewood, R., 'Ideology, Camouflage or Contingency? Racism in British Psychiatry', *Transcultural Psychiatric Research Review*, XXX:3 (1993), pp. 243–90.

Lupton, D., 'The Embodied Computer/user', in M. Featherstone and R. Burrows, *Cyberspace, Cyberbodies and Cyberpunk: Cultures of Technological Embodiment* (London: Sage, 1995).

McGuigan, J., *Modernity and Postmodern Culture* (Buckingham: Open University Press, 1999).

McLuhan, M., 'Effects of the Improvements of Communications Media', *Journal of Economic History*, 20 (1960), pp. 566–75.

McLuhan, M., *Understanding Media* (London: Routledge and Kegan Paul, 1964).

Mann, C. and Stewart, F., *Internet Communication and Qualitative Research: A Handbook for Researching Online* (London: Sage, 2000).

Mellor, P. A. and Shilling, C., *Re-forming the Body: Religion, Community and Modernity* (London: Sage, 2001).

Miller, J. D., 'Who is Using the Web for Science and Health Information?' *Science Communication*, 22:3 (2001), pp. 256–73.

Muncer, S., Burrows, R., Pleace, N., Loader, B. and Nettleton, S., 'Births, Deaths, Sex and Marriage...but Very Few Present? A Case Study of Social Support in Cyberspace', *Critical Public Health*, 10:1 (2000), pp. 1–16.

Office for National Statistics, 'Results from the July National Statistics Omnibus Survey (online), available at www.statistics.gov.uk/pdfdir/inter0900.pdf; accessed 12 May 2002 (2001).

Ogan, C., 'Listserver Communication during the Gulf War: What Kind of Medium is the Electronic Bulletin Board?' *Journal of Broadcasting and Electronic Media*, 37:2 (1993), pp. 522–56.

Parker, I., Georgace, E., Harper, D., McLaughlin, T. and Stonewell-Smith, M., *Deconstructing Psychology* (London, Sage, 1995).

Parsons, T., *The Social System* (London: Routledge, 1951).

Plant, S., *Zeros + Ones* (London: Fourth Estate, 1998).

Pleace, N., Burrows, R., Loader, B., Muncer, S. and Nettleton, S., 'On-line with the Friends of Bill W: Social Support and the Net', *Sociological Research Online*, 5:2 (2000).

Plummer, K., 'The "Ethnographic Society" at Century End: Clarifying the Role of Public Ethnography', *Journal of Contemporary Ethnography*, 28 (1999), pp. 641–9.

Plummer, K., *Documents of Life*, vol. 2 (London: Sage, 2000).

Polkinghorne, D., *Narrative Knowing and the Human Sciences* (New York: University of New York Press, 1988).

Poster, M., *The Second Media Age* (Cambridge: Polity Press, 1995).

Poster, M., 'Cyberdemocracy: Internet and the Public Sphere', in D. Porter (ed.), *Internet Culture* (London: Routledge, 1997).

Rheingold, H., *The Virtual Community: Finding Connection in a Computerized World* (London: Secker and Warburg, 1994).

Roberts, L. D. and Parks, M. R., 'The Social Geography of Gender-switching in Virtual Environments on the Internet', in E. Green and A. Adams (eds), *Virtual Gender* (London: Routledge, 2001).

Saks, M., *Professions and the Public Interest* (London: Routledge, 1995).

Selvin, J., *The Internet and Society* (Oxford: Polity Press, 2000).

Shattuc, J. M., *The Talking Cure: TV Talk Shows and Women* (London: Rouledge, 1997).

Shields, R. (ed.), *Cultures of Internet: Virtual Spaces, Real Histories, Living Bodies* (London: Sage, 1996).

Shilling, C., *The Body and Social Theory* (London: Sage, 1993).

Shilling, C., 'Emotions, Embodiment and the Sensation of Society', *The Sociological Review*, 45:2 (1997), pp. 195–219.

Slater, B., 'Who Rules? The New Politics of Medical Regulation', *Social Science and Medicine*, 52 (2001), pp. 871–83.

Social Exclusion Policy Action Team, 'Action Report on Social Exclusion', *Department of Culture, Media and Sports* (2001).

Stone, A. R., *The War of Desire and Technology at the End of the Mechanical Age* (Cambridge, MA: MIT Press, 1996).

Vincent, J., 'Benefits of Self-help Groups', in M. Saks (ed.), *Alternative Medicine in Modern Britain* (Oxford: Clarendon Press, 1992)

Wiley, J., '"No Body is Doing it": Cybersexuality as a Postmodern Narrative', *Body and Society*, 1:1 (1995), pp. 145–62.

Winston, B., *Media Technology and Society: A History from the Telegraph to the Internet* (London: Routledge, 1998).

Part III

Unruly Bodies and the Media

All of the authors in this section are concerned, in one way or another, with the ways in which the media can reflect and construct certain embodied identities as unruly, polluting, deviant and/or 'grotesque'. By way of introduction, therefore, it might be useful to outline some of the key debates that have allowed for the sort of analysis we see in the following chapters. These debates require a certain amount of understanding of a variety of historical and philosophical developments not only in biomedicine, but also in broader debates about what constitutes 'truth' and 'knowledge' (i.e. debates about epistemology).

How we understand and experience our embodied identities is very much influenced by these ideas, which have become largely naturalised (and neutralised) as 'common sense' supported by the 'facts' of science. In other words, the authors in this section recognise the 'constructedness' of bodies and identities – that bodies are brought into being via narratives, some of which (for example biomedical narratives) are given more authority than others. Contested versions, i.e. different 'body stories' (people with impairments; transsexuals; those engaging with alternative bodily practices, etc.), tend to be silenced or misrepresented in favour of a dominant narrative which ultimately supports a heteronormative bias. As Leach Sculley states:

> By opting to see the 'human body as a vast, elaborate and sometimes mysterious machine' (Elliot, 1999, p. 64), modern medicine committed itself to conceptual models that could only be used with confidence by experts and which excluded the sick or disabled person's own comprehension of his/her state. (Leach Sculley, 2002, p. 49)

Foucault (1978), again, has been very influential in our understanding of how bodies became 'mapped' through enlightenment and scientific means. Via the clinical 'gaze' bodies were, at a certain point in history, brought into being, and by the end of the nineteenth century, the 'anatomical atlas' had been constructed which laid down the template for understanding bodies, illness, health and disease.

With this template, bodies that (socially and culturally) deviated from the 'normal functioning' body of biomedicine, could also be identified, mapped and categorised according to physiological or psychological 'faults'. Foucault argued that this development was an effect of power or 'biopower' – where science and medicine engage in minute calculations of the body.

The systematisation of disease categories from governments and public health officials, and employed by medical scientists, became a social preoccupation from the end of the nineteenth century:

> In the interests of the 'surveillance' of society, what formerly had been an interest in variation around the norm was gradually reformulated so as to make categorical, classifiable distinctions between normal and pathological. Normal and abnormal were now conceptualised as dichotomy.   (Lock, 2000, p. 260)

Biomedicine thus accords special status to some kinds of embodiment over others. There is only one or a very limited number of 'valid' embodiments, whereas the repertoire of pathological embodiment is large and becomes larger as we identify even finer distinctions.

For example, bodies became sexually deviant in complexly delineated ways. For many theorists, homosexuality was created by nineteenth-century doctors (Terry, 1995; Weeks, 1985). 'Normal' (heterosexual) sexuality came to be set against sexual aberrations that were constructed as inherently biological. Prior to the anatomical map created by medical men (and later psychologists), sexuality was not seen as a biological feature of the person. Same sex sexual acts were criminalised (for men), but there was no such thing as *the homosexual*.

Theorists have debated why sexology became so prominent in this period of history and what effect it was to have on later perceptions of sexuality. Late nineteenth-century European society became obsessed with the moral issue of sexual perversion characterised by the 'purity crusade'. An area that had previously been ambiguous and non-individual, became problematised in the light of a fragile and unpredictable environment (the still infant, industrial, urban society) and the need for classification became paramount to maintain control and consensus.

With the gradual effect of the Enlightenment securing ideas of sexual individualism, there also emerged a link between morality and medicine, whereby doctors became the new 'high priests' of the state (Mort, 1987; Turner, 1995). Areas not previously considered as medical, now came under the jurisdiction of a biomedical discourse and, thus, the medical gaze extended into the bedroom (Foucault, 1978). Sexuality and sex started to enter into the medical realm as a result of what Hawkes terms the 'negative interface between morality and medicine' (Hawkes, 1996). The link between state regulation and medicine has been well documented (Mort, 1987; Porter, 1982; Porter and Hall, 1995; Turner, 1987). Medical men assumed the mantle of state arbiters in the regulation of society, and the dangers of sex to health were used to enforce bourgeois moral values against the decadence of the aristocracy and the over-indulgence of the urban poor (Hawkes, 1996).

Recent research into the mapping of the human body in the late nineteenth century has illustrated the fascination that scientists and doctors had with constructing typologies of human characteristics from race (Butchart, 1998; Jahoda, 1999); sex (Butler, 1990; Lacqueur, 1990) and sexuality (Terry, 1995). As Davenport-Hines states: 'in nineteenth century Britain there was a craving for the certitude of universal rules and axioms' (1990, p. 115).

The research conducted by the sexologists provided society with taxonomies of sexual behaviour and essentialised sexual identities, which served as a basis to regulate behaviour and set a standard for the 'norm'. The lasting legacy of sexology, reflected in its use of unyielding positivistic methods, has been the production of timeless 'truths' about sex and sexuality, evidenced in the discourses explored in the following chapters.

Anthony Pryce's chapter explores notions of moral regulation and social purity in early twentieth-century public health posters. By situating the texts against an analysis of the discourses of purity and pollution regarding sexual bodies, Pryce manages to illustrate not only the reinforcng of these notions, but also the increasing emphasis placed by health promotion strategy on the 'self' and monitoring of the self (i.e. the individual being accountable for his or her own health trajectory). As Pryce states in the chapter, 'In postmodern sexualities, diversity is becoming a "given"; it is lack of responsibility for healthiness that has become deviant!' – echoing one of the themes of this book; morality and health and the governmentality of the individual.

Watson and Whittle look at some of the different themes that shape news reporting (print media) of transsexuality. As with Pryce, the chapter affords some theoretical discussion about how different froms of body modification elicit different responses. Set against the dominant discourses of gender (and gender performance), sex, 'cosmetic' surgery, and economy, the chapter illustrates how transsexuality is situated in a variety of ways, most of which undermine any idea of an 'authentic' transgender body.

In the final chapter of this section, Andrea Beckmann discusses the social construction of bodies and the discourses of 'normality' and 'abnormality' which position some bodies as acceptable and some as 'grotesque', by comparing disability with 'sadomasochism'. Through her analysis of popular advertising, she illustrates how these grotesque bodies are constructed as without agency, being associated with animality. Tom Shakespeare (1999) has argued that whilst the discourse of 'eugenics' is publicly avoided in the medical literature on genetics, a clear set of values emerges implying that disability is a major problem and should always be prevented (e.g. narratives of tragedy). Constructed as preventing a 'disaster': the geneticists in his study talked about the 'miserable lives of disabled people'. Interestingly, the advertising text analysed by Beckmann draws on a similar discourse. Later on in the chapter, Beckmann explores the potential 'freeing' from genital sexual fixation offered by 'bodily practices' (SM), which also potentially enables disabled individuals, drawing on her own research with the SM community.

REFERENCES

Butchart, A., *The Anatomy of Power: European Constructions of the African Body* (London: Zed Books, 1998).

Butler, J., *Gender Trouble* (London: Routledge, 1990).

Davenport-Hines, R., *Sex, Death and Punishment: Attitudes to Sex and Sexuality in Britain since the Renaissance* (London: Collins, 1990).

Elliot, C., *A Philosophical Desire: Bioethics, Culture and Identity* (London: Routledge, 1999).

Foucault, M., *The History of Sexuality*, vol. 1: *An Introduction* (New York: Pantheon, 1978).

Hawkes, G., *A Sociology of Sex and Sexuality* (Buckingham: Open University Press, 1996).

Jahoda, T., *Images of Savages* (London: Routledge, 1999).

Lacqueur, T., *Making Sex: Body, Knowledge and Gender from the Greeks to Freud* (Cambridge: Harvard University Press, 1990).

Leach Sculley, J., 'A Postmodern Disorder: Modern Encounters with Molecular Models of Disability', in M. Corker, and T. Shakespeare, *Disability/Postmodernity* (London: Routledge, 2002).

Lock, M., 'Accounting for Disease and Distress: Morals of the Normal and Abnormal', in G. Albrecht et al., *The Handbook of Social Studies in Health and Medicine* (2000), pp. 259–77.

Mort, F., *Dangerous Sexualities: Medico-moral Panics in England since 1830* (London: Routledge, 1987).

Porter, R., *English Society in the Eighteenth Century* (Harmondsworth: Penguin, 1982).

Porter, R. and Hall, L., *The Facts of Life: The Creation of Sexual Knowledge in Britain, 1650–1950* (New Haven, CT: Yale University Press, 1995).

Shakespeare, T., 'Losing the Plot? Medical and Activist Discourses of Contemporary Genetics and Disability', *Sociology of Health and Illness*, 21:5 (1999), pp. 669–88.

Terry, J., 'Anxious Slippages between "Us" and "Them": a Brief History of the Scientific Search for Homosexual Bodies', in J. Terry and J. Urla (eds), *Deviant Bodies: Critical Perspectives of Difference in Science and Popular Culture* (London: Routledge, 1995).

Turner, B. S., *Medical Power and Social Knowledge* (London: Sage, 1995).

Weeks, J., *Sexuality and Its Discontents: Meanings, Myths and Modern Sexualities* (London: Routledge, 1985).

'Planting Landmines in their Sex Lives': Governmentality, Iconography of Sexual Disease, and the 'Duties' of the STD Clinic

7

Anthony Pryce

Introduction

Infections such as syphilis, gonorrhoea, chlamydia, herpes, or HIV/AIDS have emerged and re-emerged in history and have been socially constructed in the image of the historical moment when they appeared. This chapter concerns the attempts by the state to control sexually acquired infections using public health campaigns in the twentieth century. These campaigns have relied on visual images to tell a medico-moral story that both reflected and shaped discourses around sexual diseases, social roles, sexual identity, and sexual citizenship.

In the years following the First World War, a network of 'special' or VD (venereal diseases) clinics was developed as a response to the problem of an

Acknowledgement: An earlier version of some of this material was published in *Nursing Inquiry*, 8: 3 (September 2001), pp. 151–61.

increasing incidence of syphilis within the population. These clinics were intended to be the locus of formal medical treatments and sexual health surveillance, as well as the means of collecting epidemiological data and providing education within wider public health campaigns. Such campaigns increasingly exploited the new media techniques to construct powerful poster images to convey the medico-moral message of sexual hygiene. Through much of the twentieth century, these images reflected popular discourses that located sexual diseases as symptomatic of not only a medical, but also a social threat. Such threats and constraints were represented through an iconography of *social diseases* that tells a story reinforcing heteronormative gendered, sexual roles and social expectations. Especially when associated with 'deviant' or 'illicit' activities such as premarital sex, erotic encounters are constructed as a conduit for moral as well as bodily contagion, to be controlled through social surveillance, political control and medical purification. However, public health campaigns do change to reflect the social and sexual discourses of the day. Through the Second World War, the postwar period, the imperatives of the AIDS pandemic, and up to the present, it is clear that posters and images now underscore the individual's responsibility and education regarding their conduct of sexual activity. This emphasised both the function and duties of the clinic, where medicine becomes an agent of social purity, and marked a paradigmatic statement of the panoptic role of medicine in the mapping of the social and psychological spaces between individuals.

This chapter will explore the role of public health posters and the construction of iconography of sexual diseases in sexual health campaigns from the early twentieth century to the recent past. I shall briefly delineate what I mean by the term 'iconography', then outline how Foucault's (1978) notion of the *Ars Erotica* can be linked with the recruitment of the individual as a self-observing *active patient* (Armstrong, 1983a). The *active patient* is the result of the deployment of disciplinary practices to the citizen, resulting in individuals who are recruited to examine themselves for signs of disease, and increasingly to maintain a bewildering array of 'good' health regimes. The emphasis on self-care and self-improvement constitutes core practices of the self and creates a form of governmentality. In other words, the individual internalises the way of seeing defined by medicine, and monitors the conduct of his/her own body and self. The individual as an active patient is acting as the locus of health promotion strategies that have increasingly moved from the communitarian ideological assumption of the state protecting the health of the body of the population, to becoming the responsibility of the individual. This is a key factor that will be explored through the use of historical twentieth-century media images surrounding the control of syphilis and other infections. These images work to reinforce modernist rhetoric on medicine and governmentality whilst frequently failing to problematise sexuality.

Armstrong (1983a) used the history of venereal diseases (VD) to illustrate the development of the clinic or dispensary as the later manifestation of Foucault's concept of the Panopticon. He argues that the outpatient STI (sexually transmitted infections) clinic and its practices display characteristics of surveillance medicine *par excellence*. I shall explore how the sexual regulation and governance operates, notably through the illustrations used in campaigns that draw on the iconography of moral and sexual codes. Some of the illustrations used in public health campaigns demonstrate this increasing emphasis placed on the individual in two key ways. The first injunction calls on individuals to avoid illicit sexual activities, by appealing to their moral and social duties as citizens. The second, if they fail in that restraint, is that the individual is required to attend a clinic, confess and reveal the source of infection, and accept the examination and penetration of his/her body before complying with the treatment regime prescribed by the doctor.

I shall conclude by suggesting that health promotion and AIDS campaigns have reflected changing popular and professional discourses, and that the dominant mode of anti-STI propaganda has shifted significantly. In the early twentieth century, the pervasive message was clearly rooted in an unproblematic, heteronormative moral proscription that drew on notions of 'duty' and social (class, sexual and racial) purity. However, by the end of the century, the influence of individualistic, consumerist culture had replaced these notions of the duty to, and of, the State with greater emphasis on individual responsibility. This signals the shift to a more sophisticated identification of sexual diversity as *lifestyle*, but also a deeper level of governmentality, where the duty lies in the self-monitoring of the actor's 'informed' practice and a new interpretation of restraint.

Method: key themes

The role of iconography

The term 'iconography' most often refers to imagery used in sacred art. The word draws on art-historical references to the knowledge required by the viewer to 'read' the meanings attached to pictorial representations. The common usage refers specifically to 'icons' in the Eastern churches, where often-static images carried mystical, spiritual meanings. For example, in most Christian traditions of sacred art the conventions of a lamb and flag represent Christ's sacrificial role, or a scallop shell worn as a brooch signifies a pilgrim. Another interpretation of the word 'iconography' is a collection of portraits (Murrey and Murrey, 1989). In both cases, the essential condition is that the meanings are known, or can be deduced. The key feature of any iconography is that the images can be 'read' by the viewer, where signifiers such as a skull or a pair of handcuffs may be interpreted both literally and symbolically. This also requires the images to be 'current' (for example, much Christian or pagan iconography would be unintelligible to many modern people). For such images to work, particularly in the context of a mass campaign, they need to reflect contemporary meanings and to be read against shifts in the discourses. The images used in this chapter are secular, medicalised and part of public health campaigns of the 1940s and 1950s, with some examination of the HIV/AIDS campaigns of the 1980s. The illustrations in public campaigns are full of rich imagery that obviously reflects and shapes sexual mores, health and hygiene discourses. However, central to the iconography are recurring themes around moral as well as physical purity, the individual's sexual restraint and the State's responsibility for the monitoring, treatment and education involving STIs.

Interestingly, there is little sustained interest by sociologists in charting these images. Gilman (1988a; 1988b; 1989) has been concerned with the iconography of syphilis, but otherwise there is surprisingly little sociological literature on sexually transmitted diseases except where it is incidental to AIDS. It may be that STIs are a less attractive topic for research, where even in texts entirely concerned with the sociology of sex, such as Hawke's (1996), there are only six passing references to venereal diseases. This is particularly interesting given the extent of the social impact of these diseases in pre-modern and contemporary societies. The body and sexualities are both the object and subject of the images explored in this chapter. It will become apparent that the changing use of such images reflects changing attitudes, forms of sexual consumption, commodification of sex and the increasing individualism of health and social discourses. However, before considering the ideological work of the media in the history of public health campaigns around sexual health, it is important to consider the ways in which sexualities have been increasingly problematised.

Sexual sciences or erotic arts?

The control of sexual activities that result in diseases, teenage pregnancies or the destabilising of supposedly rigid sexual categories and roles reveals a number of tensions at the social and individual level. In contemporary cultures, this remains apparent in continuing public virtue/private vice discourses. Individuals are urged both to be liberated and to explore their erotic bodies and emotions as a project of identity formation, whilst being subjected to competing, sometimes conflicting theories, or to explain or talk of sexual processes through psychoanalysis, counselling or simply talk. Michel Foucault (1978) outlined his thesis that the emergence of the *Scientia Sexualis*, or scientific knowledge of sex, appeared, in western culture at least, to replace earlier 'procedures for producing the truth of sex'. These earlier procedures were, he argued, evident in ancient Greek and Roman and Indian cultures and rooted in the knowledge gained from the refinement of the individual's own experience of erotic pleasure or *askēsis*. Particularly for men, this was a model of 'ethical subjectivity' as opposed to the later Christian ethos of a moral, ascetic regime. It presents the possibility for the individual to enjoy types of sexual pleasure without reference to exterior laws of the permitted and the forbidden, but first and foremost in relation to pleasure itself. In other words, the individual is engaged in the project of refining and developing the appreciation of sexual pleasure or *askēsis*.

A clear problem for society and for the individual citizen is how to engage with the exploration of the sexual self, whilst also being informed and able to calculate risk and monitor the self for signs of disorder. Governmentality, operating through the body of public health knowledge specifically relating to sexual diseases, privileges scientific truths of sex over the lived truths of erotic pleasure and sexual freedom. As Bristow (1997, p. 186) summarises, 'the self-regulation of desires constitutes a liberating autonomy, for such *askēsis* creates a realm of freedom over which the male citizen at last maintains control'. This has been particularly evident in communities that have been organised around sexual identity and/or transgression. In relation to contemporary gay culture in particular, Foucault (1989, p. 228) remarked that what most 'bothers those [people] who are not gay about gayness is the gay lifestyle, not sex acts themselves'. In other words, how notions of transgressive sexual identities challenge stabilised sexual categories. For example, in the AIDS campaigns of the 1980s and 1990s sexual categories and identities began to be problematised – to assume a married man is exclusively heterosexual is naive, and regarding a man who has sex with men as 'gay' is clearly insufficiently nuanced. Similarly, this challenging of assumptions of sexual polarities was reflected in significantly greater penetration of sexual subcultures by health agencies in the context of an increased emphasis on the quest for the 'authentic' self and the healthy body.

In the late twentieth century, this 'healthy' body was being (re)constructed through the problematising of heterosexuality itself, as well as other sexual identities and 'lifestyles' (Richardson, 1996). The 'taken-for-granted' status of heterosexuality as being privileged as 'natural' and institutionalised in social policy, was clearly challenged through feminist discourses (Jackson, 1996). Similarly, as Petersen (1998) and others have explored, notions of male health, identities and bodies are also being reconfigured through the apparent threats to hegemonic masculinities brought about by changing work patterns, and by economic and other social drivers for change. From a predominantly metropolitan, liberal perspective, the healthy body is now defined less by signifiers of 'deviance' such as homosexuality, but rather by the knowledge and practices that maintain and demonstrate 'health'. In postmodern sexualities, diversity is becoming a 'given'; it is lack of responsibility for healthiness that has become deviant!

The 'active' body and governance

At the intersection of the two discursive formations of 'scientific' sex and the erotic, individuals are required to observe their own conduct in the complex public/private spaces of the social world. Governmentality is achieved through the identification of orthodoxies being assimilated into the conduct of everyday life, and these are predicated on the (re)invention of taboos, 'unhealthiness' – impurity. Most religions have constructed strong associations of bodily functions such as sex, with dirt, danger, sin; and these have become interwoven in the psycho-social and medical assumptions of daily life. Mary Douglas (1966) proposed that 'dirt is matter out of place', thereby suggesting that what is appropriate in one setting may take on very different symbolic meanings when located elsewhere. She traced how cultural beliefs about dirt and contamination have been central to the construction of dangers such as disease, and the formation of 'otherness' in practices, individuals or populations that are surrounded by boundaries of taboo and ritual. For example, there are widespread belief systems and taboos surrounding the magical, dangerous, polluting powers of menstruation, or the weakening of the young (particularly) male through masturbation. Similarly, a recurring theme in the iconography of sexual disease is the 'loose' woman, who appears 'clean' but acts as the locus of infection. Therefore, drawing on Douglas (1966), the discursive device that is provided by notions of pollution, and by mechanisms of control in the social construction of sexual disease as risk or threat, is helpful in exploring instrumental and symbolic sexual activities. One key element here is the construction and governance of the sexual citizen, faced with the risk of 'pollution', and how the healthy body is transformed by sexual contamination.

The 'healthy' body that attends the STI clinic is the body that *outside* has embraced; that penetrates or was penetrated; that kissed; cruised; role-played erotic games; was inscribed by tattoos or pierced; spoke and ejaculated. This is the body that is socially located in time and space, transformed from lover to patient; from subject to both object and subject; from knowledge of desire to knowledge of sickness. *Inside* the clinic this (postmodern) body is symbolically stripped of the eroticism of its outside life whilst retaining its potentiality, in an environment that is saturated with sexuality whilst operating within models of (modernist) medical and organisational rational-ities. This also sets up another important potential arena of inquiry. The contemporary notions of risk and scientific sexuality permeate the actor's sexual activities and identity through his or her recruitment into the active patient role.

Associated with this active patient role and central to the contemporary context of health policy, particularly in safer-sex discourses, is the construction of risk and the *risky self*, of which there are four main models (Bloor, 1995). This is axiomatic to calculating the social costs and dangers of undesirable individuals and more especially, populations. Castel (1991, p. 287) suggests that,

> a risk does not arise from the presence of particular danger embodied in a concrete individual or group. It is the effect of a combination of abstract factors which render more or less probable the occurrence of undesirable modes of behaviour.

This creates moral environments where the construction of risks that become the target of 'witch-hunts' and moral panics (such as the inflaming of public concern in the UK with paedophilia, underage pregnancies or internet porn) is a more subtle and effective mode of regulation than simply that of identifying 'aberrant' individuals. Petersen and Bunton (1997, p. 191) locates this within the emergence of *neo*-liberal regimes that create a sphere of freedom for subjects. Thus, they can exercise a regulated autonomy, where self-conduct is linked to a consciously contrived style of conduct (Rose, 1994). Here, the entrepreneurial individual is endowed with freedom, autonomy and the capacity to care properly for him/herself within 'a market governed by the rationalities of competition, accountability and consumer demand' (Rose, 1994, p. 285).

Following Armstrong's proposition, this is contingent on individuals endlessly examining themselves; self-care and self-improvement being core practices of the self. This constitutes the 'active patient' and is the vehicle whereby health promotion strategies have increasingly moved from the communitarian ideological assumption of the role of the state protecting individual health, to the responsibility being assumed by the individual. Higgs's (1998) lucid review of the conceptualisation of citizenship draws on Turner and locates risk and governmentality as tensions in modern society, between 'the deregulation of the macro-level and the micro-level requirement for a continuing micro-politics of surveillance and control'. This has particular resonance in relation to sexuality and sexual health when he goes on to argue (Higgs, 1998, p. 193) that:

> the imagery of risk is incorporated into the practicalities of everyday practice as more and more knowledge is disseminated and more and more risk is identified. Health promotion steps into the public domain as a virtuous activity not only promoting public health but also the person. While this seems to accord with the modern conception of the agentic individual who can mould himself or herself, it also provides the basis for the new relationship between state and citizen – one concerned with demonstrating the appropriate 'technologies of the self'.

For Douglas (1966), the ideas of purity, contamination and pollution that may culturally confirm or refute perceptions of danger or risk to the individual do not simply disappear but may be reconfigured.

Sexual infections have come to occupy a different social space over the last hundred years. Venereal diseases, particularly syphilis, have been part of the ideological work of modernity. In other words, heteronormative stories of purity and restraint were incorporated to maintain and reinforce the project of class, race and gender formation. In the early twenty-first century, attitudes and behaviours surrounding sex seem more complex and interwoven with subtle reworking of the social construction of gender and sexualities. Clinic patients and practitioners explore tensions between professional and personal identities whilst policing boundaries of sexual practice. The newer 'liberal' approaches to sexual health signify the deployment of professional, disciplinary powers that penetrate the individual and the population's everyday theory and practice of sex. The *untouchable* element of venereology as a low-status medical speciality may appear to have been challenged through changing social *mores* and the discourse of post-AIDS health rhetoric. Yet, the increasingly high incidence of STIs and unwanted teenage pregnancies might signify a failure of safer-sex promotion strategies. Such strategies have an important role in revealing how the iconography of disease has moved from purity to the consumption of desire, and where the regulation of disorder has moved from moral proscription to governmentality.

The texts

Governmentality and the clinic duties

At the heart of the discussions around governmentality, surveillance and medical power, it is essential to consider *how* such abstractions are deployed in everyday life. One way, which is explored here, is in the use of a number of posters developed to control the spread of syphilis and other sexual diseases, and increase the effectiveness of measures to prevent them particularly during the 1940s and 1950s and again as a response to HIV/AIDS. These posters appeared from the early 1920s up to the early 1990s. These have been selected because they vividly illustrate how the discourses have developed around the moral and social regulation of sexualities, surveillance, and the project of governmentality.

As Foucault argues (1978), during the nineteenth century the 'family as Panopticon' became one site and unit of surveillance. The STI or *clap* clinic is most definitely another. The sexual health clinic (or indeed virtually any clinical environment where the sexual body is regarded by medicine) is located at the interpenetration of two discursive formations – where medicine and the erotic engage. One concerns scientific disciplinary knowledge(s) and praxes of medicine (*Scientia Sexualis*); and the other is engaged with the embodied pleasure (*Ars Erotica*) of the client. They constitute discursive arenas within which the relationship of sexualities and disease; clinical knowledge and practices; lay and professional dangers, power and resistance, may be explored, interrogated and mapped. The iconography of modern medicine, sex, and the role of the state was clearly delineated in a poster that used small illustrations of the five 'duties' of the clinic and the role of the citizen 'you' (see Figure 7.1).

These five domains provide a robust basis for a reading of the clinic as Panopticon and the increasing governmentality through medicine of the individual and his or her sexuality (see Table 7.1). In the five *Duties* portrayed in the poster, the text reinforces its emphasis on the State being responsible for controlling syphilis, but '*You*' the individual are responsible for acting on that. Here, as Armstrong (1983b) had suggested, was an exemplar of the clinic or *dispensary as Panopticon writ large*. The five duties identified in the poster may be explicated as described in Table 7.1.

The clinic is clearly a lumen of the disciplinary gaze and the arena of local power/knowledge. However, what is absent from the medical project of sexual health rationalities is the social context(s) and the power of sexual practices and desires – in other words the *Ars Erotica* is dissolved. The 'duties' outlined here represent a most florid example of Foucault's *Scientia Sexualis*.

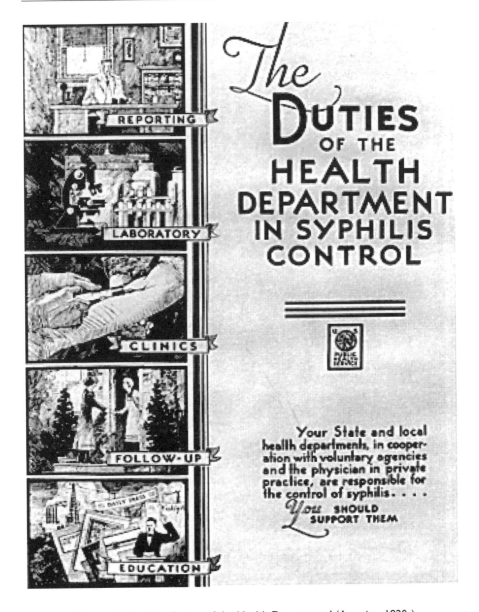

Figure 7.1 'The Duties of the Health Department' (America, 1920s)

Table 7.1   The modern role and duties of the STI clinic as Panopticon

The medical duties of the clinic	The clinic as Panopticon
Reporting	The routine penetration of bodies for the collecting of data and their translation into the statistical epidemiological drawing of populations: but also at the capillary (individual) level through disclosure and confession.
Laboratory	The exposition of the power of disciplinary knowledge where the collected data and specimens are *visualised*, constructed as images of disease processes and representations of a *dissolved* body, i.e. the bacteria or virus is made visible, whereby the whole body of the patient is rendered almost invisible.
Clinics	The location where the doctor–patient relationship is central to the subjugated knowledge and practices of the self, and to the interrelation of institutional and localised power (Lupton, 1997, p. 105). The expert, the doctor, nurse or health adviser, is the instrument of normalising judgement and arbiter of deviance.
Follow-up	Surveillance through contact tracing, illustrating the mapping of the social domain for the locus of illness (Armstrong, 1983a, p. 58) and networks of sexual relationships in the community.
Education	The recruiting of individuals to monitor their own bodies, and their transformation into *active patients*. Governmentality and increased self-monitoring through penetration of sexual sites, spaces and praxis by medicine, social science and *askēsis*.

As Armstrong (1983a) suggests in a strong echo of Foucault's hypothesis of the deployment of *Scientia Sexualis*, there is a symbiotic relationship between sexually transmitted diseases on the one hand, and the social construction and proscription of dangerous sexualities (Mort, 1987) on the other. Within such discourse a powerful array of elements may be easily detected, such as the opportunity historically provided by disease for ascribing blame to nations (Jochelson, 1996), or races (Henriot, 1996); gender (Spongberg, 1996), or sexual groups (Davenport-Hines, 1990). For example, scapegoating of marginalised and vilified groups such as prostitutes, drug injectors, lesbians and gay men, or Black Africans has been well documented in the HIV/AIDS pandemic (Bloor, 1995). This reproduces earlier cultural and national disputes on the origins and the dissemination of syphilis (Quétel, 1990) and also to some extent socially locates and reinforces the expert as the arbiter of sexual knowledge and health.

A key historical moment, which produced a shift in the popular notion of sexual disease, was thereby associated with the development of antibiotics in the treatment of VD. Quétel (1990, p. 7) suggests that the 'miraculous' cures using antibiotics created a social phenomenon at least as astonishing as the fear and loathing that preceded them. In relation to syphilis, he suggests there was

> an instantaneous shift from a frenzy of fear to a complete lack of concern . . . all that was required to destroy this fragile trepenoma (although it is impossible to produce a laboratory culture of it and therefore a vaccine) was a few hefty doses of penicillin; consequently syphilis became no more than an unpleasant memory, and folk could resume their depravities without fear.

Quétel does not go on to suggest how this 'instantaneous' transformation came about, allowing people so quickly to discount the danger of such a powerful disease. The incorporation of scientific images to public health material clearly provided substantial support for the dissemination of the medical gaze and the ideological work of the production and reproduction of medical heroism in the postwar period. It is also contemporary with the construction of a new (poorly regulated) market for the powerful drugs companies, which given the extent of sexual infections would greatly benefit from the scientific endorsement of the efficacy of their product. Here for example, in the presentation of the medical semiotics, the visual imagery of disease is increasingly represented graphically. It is supported by extracts of research evidence undertaken by referenced 'experts' within a health market that is already using the individualised market language of 'choice'.

Medicine increasingly was portrayed as both the route to confirming diagnosis and the means of effective treatment. It was also more able to create new, more accurate and penetrating degrees of observation and mapping of the threads of relationships between individuals and populations. The advertisements and populist, street-level health campaigns alerted the population to new wonder cures and a 'magic bullet' that renders disease less miasmic. The doctor as privileged expert is the gatekeeper of both the means of diagnoses and the treatment. Another problem in Quétel's analysis is that he disregards the continuing importance of VD in the iconography of public morality discourses throughout the 1940s, 1950s and early 1960s. The pervasive and recurrent imagery of VD sustained by moral injunctions that privilege heteronormative monogamy also draws on notions of national purity. It promotes the observation of self within sexual actions, regimes of physical and moral *clean-ness*, reproducing anxieties of *otherness* within formations of medical surveillance.

In ascribing blame and creating *otherness* the disease has provided the basis for moral signifiers of criminality, decay, degeneracy, decadence, the construction of social standards, identities, class and racism. Such signification thereby legitimises the imperatives for social policy and moral bases for surveillance, segregation, regulation and discrimination of populations and surveillance of the body itself. Sexually transmitted infections and the individual have been discursively reconstructed from dangerousness to risk (Castel, 1991). Petersen (1998, p. 192) explores this from a Foucauldian perspective, proposing that:

> Over the last hundred years there has been a shift in emphasis from controlling the dangerous individual, via face-to-face interventions of preventive medicine and use of confinement, to an emphasis on anticipating and preventing the emergence of undesirable event, abnormality and deviant behaviour.

In other words, the history of health policy and of the regulation of disease and danger has created new roles for experts and expert knowledge in the government of populations and the regulation of personal identity. Whilst this may refer to the processes of reconstructing threats of any disease, it most commonly refers to those iatrogenic factors in lifestyle such as food additives, alcohol or tobacco, and lack of exercise. However, we might add sex or erotic desire to this list and such a model is particularly useful when applied to the history of VD over the last 60 years.

Wartime lay beliefs and the deployment of iconographies of contamination

War has often been associated with apparent increased sexual activity and the spread of sexual infections. The onset of the Second World War coincided with a vigorous deployment of public health campaigns that utilised the media and martial imagery of the time. Partly through the introduction of STI clinics, the incidence of syphilis was, by 1939, at an all time low, and the incidence of early-detected syphilis in the UK civilian population was 5000 (Porter and Hall, 1995, p. 240). Evidence from contemporary records suggests that by the time of the Second World War there was a significant shift in the sense of otherness which had characterised the earlier public views of both the army and the distance of civilians from the field of warfare. First, the troops were predominantly conscripts or volunteers, not career soldiers. Secondly, the theatre of war was now very explicitly inclusive of Home Territory through the *blitzkrieg* and the new forms of enemy propaganda such as radio and films. There had been improvements in the treatment of gonorrhoea with early antibiotics, and syphilis could be controlled by penicillin in 1943 (Hicks, 1994, p. 33). However, as Hall (1996, p. 5) reports, the Mass Observation (MO) survey of 1942/3 suggested that there was still widespread ignorance of the causes and modes of transmission of VD (Stanley, 1995). In responding to the MO interviewers, it appeared that men were rather more rigidly dogmatic, and more embarrassed about discussing the issues in their attitudes towards VD and its control, than women. However, it was reported that most respondents welcomed the opportunity to discuss the issue and wanted to know more (Stanley, 1995).

Of particular concern were prostitutes and 'easy' women (see Figure 7.2). Most respondents assumed that prostitutes were the main source of infection, although this was extended to incorporate 'bad women', 'loose-living women' and, some went so far as to suggest, women in general. In Figure 7.2, the jaunty hat on the skull provides a potent image that suggests the proximity of disease (and of course death) even in familiar people or situations – including sex. Consistent with other historical discourses, it is women who are primarily to be blamed; the notion that men could or should take responsibility for the avoidance of infection (or pregnancy) was not addressed. The other objects of blame were 'the troops', 'West End night-clubs', 'foreigners' and 'Americans'. There was still an element of belief that VD was miasmic, all-pervasive, and that infection was not confined solely to sexual contact, but could be 'caught' from a range of public facilities, such as from using public lavatories! Another element in the context of the MO responses was of course the war, where despite the tendency to locate disease in 'known' bodies, anxiety was expressed about the difficulty of identifying carriers. In other words, who is the enemy? Numerous VD posters provide an example of how this represented the linking of wartime anxieties and imagery with the war against hidden disease.

To some extent, not being able to locate the specific 'other' body metamorphoses infection into a sinister fifth columnist contaminating and sabotaging the Home Front, and contributes to the construction of new risks. Posters and propaganda depicted militarised disease located in women, as being far more insidious and dangerous than the enemy Axis. The notion of running 'the risk' of disease by having sex with an 'easy' girlfriend is underpinned by the text, which outlines the dreadful consequences of taking a risk in the first place and then compounding the danger by not seeking treatment.

There was considerable emphasis on 'cleanliness', 'hot baths' and, particularly for the woman, the admonition that she should not use public lavatories. There

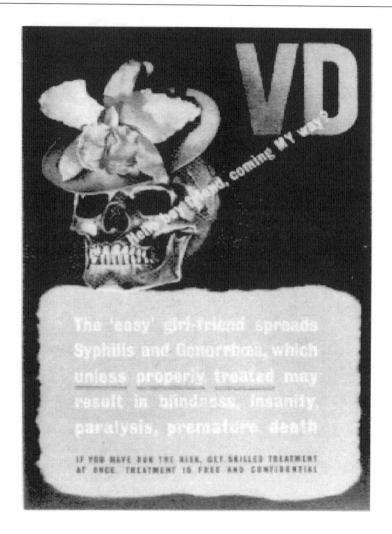

Figure 7.2 'Easy' (1940s)

were injunctions that 'every woman should keep herself clean, scrub herself, not sit on any lavatory seat' (Hall, 1996, p. 6), and 'cleanliness' was as much a moral imperative as a statement of hygiene.

The appearance of cleanliness, however, is a guarantee of neither moral purity nor freedom from disease. In terms of ideas to control infection, the public appeared to favour extreme regulation, with compulsory monthly exam-ination of prostitutes being one suggestion that echoed notions of legalising brothels and prostitution. The state and the citizen were activated and regulated by a combination of moral order, relentless self-control and vigilance, and social taboo. The role of the state and the operation of its gaze through medicine were particularly favoured. Examples of ideas from the Mass Observation (Hall, 1996, p. 6) included those by a middle-class woman who proposed that it would be:

> a very good idea if the State made everybody have a medical examination every so often. Say every five years. Many things would be found out which should be attended to, and are not.

Many male and female respondents deemed compulsion, as an element in the state surveillance of the eroticised body of the population, crucial. Some of them proposed that medical examinations should be annual and ought to include 'instruction'. As in the later public response to HIV, there was some opposition to these draconian levels of observation. There were recommenda-tions to improve education using plain language rather than euphemisms, and to provide free prophylactic condoms like those supplied to US troops in a pragmatic recognition of the need for precautions. It was widely believed in the MO that these should also be on sale to civilians through chemists' shops. As Hall (1996) points out, these observations were expressed very much in the context of a militarised frame of mind, where those who were at home as well as the troops were in danger of sexual disease. Danger was both random and all-pervasive and much use was made, in poster campaigns, of euphemism and suggestive phallic imagery such as tank guns and torpedoes. Some precautions had to be taken, and enforced – like the air-raid precautions – but ideas about public education and advances in scientific medicine reflect sometimes contra-dictory contemporary discourses. One such tension was located between the belief in the therapeutic value of antibiotic regimes, and the anxiety that new drugs and condoms giving freedom from the fear of disease would promote licentiousness. Such arguments are recurrent and resurfaced forty years later in the debates around measures to limit the transmission of HIV.

The emphasis in posters often underscored the message that the curative potential of drugs does not erase guilt (see Figure 7.3). Despite the traditional admonishment to restraint, some conditions are assumed to lead to greater temptations. For example, servicemen away from home are at greater risk of sin, partly because they are male and therefore subject to greater sexual urges, which need relief through commercial sex or 'easy' transitory relationships!

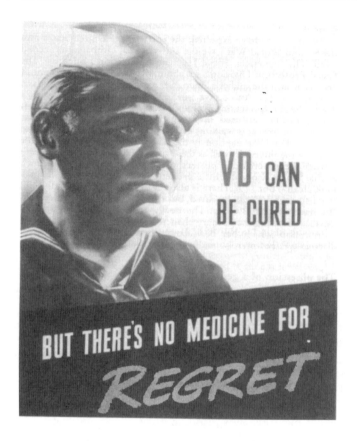

Figure 7.3   'Regret' (America, 1940s)

Postwar moral conservatism reinforced the necessity of social–psychological and moral self-monitoring by the individual, despite the availability of condoms for US servicemen and the increasing use of antibiotics. This neo-conservatism privileged notions of physical as well as moral purity and enabled the further penetration of the panoptic clinical gaze into the population, where guilt and regret act as reinforcers of restraint, if not abstinence.

Postwar surveillance and the penetration of modern social spaces

In the postwar years, disruption to the natural order caused by war and the upheaval in the social order, was interwoven in discourses that reconstructed

VD in the imagery of the family and the government of the body. It is not surprising then, in this new scenario of professionalised sexual health care in the 1940s and 1950s, that Mort (1987, p. 208) goes on to suggest:

> Sex education firmly reinstated normalising hierarchies of knowledge, which set teachers above parent, medics over patients and dismissed competing feminist and popular understandings as lunatic, amateur and irregular. Instruction from above was the keynote. There was none of the emphasis on active self-determination which had characterised the positive side of purity feminism. With the renewed expansion of social policy and state provision in the 1940s and 50s, social hygiene became written into the rubric of the welfare state.

This was obviously reinforced in the UK by the creation of the NHS and the increased provision of free treatments in VD clinics. The sexual health policies were also consistent with the representation of conventional gender roles, the family, and the construction of postwar medical knowledge and the role of the State. The clinics themselves remained sites of stigma, often being located in inconvenient, poorly maintained parts of old hospitals, but became increasingly successful in terms of the number of patients seen and treated (Porter and Hall, 1995, pp. 234–6 and 239–40).

Even after the war, the UK civilian incidence of syphilis in 1946 was 17,000 and there were nearly 48,000 cases of gonorrhoea (Felstein, 1974, p. 35). The drive to eradicate syphilis was appropriated as part of the ideological work of reconstructing the roles of marriage and the family. The imagery still drew on the *invisible* contagion: appearances being deceptive, where the loose woman, with her unblemished face or jaunty hat that masked disease, would infect and permeate the nation's manhood. Authoritative, scientific, medical texts reinforce images where women remain the locus of sexual anxiety and pollution. The only *proper* treatments being, of course, the result of medical inspection and investigation. The injunction to be examined invokes the companion stigmas of twentieth-century *otherness* – disability, insanity and premature death. Treatment is only 'proper' when conducted by 'skilled' practitioners, but importantly is free and confidential.

Acting also within a discursive polarity with such proscription of the 'easy' girlfriend, is the construction of *purity* located in notions of the bride and marriage. In one poster, 'Here comes the Bride' (Figure 7.4), the sanctification of marriage is appropriated to admonish the man to avoid infection so that he doesn't commit a *personal* sin of infecting his bride, who is assumed to be virgin.

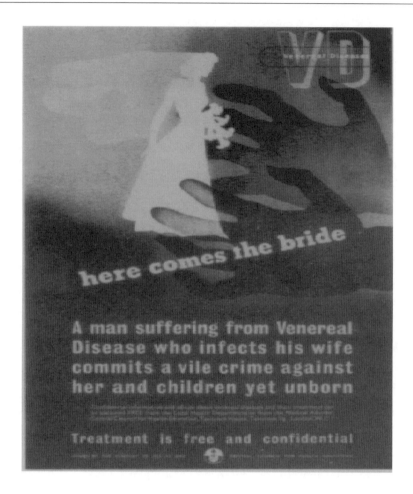

Figure 7.4   'Here Comes the Bride' (1950s)

Disease was seen as a threat to the family, and crucially, infecting a partner was now being constructed as a (vile) crime. Disease was no longer a miasmic, haphazard event but now personalised, and cure was within the power of the individual, who should subject himself (*sic*) to medical examination and treatment. Thus, the iconography within the poster combined *film noir*-influenced graphics from crime/detection movies with polemic text to engage with the 'man in the street'. Actually, the most common place for such posters was in public toilets, so yet again underscoring the relationship between 'dirty' body functions and the risk of sex and disease. As with many cultural beliefs and practices, the shifts in discourses do not mean that the earlier ones disappear, they are merely subsumed!

The domestic ideology firmly located women in the home, where gender roles were clearly defined, and moral injunctions to purity were concerned with personal happiness but also with the health of the nation's gene pool (see Figure 7.5). The social and sexual spaces beyond the home were surrounded by dangers, which in some posters were depicted with the same lurid, *noir* imagery operating in pulp fiction and 'B' movies. The theme continued in anti-VD campaign posters, where responsibility for helping to ensure the purity and health of the future populations was placed with parents. Here, both men and women as future parents are equally identified as being responsible not just for their own pleasure but for the happiness and health of their offspring. The notion of 'clean living' recurs, but a change appears evident. The admonition is less to do with the morality of sex (premarital or extramarital) and celibacy, but whether people are sufficiently educated and informed to know how to avoid infection. In other words, 'clean living' moves from restraint in sexual activity to a position where the individual may experience sexual activity but must take responsibility to ensure that the interaction is clean and safe.

Other campaigns (e.g. Figure 7.6) utilised images of marriage, with happiness predicated here on axes with two central assumptions. First, that sexuality is co-terminous with the social status of marriage. There is no acknowledgement of any risks or dangers other than through heterosexual modes of transmission: any other sexual orientation or identity remaining invisible in health promotion imagery until the late 1970s. The iconography clearly indicates the subtext of marriage being the only legitimate social state for the enjoyment of sex; the marriage contract also being the public rite whereby a virgin bride is transformed into a married sexual partner – albeit within a restricted, gendered social role.

A second axis of health promotion provides the delineation between the healthy and the diseased. This underscores both the moral and the social purity of the couple, who may be absolved of any earlier premarital impurity, uncleanness or *sin*, through confession and absolution via the inspection of the medical gaze. More particularly, scientific medicine is the means by which lucky couples achieve knowledge of their health. If they are clean, uninfected, theirs is a union that is sanctified not only by the Church and State, but also by medicine (Turner, 1984). It became a truism in relation to AIDS (Sontag, 1989), but also in the rise and rise of laboratory medicine in the 1940s and 1950s, how the triumphalist medical discourses were constructed through the rhetoric of science, purity, warfare and military metaphor.

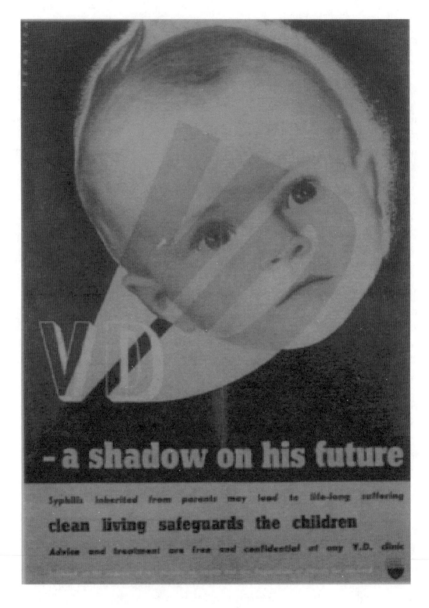

Figure 7.5 'A Shadow on his Future' (1950s)

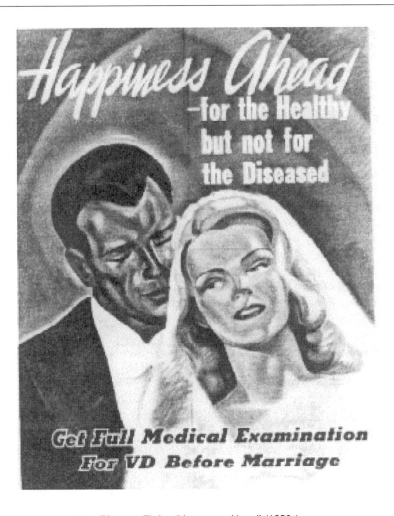

Figure 7.6   'Happiness Ahead' (1950s)

The educated consumer as active patient

It has been commonly assumed that sexually transmitted diseases were inconvenient but not life-threatening. For the postwar generations, the belief that cure is better than prevention has proved chimerical. Certainly, the introduction and production of penicillin coincided with a transition in the development of several issues: the ascendancy of medical heroism and laboratory science; the wartime sexual 'liberalism'; and the increasing therapeutic optimism offered by drugs against infectious diseases. Such a position later supported the brief growth of sexual liberation and gay culture in the 1970s and early 1980s. It also tended to reflect the assumption that medical power was able to overcome the most feared of the venereal diseases, such as syphilis. The safer-sex campaigns of the 1980s and 1990s used imagery that succeeded in utilising the aim of avoiding the older sexually transmitted diseases (STDs) as a secondary benefit to being able to enjoy sex whilst not putting the person at risk from HIV.

The use of fetishised, hypermasculinised gay imagery demonstrates the transformation of the individual body as the consumer of sexualities, which is no longer under moral restraints. It has become an arena where the actor has responsibility; as the site for educated pleasure (*askësis*), the body is a site of desire but also danger. In one such poster ('Tom of Finland'), a very muscular and übersexualised man, partially dressed in rubber, stands beneath a banner that orders the viewer to 'Use a rubber!' Yet there is no visible source of danger or visualisation of the disease organism. The injunction to 'Use a Rubber' is unsupported by any medicalised rationale. Rather, the slogan 'Use a rubber' is located in discourses of mastery, power and domination, with references to subcultures of difference, and the observer is meant to obey and comply with the order.

Health education appropriations of gay imagery are of course very specifically focused at a particular (sub)cultural group, but other campaigns similarly target gendered and other ethnic or cultural groups. They demonstrate how health education increasingly operates on the basis of governmentality, deploying carefully delineated elements of a particular population under focus. There is a greatly increased use of consumer 'types' and marketing practices, which have been injected into medical discourses to refine, focus, and be more productive of the active patient. It is thereby assumed that individuals are informed through their subcultural references, not just the health education posters themselves. In so doing, these campaigns also mask the medical message whilst also relying on the 'knowledgeable' person being all too aware of the 'silent' message contained in such a poster! The discursive practice here is intertextuality, where intersecting discourses are used to facilitate the 'message'.

In the 'Safe SM' [sadomasodism] poster (Figure 7.7), the handcuffs signify other restraints which are both the instruments of power, for use to exert or experience consensual submission, and the semiotics of sexual drama.[1]

The handcuffs are part of a lexicon of non-verbal signifiers of modality and sexual behaviours. Whilst the image signifies restraint as holding back, it engages with notions of delay in gratification that are far removed from the purity discourses surrounding images of moral 'clean-ness' and the virtue of celibacy until marriage (e.g. Figure 7.6).

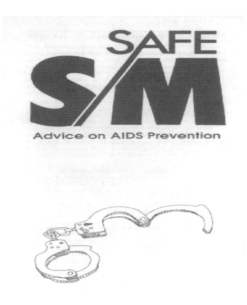

Figure 7.7   'Restraint'

Just from these examples it is clear how the *askësis*, the *Ars Erotica*, is co-existing in the spaces that the clinical gaze seeks to survey. The observation of the body for signs and symptoms of disease is located in discourse where the body is the site of pleasure, the concern is less with the deviance of that behaviour than with the practices of the pleasures. Like the clinical medical samples that reveal the pathology beneath the surface veil of skin, cell or gene, it is now recruiting *difference*, *danger* and *desire* to new atomic levels in the spaces of social intercourse. A paradox here is that communities may feel more *empowered* by the visibility of health material that appropriates such iconographies of sleaze, fantasy and fetishism, but in the process the *gaying* of the message renders it *less* Queer.

Such inversions of the apparent order are of course not universal. It is valuable to take some note of how different cultural formations of health and the sexual are represented, and how they reproduce national and cultural, moral and structural values.

Conclusion

In this chapter the aim has been to show how sexually acquired infections, and particularly syphilis, have been central to wider social discourses surrounding the dangerousness of sex and sexuality, controlling populations of *others*. Similarly, the frenzy of moral panic and concern about the cleanliness of the urban, human spaces echoes the intensifying focus of the clinical gaze and the pervasive surveillance possibilities of the colonisation of sex and the production of scientific sexualities since the early to mid-twentieth century.

There is little doubt that the posters themselves utilised iconography that was easily read by the population. To that extent, they can be seen as successful in terms of reduction in disease rates and the consistency with many social mores of the period. It is important to note here though that extra- or premarital sex and also same-sex encounters happened, but these were invisible in the public literature or the iconography of the campaigns. However, in the post-AIDS environment of the early twenty-first century, there is clearly some shift, in that there is no longer the automatic 'fit' between image and social attitudes, public virtue and private practices. Questions remain about the effectiveness of such campaigns and the role of the images and text in cultures that are saturated in a postmodern Babel of media signs and signifiers. The contemporary resurgence of sexually acquired diseases suggests that the mass education campaigns are no longer appropriate, or are insufficiently nuanced with regard to the potential audiences, or that political will lags behind public practice. In the UK between 2001 and 2002, chlamydia was the most commonly diagnosed STI, and had increased by 14%. Syphilis rose by 67% in males and 33% in females. Overall, cases of gonorrhoea rose by 8% in males and 10% in females. The rise in viral infections was less, with genital herpes up by 1% in males and 4% in females, and genital warts up by 3% in males and 1% in females (Public Health Laboratory Service, 2003).

The processes of locating the body as a site of self-observing pleasure and responsibility were represented through visual imagery. The medico-moral discourses appropriated the iconography both of medical science, such as pathology, and of the construction of the family as a site of moral surveillance and governmentality. By the 1930s, the duties of the STI clinic were clearly defined and marked a paradigmatic statement of the panoptic role of medicine in the mapping of the social and psychological spaces between individuals in the community. Just as psychiatry gained power in relation to the mind and social behaviour, sexual sciences claimed privileged status through the deployment of expert, clinical knowledge to penetrate the sexual practices of populations. In so doing, it emphasised the individual's roles and responsibilities through the changing constructions of sexual citizenship from moral purity to *Ars Erotica*. The visual imagery used in public health campaigns around sexually acquired infections seems to suggest continuing professional and social stigma, low status, and isolated clinical 'otherness'. However, much of the imagery that was appropriated reproduced other, wider social discourses acting on the formation of gender and sexual citizenship. A key example was in the postwar ideological work of the moral (re)construction of the family. This was reflected in the rise of medical triumphalism and therapeutic optimism. It also enmeshed in the creation of beliefs concerning the power of treatment and knowledge, as well as the increasing intervention of the State in reproduction and the control of sexualities.

The iconography of sexual health in public health education campaigns over the last century produce and reproduce social and moral constructions of disease and the erotic, as well as demonstrating the growth of medical surveillance in 'private' spheres of desire. The role of panoptic surveillance is evident now in the way that disease discourses have moved away from control over behaviour reinforced by stigma and social control. In many ways such discourses have revisited notions of 'restraint' and reinterpreted regulation. This is increasingly being marked, in developed countries at least, by reflecting on the increasing withdrawal of the State from the provision of welfare, where the locus of responsibility lies with the individual being 'educated'. Whilst moral panics recur, the images that remain increasingly dominant are drawn from discourses that emphasise negotiation of risk. These neo-liberal consumerist pressures reinforce the message that the individual must engage in educated calculations that direct and control his or her sexual health responsibilities. In westernised cultures that continuously celebrate the body through visual imagery and media, the 'ethical' element is the condition of being informed in the practice of erotic pleasure(s) rather than moral restraint.

NOTE

1. This is explored in more detail in Coxon (1996, pp. 118ff.).

REFERENCES

Armstrong, D., *Political Anatomy of the Body: Medical Knowledge in Britain in the Twentieth Century* (Cambridge: Cambridge University Press, 1983a).

Armstrong, D., 'Public Health Spaces and the Fabrication of Identity', *Sociology*, 27:3 (1983b), pp. 393–410.

Bloor, M., *The Sociology of HIV Transmission* (London: Sage, 1995).

Bristow, J., *Sexuality* (London: Routledge, 1997).

Castel, L., 'From Dangerousness to Risk', in G. Burchell, C. Gordon and P. Miller (eds), *The Foucault Effect: Studies in Governmentality* (Hemel Hempstead: Harvester Wheatsheaf, 1991).

Coxon, A. P. M., *Between the Sheets* (London: Cassell, 1996).

Davenport-Hines, R., *Sex, Death and Punishment* (London: Collins, 1990).

Douglas, M., *Purity and Danger* (London: Routledge & Kegan Paul, 1966).

Felstein, I., *Sexual Pollution* (Newton Abbot: David & Charles, 1974).

Foucault, M., *The History of Sexuality*, vol. 1 (London: Penguin, 1978).

Foucault, M., *Foucault Live (Interviews, 1966–84)* (New York: Semiotext, Columbia University, 1989).

Gilman, S. L., *Disease and Representation: Images of Illness from Madness to AIDS* (Ithaca, NY: Cornell University Press, 1988a).

Gilman, S. L., 'AIDS and Syphilis: the Iconography of Disease', in D. Crimp (ed.), *AIDS: Cultural Analysis, Cultural Action* (Cambridge, MA: MIT Press, 1988b).

Gilman, S. L., *Sexuality: An Illustrated History* (New York: John Wiley, 1989).

Hall, L. A., '"War always brings it on": War, STDs, the Military, and the Civil Population in Britain, 1850–1950'. Paper presented at 'Comparative Perspectives on the History of Sexually Transmitted Diseases', 6–9 April 1996, University of London (1996).

Hawkes, G., *A Sociology of Sex and Sexuality* (Milton Keynes: Open University Press, 1996).

Henriot, C., 'STDs and Prostitution in Colonial Shanghai'. Paper presented at 'Comparative Perspectives on the History of Sexually Transmitted Diseases', 6–9 April 1996, University of London (1996).

Hicks, D., 'A Brief History of STDs', *British Journal of Sexual Medicine*, July/August (1994), pp. 32–3.

Higgs, P., 'Risk, Governmentality and the Reconceptualisation of Citizenship', in G. Scambler and P. Higgs (eds), *Modernity, Medicine and Health* (London: Routledge, 1998).

Jackson, S., 'Heterosexuality and Feminist Theory', in D. Richardson (ed.), *Theorising Heterosexuality* (Buckingham: Open University Press, 1996).

Jochelson, K., 'Healthy Tribes and Corrupting Cities: Racism and Medical Discourse in South Africa, 1880–1950'. Paper presented at 'Comparative Perspectives on the History of Sexually Transmitted Diseases', 6–9 April 1996, University of London (1996).

Lupton, D., 'Foucault and the Medicalisation Critique', in A. Petersen and R. Bunton (eds), *Foucault: Health and Medicine* (London: Routledge, 1997).

Mort, F., *Dangerous Sexualities: Medico-moral Politics in England since 1830* (London: Routledge & Kegan Paul, 1987).

Murrey, P. and Murrey, L., *Dictionary of Art and Artists* (London: Penguin, 1989).

Petersen, A. and Bunton, R. (eds), *Foucault: Health and Medicine* (London: Routledge, 1997).

Peterson, A., *Unmasking the Masculine: 'Men' and 'Identity' in a Sceptical Age* (London: Routledge, 1998).

Porter, R. and Hall, L., *The Facts of Life* (London: Yale University Press, 1995).

Public Health Laboratory Service, 'Sexually Transmitted Infections' – Press release (2003) www.hpa.org.uk/news/030703_sti.htm

Quétel, C., *History of Syphilis* (Cambridge: Polity Press, 1990).

Richardson, D. (ed.), *Theorising Heterosexuality* (Buckingham: Open University Press, 1996).

Rose, N., 'Medicine, History and the Present', in C. Jones and R. Porter (eds), *Re-assessing Foucault* (London: Routledge, 1994).

Sontag, S., *AIDS and its Metaphors* (London: Penguin, 1989).

Spongberg, M., 'Written on the Body: the Congenital Syphilitic as Moral Degenerate'. Paper presented at 'Comparative Perspectives on the History of Sexually Transmitted Diseases', 6–9 April 1996, University of London (1996).

Stanley, L., *Sex Surveyed 1949–1994* (London: Taylor & Francis, 1995).

Turner, B. S., *The Body and Society* (Oxford: Basil Blackwell, 1984).

Slicing Through Healthy Bodies: Transsexuality and the Media Representation of Body Modification

8

Katherine Watson and Stephen Whittle

Introduction

Going to extremes

In February 2001, Dr Robert Smith of the Falkirk and District Royal Infirmary in Scotland removed healthy legs from two men, one a UK citizen, the other from Germany. Both men paid around £3,500 for the amputation of perfectly healthy limbs. Both patients had been diagnosed as suffering from a psychological condition termed 'apotemnophilia'. Generally, sufferers of apotemnophilia cannot achieve sexual pleasure without fantasising about becoming amputees, or by becoming amputees. Many will seek medical intervention to remove a limb, and some, without intervention, will go to extremes, removing the limb for themselves by means such as shooting or lying down on railways to have a passing train remove it. The disorder is seen medically as a severe form of Body Dysmorphic Disorder, which takes the normal tendency to compare oneself with others in appearance to an obsessive level.

The media response to these surgical procedures was the raising of a 'public' outcry, not just in the UK but worldwide. The view that the operations were ethically wrong and that 'this was not real medicine' prevailed. Interestingly, although the procedures could have been compared with many other types of elective surgery, what was chosen for comparison by almost all media coverage was gender reassignment procedures, the 'sex change'. One article regularly quoted was that of Paul McHugh, who in 1992 had said when writing about gender reassignment treatment: 'We don't do liposuction on anorexics. Why amputate the genitals of these poor men? Surely the fault is in the mind, not the member' (Leo, 2001). Earlier, in 1979, McHugh, a doctor, had been instrumental in closing the USA's first major gender reassignment programme at Johns Hopkins Hospital in Baltimore. Since that time gender reassignment clinics have faced an uphill battle in the medical, and media, worlds to regain their reputations as the centres of medical excellence that many of them are.

This chapter analyses the media construction of transsexuality (popularised as 'sex change') in the UK newsprint media and offers some critical thoughts regarding the effects of such constructions. Whilst much work is being done in the fields of cultural studies and sociology to deconstruct psycho-medical constructions of sexuality and indeed to challenge dichotomous ideas of sex/gender, transsexuality is still being constructed as an 'inauthentic' alternative to the binary representations of 'man' and 'woman'. We have used critical discourse analysis (CDA), therefore, in order to unpick some of the devices used by journalists in both constituting as well as reflecting popular ideas about the 'authentic' body in relation to sex and gender.

Background

Since the story of Christine Jorgenson headlined the New York papers in 1952, transsexual people have lurked on the edge of public imagination in a myth that goes something like this: Due to a mistake in nature or biology, a woman is born trapped in a man's body. After years of denial and mental torture, he has a sex change operation and goes on to live life as a traditional heterosexual woman, revealing her past only as the result of a medical emergency or as a guest on some prurient chat show. But in 2004, that scenario is outdated, if not obsolete. 'Gender identity disorder', as defined in medical diagnostic manuals, is characterised by a 'persistent discomfort about one's assigned sex'. It's aetiology is unknown, and there is no known cure, in that the only successful treatment (Pfafflin and Junge, 1998) appears to be for the sufferer to undergo gender reassignment, including life-long hormone therapy and surgical procedures to make the body resemble more that of the opposite natal sex.

The international guidelines on the treatment of transsexual people require that hormonal or surgical gender reassignment is not made 'on demand' (HBIGDA 2001), and that a period of assessment and psychotherapy should be undergone before hormone treatment is provided. Before any referral for surgical intervention there should then be a further period in which the patient lives for 12 months in the chosen gender role (the real-life test). Similarly, the requests of Smith's patients with apotemnophilia were not met 'on demand'. Before the operations two psychiatrists and a psychologist had assessed both patients, and the surgeon consulted the hospital's medical director and then further obtained written permission from the facility's chief executive (Cue and Benkoil, 2001).

Many surgical procedures are concerned with improving mental well-being; sometimes this may be the side-effect of an operation but it can also be the primary purpose. However, regardless of the benefits of gender reassignment surgery (currently viewed as 96–8% successful in achieving enhanced social well-being), the media attack on transsexual people has continued unabated throughout the history of the treatment. As long ago as 1929, the father of gender reassignment treatment Magnus Hirschfeld was vilified in the Nazi press as the 'Apostle of Indeceny' (in *Der Stürmer*, July 1929, p. 1), a charge that was to result in his becoming exiled after being attacked several times in the street. Since then hundreds of pages of newsprint, legal documentation, academic articles, and textbooks have been published each year around the transsexual phenomenon, many of them derogatory.

'Trans' has become a particular cultural obsession in recent years. Television, film and the news media all seek out new angles and storylines that include people who have 'changed sex'. In our daily lives, we cannot escape being reminded that many people in our society have now undergone this drastic life-changing process. Popular images include 'Hayley' on *Coronation Street* (see Figure 8.2) and 'Dil' in Neil Jordan's successful film *The Crying Game*. And of course the true-life transsexual woman Dana International won the Eurovision Song Contest for Israel in 1998 (see Figure 8.1). Interestingly, more members of the UK population watched the 'marriage' of *Coronation Street's* transsexual character 'Hayley' to Roy Cropper than watched the Royal Wedding two months later of Prince Edward and Sophie Rhys Jones (16.4 million people watched *Coronation Street* on the night of Hayley's wedding as compared with 14.3 million people who watched the Royal Wedding [figures from Broadcasting Audience Research Board]).

Yet, few media representations of trans people are positive. The overriding images still come from *Jerry Springer* and the Sunday tabloids. Transsexual people are portrayed as fraudulent deceivers. The classic example is the 1997 Sauza Tequila advert that featured a picture of the transsexual woman

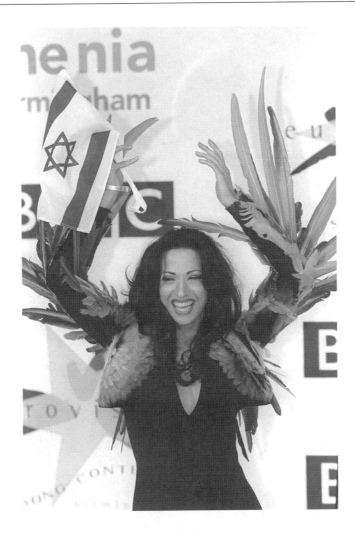

Figure 8.1   Dana International: this and Figure 8.2 are popular images of transsexuals in contemporary media

and model Tula (Caroline Cossey). Under the picture of Tula is the moto 'Life is Harsh: Your Tequila Shouldn't Be', and across her breasts is written 'She's a He'. Similarly in 1997, Holiday Inn's Super Bowl commercial featured a sexy, post-op transsexual at her high school reunion, who is recognised with staggering shock and horror by a former classmate. This

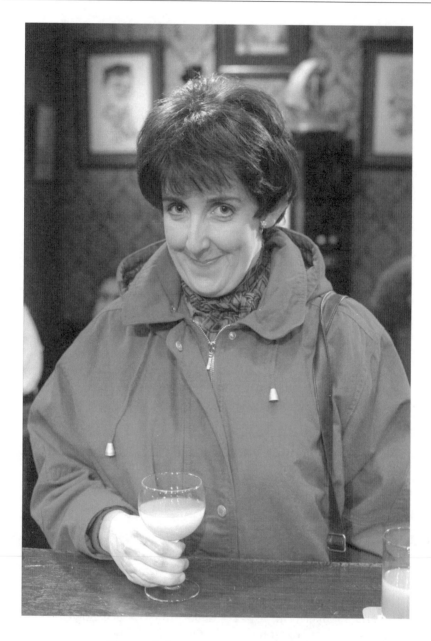

Figure 8.2 Hayley from *Coronation Street*

hugely unoriginal 'joke' has been repeated endlessly since then in all types of advertising medium. In 2001:

> 24 transgender-themed television and print ads [were] counted worldwide this year, an all-time high, up from 11 such ads found for 2000 and 1999. But very few come off positively for the transgendered.   (Wilke, 2001, p. 52)

According to Gwen Smith:

> The media is rife with themes of transgendered people being out to deceive others. It happens nearly every day on Jerry Springer or Maury Povitch. Movies such as 'Some Like It Hot', 'Tootsie', 'Mrs Doubtfire', 'One of the Boys', 'The Birdcage' and the recently-released 'Sorority Boys' thrive on the deception angle. In fact, I would dare say that there is no single idea equated more with transgender media representations than that of deception.   (Smith, 2002)

Yet this is not the only representation. Transgender and transsexual people apparently 'choose to change sex' even though all trans people deny that repeatedly. Sometimes they are simply portrayed as unwelcome additions to life, one advertisement which listed 'Life's Nasty Surprises' included 'transsexuals' alongside spiders in your soup and snakes in your bed. Vivien Namaste (2000) has criticised representations of transsexual people, even by transsexual people themselves, as limiting, offensive, and unrealistic.

The study

We have chosen for this particular study to analyse the discourse of transsexuality or 'sex change' in the UK newsprint media in order to illustrate some of the underlying normative notions of gender and sex that inform journalists' narratives and which are used as a springboard to constitute a 'trans' identity as 'undeserving'. These narratives, however, are often complex, interweaving a number of diverse ideologies in a way that could be termed 'polydiscursive' (Fairclough, 1995). By this, we mean not only that narratives of transsexuality in the newsprint media draw on normative notions of sex and gender (and the sorts of authentic relationships assigned to these constructions), but that these are framed within broader debates such as the state of the NHS and the debate about funding. Clearly then, newsprint narratives of transsexuality are not unchanging entities, but 'shape shift' and change tone according to the specific concerns at any given time. 'Trans' narratives in the newsprint media are always layered and require some 'peeling away' to understand the discourses that operate to sustain their constitution as 'newsworthy' stories.

There is a long history in cultural and media studies of newsprint analysis (Gamson and Modigliani, 1989; Hartley, 1982), which has helped us understand 'News' as a form of storytelling shaped by the conventions of 'narrative' (beginnings, middles, ends, plot, scene and characters, etc.). As Potter (1998, p. 112) states: 'news is not something that happens; instead news is what gets presented'. Moreover, whilst there are complex debates about audience readings of texts (see the introduction to Part I of this text), many theorists have analysed news texts particularly in relation to how those constructing the stories offer a particular 'version' of a narrative: 'By (re)producing symbols familiar to their audience, reporters and editors proclaim the "preferred reading" of a text' (Tuchman, 1991, p. 90). In this study therefore, we aim to utilise a critical discourse analytic approach to analyse the texts (outlined below), and then to situate the emerging themes within a broader discussion of 'moral panic', assessing whether transsexuality can be constituted as an example of moral panic, and if not, which elements disqualify it from this category of analysis.

Method

In order to analyse a 'representative' sample of reporting on transsexuality in the British newsprint media, we conducted a search using a library facility, 'Custom Newspapers' (*Mirror, Guardian, The Times, Independent*) and library CD ROM (*Daily Mail, Mail on Sunday, Telegraph*). The search was limited to the period between 1995 and 2003, and the key words 'transsexuality' and 'sex-change' were used to refine the area. A total of 52 articles were chosen for analysis, representing a variety of formats ranging from reports of legal 'gains', human interest stories, editorials, articles focusing on a central narrative of NHS funding and delivery, and stories that highlighted issues of community (living/workplace, etc.). There were a disproportionate amount of articles attributed to certain newspapers (the *Daily Mail*, for example, totalled over 20 articles), which perhaps reflects the volume of coverage per paper, but only a selection of all the articles that have been published were used, because of repeat stories or similarity of themes.

The articles were then analysed using critical discourse analysis (CDA), the underlying principle of which, understands language as a form of social practice (i.e. performs actions) and that language both socially shapes (i.e. it is constitutive of) discourse, and is socially shaped by popular ideologies (Fairclough, 1995; Wodak, 1996). CDA therefore analyses the relationship between these two elements in relation to how 'the world' (events, relationships) are represented and what identities are set up between, and for, those involved in any given story. In this respect, CDA is particularly interested in the effects of power and how language can be ideological (Titscher et al., 2002).

Practically, then, CDA examines the language used in texts in order to illustrate how it connotes or conveys meaning, linking this to a broader analysis of ideologies and discourses that may be neutralised in social and cultural practice and belief. For instance, certain devices and terms are frequently used as shorthand, in order to convey a particular 'reading' of an identity (for example, 'traffickers', 'pushers' etc. connote a particular position in relation to how we should 'read' the identity of 'drug-dealer'). This sort of technique, it is argued (Fairclough, 1995), such as using colloquial language, has ideational and interpersonal functions in that it draws on particular representations of the social reality in question as well as claiming co-membership with the audience.

Transsexual people as 'undeserving'

One overriding theme that emerged from the analysis of the articles was that of transsexual people as undeserving, underpinned by a general narrative that assumes the surgery associated with transsexuality (the 'sex change') to be implicitly (and as a matter of common-sense) 'unnecessary'. This returns us to the title of this chapter, 'Slicing Through Healthy Bodies', where the transsexual person is modifying a perfectly 'healthy' body in order to create an inauthentic parody of the 'opposite sex'. This overriding theme, however, does have a number of complex sub-sections that need unpacking in order to illustrate the underlying discourse/ideologies at work.

Deserving/underserving no. 1: Pantomime dames

Transsexual people are positioned in the vast majority of articles as undeserving, because of their 'gender deviance'. Drawing on the ideology of the 'two-sex model' (i.e. only recognising the categories 'men' and 'women', and specifically, in relation to genitalia), the articles emphasised the transgression of transsexuality. This was actualised through a variety of narrative devices.

(a) Occupation

In the majority of articles, transsexual occupation was headlined (or mentioned, for no particular reason as a descriptor) in order to reinforce the extremes of the gender polarity. Very rarely were transsexual people reported as being in non-gender specific jobs, but instead the occupations followed a highly gendered narrative: RAF pilots, bus drivers, truck drivers and merchant seamen were consistently used as 'previous' job descriptors. Tag lines such as 'How an army colonel became a prima ballerina' (*Mirror*, 19 May 2001) and, in another article, a description of a 'former' mechanic who 'wore a blonde wig and stockings under his mechanics overalls' (*Daily Telegraph*, Oct. 2000), juxtapose the extremes of gender identification, with a class narrative also reinforcing the 'maleness' of certain (working-class) occupations (the latter also denoting a 'pantomime' theme worthy of a 'Carry On' film, an issue we will return to later). In that there was no 'information gain' to reporting such former occupations, clearly this was a device used to position transsexuality at the *extremes* of the gender continuum, assigning a former highly stereotyped identity that would very rarely be recognised by members of the trans community.

(b) Transsexual people as 'ridiculous'

Linked to the above, the positioning of transsexual people as 'ridiculous', is a theme that runs throughout the stories underlining the difference between 'the real thing' and the inauthentic body and performance of the transsexual person. In many ways, the 'character' of the transsexual person is positioned as 'ridiculous' by virtue of the attempt to 'mimic' women. In more than a few articles, m–f transsexual people were said to now enjoy 'knitting', 'crocheting' and 'sewing', in stark contrast to their previous 'high flying' or 'manly' occupations. Interestingly, in none of the articles we analysed did f–m transsexual people appear, which illustrates the media's co-option of the narrative of the 'pantomime dame' in their construction of transsexual identity (and the British obsession with the comedic elements of cross-dressing). In one story, for example, the two 'burly male' transsexuals are to be read as unaware of how ridiculous they (clearly) looked as they stood 'proudly in skirts and silk scarves' (*Independent*, 22, Feb. 1997).

Other devices infantilise and ridicule the personae of the transsexual person. In many articles, m–f transsexual people were given the pre-fix 'Miss' (regardless of their marital status) to reinforce, through the utilisation of the authentic gender narrative, the ridiculous attempted parody of the transsexual person. In one article: 'Miss Goodwin, who left court with two of the four children she fathered in a relationship before her operation, said she was euphoric at the decision' (*Independent*, 12 July 2002). The technique of inserting information that leads to an effect is a popular one. In the above example, the information about 'Miss Goodwin's' four children is strategically positioned to produce a reading (the reading may of course be an oppositional one but we are invited to 'read' all the same). A very different reading would have been invited had Christine Goodwin been [simply] euphoric at the decision, and supported by her children as she left court.

Another thread of this issue is the suspicion narrative, which suspects that transsexuality is an impossibility. As Fairclough (1995) has pointed out before, journalists utilise a stock of language to question the truthfulness of what is being said: such as 'so-and-so *claimed* . . .' instead of 'so-and-so said'. Throughout our analysis we found many examples of transsexual people being not only disbelieved, but infantilised by the narrative. In one article, 'Sex-change teenager "Having a Baby"' (*Daily Mail*, 5 Oct. 1996), the columnist Charles Ferro states:

> A teenager who was brought up as a boy is to have a baby *it is claimed.* . . .
> Bo Christiansen, 18, *apparently* born hermaphrodite . . . last week married the man *she says* is the child's father.   [my emphasis]

In this example then, the hermaphroditism of the main character is viewed with suspicion because she was 'brought up as a boy'. Again, the 'transsexual' person is positioned as a fantasist and liar. Christiansen is a teenage mother, which adds another layer to the narrative (i.e. tapping into moral concerns about teenage pregnancy) and produces yet another effect.

This can be seen in other articles. For example, a convicted arsonist at Ashworth, '*claims* that the hospital authorities are infringing his human rights by stopping him wearing women's clothes and make-up outside his room'. In this story, clearly overlayed with the deserving/undeserving debate (an arsonist should not have special rights, particularly at any expense to the taxpayer), the main character is infantilised by the text:

> *He is allowed* to wear women's underwear in his room and to have his ears pierced and hair dyed, but *he has been stopped* from dressing as a woman elsewhere in the hospital. (*Daily Telegraph*, 4 Dec. 2001; my emphasis)

(c) *Failure of the heteronormative dream*

A further way in which transsexuality is written as transgressing gender is through the implicit (and explicit) effect on 'normal' (i.e. heterosexual) 'family' (i.e. wife and children) life. An interesting technique that is frequently used in this respect, is the voice of the wife of the transsexual person. In many of the articles, the wives are constructed as 'bereaved' and the children as innocents suffering at the hands of a gender-confused 'father'. The m–f transsexual person is, in most of these accounts, to be 'read' as male, owing to the inauthenticity of the female 'performance', thus reinforcing the 'crimes' against wife and children due to the unnecessary and selfish indulgence of a 'fantasy'.

This heteronormativity is often reinforced in terms of occupational and economic 'losses' for the wife. For example, in an article in the *Mirror on Sunday* (14 Jan. 2001), the wife of a transsexual person originally 'chose common-sense over hedonism and traded independence for a family' when she first married her husband, because 'after all, his career was soaring and he was regarded by a succession of employers as a superstar'; thus 'Harmanna's strategy appeared to have paid off.' According to the article, however, since her husband's disclosure, 'Harmanna faces the uncertain future she so dreaded.... She has her two sons, no money, and may soon have no home.'

Underpinning this narrative is an explicit reference to the gendering of capital. The husband's career is constructed normatively, whereas the wife's potential career is constructed as 'hedonist independence' set against a 'common-sense family' choice. When 'husband' becomes woman, she is assumed to lose both economic and cultural capital in the form of job and family.

It is no surprise that the newsprint media present transsexuality in these ways when we consider the impact of psychological discourses of sex, gender and sexuality. As Hird states, the discipline of psychology 'remains wedded to sex and gender as coherent, stable and "real" concepts' (2002, p. 578). Moreover,

> The notion of authenticity rests upon three inter-related assumptions: that sex and gender exist; that sex and gender constitute measurable traits; and that the 'normal' population adheres to the first two assumptions. (Hird, 2002, p. 581)

Transsexual people have, by virtue of their deviation from the two-sex model (or their perceived imitation of it), been confirmed as the pathological narcissists that psychological discourses have always believed them to be (Lothstein, 1988; Socarides, 1970).

Deserving/undeserving no. 2: The deviant deviants

Interestingly, another layer of this theme positions some transsexual people as *more* underserving than others. In a few articles, transsexual people are positioned as deserving according to their perceived contribution to society ('Lynda Cash, 49, was leading medical assistant Brian Waling when she was forced to leave the Navy after 15 years service, which included serving alongside the Duke of York in the Falklands' [*Daily Telegraph*, 25 Aug. 1999]); or if the 'contribution to society' issue is combined with acknowledgement of self-funding

('Flt Lt Eric Cookson, 39, paid for the operation in May and became Caroline Paige' [*Daily Telegraph*, 14 Aug. 2001]). In this last article, however, the cost of the operation (£18,000) is set against the cost to train her (£750,000) and her annual salary (£45,000), in a complex interweave of positions that balances an acknowledgement of individual responsibility and not wasting training resources already paid, but with an eye on the (perhaps undeserved) training in the first place, the annual wage and the (relatively) low cost of the operation.

However, the vast majority of articles focused on the negative 'hooks' to further discredit the authenticity of the transsexual identity. In journalistic terms, the added element of criminal outrage provides the sort of story that makes headline news. In these narratives, economic or criminal deviance is used as a hook to further highlight the atrociousness of the already undeserving transsexual person (as a gender/sex deviant).

(a) *Economic*

Economics plays a vital role in the discrediting of the transgender identity (as unnecessary 'mutilation' of perfectly healthy bodies), and here, occupations are linked with the already devious and deviant characterisation of the transsexual person. In a number of articles, transsexual lawyers and solicitors (and we are being invited to regard with suspicion these 'grabby' professions) 'swindle' and 'embezzle' their way onto the pages with headlines such as:

The swindlers secret: Solicitor fleeced his clients to raise cash for a sex change (*Daily Mail*, 28 April 1998)

Sex Change Lawyer Fails to Pay Off Debt (*Daily Mail*, 8 Aug. 1998)

When I Saw my Husband Dressed as a Woman, It was More of a Shock Than His £220 Million Fraud (*Mirror on Sunday*, 4 Jan. 2001)

In these stories, the main character is demonised in very familiar journalistic ways. In the first article, for example, the solicitor 'stole thousands of pounds to pay for a sex-change operation, using the identities of *dead children* to *launder the cash*' (my emphasis). Later the article states: 'The court heard that when police searched Challenor's home in Chichester...they found a collection of hardcore pornographic films. They also discovered birth certificates in the names of dead children', and again, towards the end, 'Glyn and Jean Jones, whose son Stephen suffered from cerebral palsy and died aged two in 1969, said they were "disgusted" at the way Challenor had "abused" their boy's memory by using his name' (my emphasis). It would seem no surprise that the *Daily Mail* is inviting its readers to make a connection between pathological transsexuality, the evil launderer of cash, and the paedophile, in a text that introduces elements of pornography, dead children and abuse in quick succession. As Critcher (2003) states, with reference to the moral panic incited by paedophilia narratives:

> [The case studies] had a single common denominator: the presence and agency of the *Daily Mail*. In Britain during the 1980s and 1990s, no other individual organisation or group has had such a profound effect on the development of moral panics. (Critcher, 2003, p. 142)

(b) *Criminal*

Perhaps some of the most interesting characterisations of the undeserving transsexual person, however, are offered in the 'sex-swap' criminal narratives that appear with unnerving frequency. Arsonists (*Daily Telegraph*, 2001), thieves (*Mirror on Sunday*, 2001), gunmen (*Daily Telegraph*, 2000), paedophiles (*Mirror*, 2000) and psychopaths (*Daily Mail*, 2001) join the role of players acting out the transsexual person's performance. Two of these articles provide a good example of some of the journalistic devices (saturated in 'popular' criminal discourse) used to guide the reading. The first, in the *Daily Telegraph* – 'Anger at NHS sex change for jailed gunman' (David Sapsted, 20 Oct. 2000), is particularly rich in discursive techniques, reflected in the narrative 'morphology' (shape); the characterisation of different identities and the reference to popular ideologies. The story moves through a variety of emphases that catalogue procedures listed as at the taxpayer's expense (including not only the 'at-the-drop-of-a-hat sex-change' operation itself but electrolysis, hormone drugs, etc.) and foregrounds a narrative that invites the audience to feel berated for allowing such a situation to occur: a representative of the Victims of Crime Trust, for example, is quoted as saying 'This country should hang its head in shame at some of the outrageous decisions like this one,' occupying a 'modal' role 'to mitigate and disclaim responsibility for a damning judgement by attributing it to unspecified others' (Fairclough, 1995, p. 5). In the last paragraph, this sorry situation is underlined by a particularly emotive reference to the crime originally committed:

> David Halberg, the postmaster, was cradling his eight-month-old son Jonathan when Cross blasted a security screen, peppering him with pellets and debris.

In another example of the use of 'innocent childhood' (see Clive Seale's chapter elsewhere in this volume), coupled with maternal references ('cradled') and 'war-like' language ('blasted'; 'peppering him with pellets and debris'), the deviance of the perpetrator is thoroughly underlined.

Similarly, an article in the *Daily Mail* titled 'Frocky Horror Show' (20 February 2000) tells the story of two 'notorious paedophiles' who had been given sewing machines in jail in order to make women's clothes. The article states that '[F]or the last year, HIV-infected Smith has said he wants to be a woman, claiming his "confused sexuality" had made him a sex offender.' An amalgam of deviant identities (paedophile; 'HIV-infected'; transsexual) come together, therefore, to push Smith to the far reaches of the undeserving spectrum.

The underlying discourse in all of these narratives focuses on the cost of this unnecessary, narcissistic and pathological obsession with wanting to be the 'opposite sex'. It is to this theme that we will now turn.

Deserving/undeserving no. 3: the cost to society

(a) *Characterisation of transsexual people*

A large number of articles, particularly relating to the legal gains of transsexual people, positioned them as money-grabbing zealots, savvy to the law and always looking for a chance to sue. Transsexual people, therefore, are seen as cold and manipulative; queue-jumpers and 'freeloaders' of the state and the NHS.

In an article from the *Daily Mail* ('Sex-swap teacher buys a Merc with her sacking payout', *Daily Mail*, 28 Sept. 2001), a woman who had received £3,780 compensation for sexual discrimination (having lost her job for fear of pupils' concentration being affected) is positioned as the undeserving squanderer of the school and council's (and by referent, taxpayers') money, which, moreover, had been awarded erroneously ('A transsexual teacher *who claimed* she was sacked because of her sex change' [my emphasis]). Numerous other articles refer to transsexual people suing companies, the prison service and the state. The implication of these 'charges' draws on a broader narrative that implicitly criticises the 'Americanisation' of social practice, designating the transsexual character as someone who flouts British liberalism and instead seeks monetary reward from agencies ill-able to afford these outrageous demands.

(b) *Footing the bill*

It is no surprise, then, that one of the most frequent positions taken by journalists in relation to transsexuality is as a taxpayer in a country where the underfunded NHS is suffering because of the demands of undeserving operations. The NHS is frequently anthropomorphised in these accounts; a philanthropic and coherent organisation, positioned outside of the decisions made by different authorities and in 'symbolic', philosophical opposition to them. In an article by Richard Littlejohn of the *Daily Mail* entitled 'Why the NHS is Bleeding to Death', the author clearly illustrates this positioning:

> The 'routine' operations being rationed by Berkshire Health Commission also include sex-change therapy, stomach tucks, breast enlargement, liposuction and tattoo removal. We are entitled to ask why on earth such treatments are being provided by the taxpayer in the first place. Are they what the founding fathers of the NHS had in mind? (*Daily Mail*, 1 Sept. 1995)

Frequently used terms such as 'footing the bill', 'on the NHS', making 'taxpayers bear the cost' neatly simplify complex decision-making processes and legal interventions to construct the audience as direct losers.

(c) *Upward comparisons and priorities*

A further device used to fuel the economic debate is that of priorities, often illustrated by *ad hoc* comparisons. In an article from 1997, for example, entitled 'Sex-swap charity is a lottery winner' (*Daily Mail*, 14 Jan. 1997), deserving charities are listed as war veterans, heart attack and stroke victims, and the Samaritans. Whilst a substantial amount of information is given about the Samaritans (how much it costs to run; how many calls it receives, etc.), no information is given about the function of the Gender Trust, and the article goes on to say:

> A further £184,929 is going to the National AIDS Trust bringing the amount of lottery cash handed over to the AIDS and HIV groups to £5.5 million: in comparison, the Burma Star Association will receive £83,454 – around £17,000 less than it wanted – to help its 18,000 war veterans. (*Daily Mail*, 14 Jan. 1997)

'Sex-change' operations, in terms of NHS priorities, are frequently subject to comparisons with therapeutic interventions such as hip replacement and drugs for MS sufferers, and instead categorised with other 'non-essential' surgery. In many of these articles, the role of players expands to include 'outraged' voices from representatives from the disadvantaged groups (pensioners, MS sufferers, etc.), health authorities, wives and politicians, who function as a 'moral barricade' (Cohen, 1972). Quite often, European law and its arbiters (judges) are set in opposition to the equally anthropomorphised health authorities, who are often 'disappointed' with the decision to allow sex reassignment to go ahead.

Discussion

Throughout all of these themes then, a recurring narrative of transsexual people as undeserving of recognition (therapeutically, socially, legally and financially) emerges as a strong unifying characteristic. The newsprint media have utilised a variety of devices to convey complexly layered accounts of the transsexual person as a manipulative impostor. When setting this analysis within the framework of 'moral panic' (see Cohen, 1972; Critcher, 2003), it is possible to see how elements of the panic model function here. For example, the techniques of exaggeration and distortion are frequently used by journalists attempting to assess the extent and cost of transsexuality (numbers vary wildly on this). Phrases such as 'opening the floodgates' and 'a number of cases are understood to be pending' are frequently employed to distort the facts and imply that the enormous numbers of transsexual people could become a viable threat to Britain's economy. Experts are wheeled in to pronounce on the pathology of transsexual people and a 'moral barricade' is provided to reinforce the transgressiveness of transsexual people. There has even been an attempt in some quarters of the newsprint media, to introduce the notion of transsexual 'sects' (see, for example, *Sunday Times*, 31 May 1998, 'Secret sect of transsexual priests shakes church'), another 'moral panic' device used to galvanise public outcry.

Ultimately, however, transsexuality evades the category of 'moral panic' primarily because it is still constructed as individual pathology and individual mutilation based on choice (similar to the 'reading' of smoking prior to the Registrar General's report on passive smoking [Brandt and Rozin 1997]) and whilst the newsprint media have attempted to construe transsexual people as a threat to the taxpayer and to heteronormative society, the overall legacy is one of moral outrage rather than moral panic. Transsexual people do not occupy the same place as other 'folk devils' (Cohen, 1972) such as people living with HIV or paedophiles, primarily because whilst the former can threaten our lives and families, the sex/gender system is so undisputed that transsexual people remain a distant and often comedic parody.

What seems to emerge from this analysis, and in conjunction with recent theorising in the field of sex and gender, is the fundamental stability of the binary sex/gender system, rendering any other performative expressions redundant. Alternative ideas about the sex/gender performative (Butler, 1990; 1993; Hird, 2002) have yet to be acknowledged in popular discourse, as Hird states:

Within our current discursive field, to exist at all means being a woman or a man; 'sex is the norm by which the "one" becomes viable at all' (Butler, 1993, p. 2). This explains in part, why individuals continue to demand sex-reassignment surgery, despite the fact that sex and gender are primarily observed and judged 'by various visual and vocal signals such as hair, clothes, body shape, and movement, gestures and facial expressions, voice and speech' rather than by the appearance of the genitals (Woodhouse, in MacKenzie, 1994). (Hird, 2002, p. 589)

Conclusion

We can start from a basic premise that surgical interventions will often improve psychological well-being, and in many non-emergency surgical procedures these are seen as positive and welcome outcomes. Further, if we step away from the idea that body 'normalising' should be the sole purpose of surgical intervention, there are some surgical procedures in which psychological health is the sole outcome, and many of these procedures are legal within health care systems. In fact, if it was suggested that the only purpose of any surgical intervention was to be the achievement of some sort of 'normalised' body, in most cases there would be outrage. However, even that is not that simple. The form the normalised body takes does not stand alone, but is mediated constantly through the media. The normalised body is not normal, it is the body beautiful and not the body natural, and beauty is a transient social, cultural concept that targets our pockets and our excess income, rather than our mental or physical health.

Body modification is, for most people, about free expression. In some cases (those of transsexual people and those who are apotemnophiliac) it is about core expression of the self, which justifies surgical intervention as part of the whole health package which modern western medicine promises. Yet it is clear that the media have obtained a victim they can target. We could think about this in terms of the puritan reaction to sex and about sexual pleasure, yet the very fact that most body-modification practices will also include aspects of self in the pursuit of sexual pleasure, and they are not targeted, means it is about something more. It is about difference and, just like racism, it is about providing a scapegoat for the 'public' to feed upon when they wish to attack health care policies (Ahmad, 1993). The scapegoat has to be an easy target, and what better than those who are clearly a very small group in society. The problem is that then this small group can easily be refused access to treatment in order to appease the 'public'.

Body modification is part and parcel of the consumption of difference, and queer difference – though it can be aspirational in providing new desires and enhancing consumerism and the capitalist process (Whittle, 1994) – unsettles boundaries. Transgender/transsexual difference unsettles the boundaries by which one 'becomes viable at all'.

Analysing the gender system is difficult because we have nothing to compare it with, no non-gender system, nor any multi-gender system. It is so embedded in our psyche, and so wedded to the binary sex model, that alternatives cannot be envisaged because we cannot envisage men without penises and women without vaginas (Nestle, Howell and Wilchins, 2002). Trans people, whether transgender or transsexual, provide that alternative, but it has to become marginal to ensure that we are not tempted to think of other gender systems.

Transsexual people do not fill that role of the scapegoat well as we have seen. Instead, they become the pantomime dame. Being the dame they are simply parts of our theatrical imagination, not real people as such. Accordingly, why is the nation state (and, in particular, the health service) spending money on them, when after all they are simply performing their sickness? What does that imply for their access to gender reassignment health care practices, and why when, considering the original question, are they painted on the same canvas as the apotemnophiliac? The performance by transsexual people of their own, and our, imaginary genders is not far removed from Raymond's early feminist thesis (1980) in which: 'Transsexualism is a very mythic phenomenon, unfolding a world view of patriarchy that explains its origins, beliefs and practices' (Raymond, 1980, p. xx). The idea that someone can live a life within the imagination takes on the gender roles of the good woman and the good man.

Queer theory takes a position in which there is no gender identity, simply performance of gender, which in and of itself becomes gender (Butler, 1993). As such, dissident genders are not of themselves subversive but recreate norms through the repetition of them. Accordingly, the role of the transsexual person becomes a sounding board through which the news media can reinforce normative roles of good men and women, by highlighting the ways in which, if they let their gender imagination run wild, they would also become 'manipulative imposters', undeserving scroungers and potentially criminal people. As Stryker has said of those who are non-trans and who exist within the gendered binary:

> To encounter the transsexual body, to apprehend a transgendered consciousness articulating itself, is to risk a revelation of the constructedness of the natural order. Confronting the implications of this constructedness can summon up all the violation, loss, and separation inflicted by the gendering process that sustains the illusion of naturalness. (Stryker, 1994 p. 250)

Apotemnophilia produces a similar reaction in the consciousness to that of Raymond (1980). Only a woman can know what it is to be a woman, thus a man who thinks he is a woman cannot be a woman, but is merely misguided. Similarly, only a limbless person can know what it is to be a limbless person, thus an apotemnophiliac who says that in order to be whole s/he needs a limb amputating is ridiculous and possibly insane. In both cases, heteronormativity demands, that other cures (rather than the surgeon's knife) must be provided. For the transsexual person it is either psychotherapeutic intervention or, more radically, the change of gender roles and demands that Raymond necessitated. For the apotemnophiliac if therapy does not work, then at least their demands should be ignored. In both cases, the hegemonic role of heteronormativity downgrades the imagination to nothing more that a phantasm. The alternative would be to unsettle the firmest bases of modern life.

That there is expressed moral outrage is not surprising. Why should those who stifle their imaginations, and are both supportive and dependant upon the 'natural' order, pay their taxes to provide the treatment of what is really not a sickness, merely a fancy parody of those who persevere with being good men and women. To do so willingly invokes a seismic disturbance of the basis of their stability. We need to know what it is to be men and women to fulfil our roles in life.

Body modifications of all types (centred as they are on the level of blood, bone and flesh) are truly real, but they are additionally expressions of the imagination, and an acknowledgement that the mind is as real as the shell in which it is housed. Social theories of pain refer to the social and emotional costs of pain and the counter-benefits of concealing pain (Bendelow and Williams, 1995). To acknowledge the violation of the gendering process would make us all become sick; instead, it is essential we ignore or conceal this pain to gain the counter benefits that arise through the 'natural' order. Yet transsexual people and apotemnophiliacs take on the gender pain of their minds and embody it, accepting that pain in the mind can be greater than pain in the body, and eased through the body. It would be irrational to suggest that all mental pain could be improved in such a way, but it could be said that gender role and sexuality are inextricably bound through the body, and as it is imagined. Halbestram (1991) hypothesised the post-human identity in which we all have the nerve to take on the fraility of our skin and manipulate it so as to become something else.

One knows one's place from the moment the midwife lifts the baby, looks to see if there is a penis or no penis, and says 'it's a boy' or 'it's a girl'. To imagine a life beyond the constraints of the body, in which sexuality is for personal pleasure rather than procreation; in which the body is not restrictive of anything, even itself; in which gender is something for the self rather than for others, bodes badly for the heteronormative hegemony which, together with patriarchy, is premised on the life-long certainty of the sexed and gendered body. It is with some satisfaction that we reflect that the route way to gender reassignment came after the publicity concerning Christine Jorgenson (Meyerowitz, 2002). The hegemonic structures create a media which 'pathologises those on the margins' (Meyerowitz, 1994), but it is also contrary in that it additionally articulates the promise of what may be possible. Moral outrage, thankfully, expresses moral alternatives.

What would be, more than anything, the most interesting and emancipatory development, is a debate about the discursive and ideological imposition of binary sex/gender polarities, evidenced in the narratives of transsexuality explored above. In fact, as Hird (2002) has already outlined, transsexuality has the potential to disrupt notions of the authentic 'woman' or 'man':

> to the extent that transsexual individuals are able to 'pass' as 'real' women or men, they reveal that sex and gender do not adhere to particular bodies naturally. In effect, transsexual renders visible the invisible signs on which society relies to produce sex and gender. (2002, p. 586)

If the performative and interactive elements of sex and gender were more widely recognised, a more frank debate about the possibilities and limits of transsexual subversion (i.e., debates about the confirmation of hegemonic, heteronormative performances of gendered identity achieved not only by surgery but aided by the 'desire' for normality [Hird, 2002]) may, at last, be possible.

REFERENCES

Ahmad, W. I. U., *'Race' and Health in Contemporary Britain* (Buckingham: Open University Press, 1993).

Bendelow, G. and Williams, J., 'Pain and the Mind – Body Dualism: a Sociological Approach', *Body and Society*, 1:2 (June 1995), pp. 83–103.

Brandt, A. M. and Rozin, P., *Morality and Health* (London: Routledge, 1997).

Butler, J., *Gender Trouble* (London: Routledge, 1990).

Butler, J., *Bodies that Matter* (London: Routledge, 1993).

Cohen, S., *Folk Devils and Moral Panics* (St Albans: Paladin, 1972).

Critcher, C., *Moral Panics and the Media* (Buckingham: Open University Press, 2003).

Cue, L. and Benkoil, D., *Surgical Questions: Questions Raised over Amputations of Two Healthy Legs* (2001).

Fairclough, N., *Media Discourse* (London: Edward Arnold, 1995).

Gamson, W. A. and Modigliani, A., 'Media Discourse and Public Opinion on Nuclear Power: a Constructionist Approach', *American Journal of Sociology*, 95:1 (1989), pp. 1–37.

Halberstam, J., 'Skinflick: Posthuman Gender in Jonathan Demme's *The Silence of the Lambs*', *Camera Obscura: A Journal of Feminism and Film Theory*, 27 (1991), pp. 37–54.

Hartley, J., *Understanding News* (London: Routledge, 1982).

HBIGDA, *Standards of Care for Gender Identity Disorders*, 6 version (2001), www.hbigda.org/soc.html

Hird, M., 'For a Sociology of Transsexualism', *Sociology*, 36:3 (2002), pp. 577–95.

Leo, J., 'The Sex Change Boom: Is Politics the Appropriate Arena for this Discussion?', *US News and World Report*, at www.transfamily.org/library/archive/200104.htm (2001).

Lothstein, L. M., *Female to Male Transsexualism* (Boston, MA: Routledge & Kegan Paul, 1988).

MacKenzie, G., *Transgender Nation* (Griling Green: State University Popular Press, 1994).

Meyerowitz, J., 'Sex Change and the Popular Press', *GLQ: A Journal of Lesbian and Gay Studies: The Transgender Issue*, 4(2) (1994), pp. 159–88.

Meyerowitz, J., *How Sex Changed: A History of Transsexuality in the United States* (Cambridge, MA: Harvard University Press, 2002).

Namaste, V. K., *Invisible Lives: The Erasure of Transsexual and Transgendered People* (Chicago: University of Chicago Press, 2000).

Nestle, J., Howell, C. and Wilchins, R., *Genderqueer: Voices from Beyond the Sexual Binary* (Los Angeles: Alyson Publishers, 2002).

Pfäfflin, F. and Junge, A., *Sex Reassignment: Thirty Years of International Follow-up Studies after Sex Reassignment Surgery – A Comprehensive Review, 1961–1991*, trans. Roberta B. Jacobson and Alf B. Meier, www.symposion.com/ijt/pfafflin/1000.htm (1998).

Potter, W. J., *Media Literacy* (London: Sage, 1998).

Raymond, J., *The Transsexual Empire* (London: The Women's Press, 1980).

Smith, G. A., *A Transgendered Deception*, Gay.com., http://content.gay.com/people/trans_gazebo/transdeception.html. 2002.

Socarides, C., 'A Psychoanalytic Study of the Desire for Sexual Transformation: the Plaster-of-paris Man', *International Journal of Psychoanalysis*, 51 (1970), pp. 341–9.

Stryker, S., 'My Words to Victor Frankenstein above the Village of Chamonix: Performing Transgender Rage', *GLQ: A Journal of Lesbian and Gay Studies*, 1:3 (1994), pp. 237–54.

Titscher, S., Meyer, M., Wodak, R. and Vetter, E., *Methods of Text and Discourse Analysis* (London: Routledge, 2002).

Tuchman, G., 'Media Institutions: Qualitative Methods in the Study of News', in K. Jensen and N. W. Jankowski (eds), *A Handbook of Qualitative Methodologies for Mass Communciation Research* (London: Routledge, 1991), pp. 79–92.

Whittle, S., *The Margins of the City: Gay Men's Urban Lives* (Aldershot: Arena, 1994).

Wilke, M., 'Transgender Ads in Transition, at the Commercial Closet': http://www. commercialcloset.org/cgi-bin/iowa/index.html?page=column&record=52(24 December 2001).

Wodak, R., *Disorders of Discourse* (London: Longman, 1996).

Representing 'Healthy' and 'Sexual' Bodies: the Media, 'Disability' and Consensual 'SM'

9

Andrea Beckmann

Introduction

This chapter will explore the ways in which 'disability' or 'broken bodies' still operate as markers of exclusion in contemporary media representations. It is either through their very absence or their specific stereotypical representation that they continue to be discriminated against. As the 'struggle over the "control of meaning" is the "medium and outcome of power relations'" (Knights and Willmott, 1999, p. 94), it becomes evident that capitalist consumer society does not appreciate and/or value different 'bodies' and different 'bodily practices' (e.g., 'sadomasochism' (SM)) that do not neatly fit into the requirements and expectations of 'normalisation' and commodification. Therefore the aim of this chapter is to analyse and challenge the selective permissiveness of representations of 'bodies' within the public sphere of the media.

Contemporary capitalist and consumer society reinforces the traditional image of the 'body' that emerged within the era of the Enlightenment, which now serves the purposes of the market. The 'body' in this conceptualisation, which is rooted in Descartes's philosophical visions of 'body as machine', serves as a tool for the construction of fantasies of eternal possession, power and desire. The 'body' is thus a site of inscription whereby signifiers of 'ability' and (predominantly 'normal/natural') 'sexuality' serve as positive markers. This chapter argues that this process of inscription/signification, which occurs in everyday life, is perpetuated by the representation of 'bodies' within the media, to the disadvantage of, for example, 'disabled' bodies as well as 'sadomasochistic' bodies that do not easily match notions of 'body' within the reductionist framework of 'commodified normality'. The 'consuming self' of contemporary society is a representational being, permanently engaged in the 'body/self'-project. The 'self' in consumer societies is in danger of being reduced to the 'body-image presented as that which "...plays the determining role in the evaluation of the self in the public arena"' (Turner, 1994, p. xiii).

Within this context, 'unruly bodies' (Foucault, 1977) and/or 'grotesque bodies' (Bakhtin, 1984) are considered, and perceived as, 'uncivilised bodies', which show the external signs of a management gone wrong and therefore are interpreted as internal failures of the agent, instead of being regarded as different and/or valid choices of human beings. As Gordon and Rosenblum (2001) state: 'impairment is socially constructed as "deficit" rather than an alternate ontology' (p. 12).

This negative 'reading' and representation of 'bodies' does apply both to people with 'disabilities' as well as to 'sadomasochists'. This chapter will thus explore some of the dominant 'normalising' representations and discourses of 'body' and point to some of the similarities of media-representations concerning 'disability' and 'SM'.

The impact of structuralism and post-structuralism as well as a renewed interest in the ancient discipline of rhetoric (Barilli 1989; Dixon, 1971; Vickers, 1988; 1990) made the study and analysis of texts (and images for that matter) acquire new relevance, and the diversity of possible ways to go about it also evolved. Within this chapter, reference will be made to semiotic, structuralist and post-structuralist approaches that allow for the analysis of media representations.

The chapter will then continue by referring to the 'lived experiences' of the alternative 'life-world' of the scene of consensual 'SM', which not only allows for acceptance of 'sexual diversities' but is also open towards and used by 'disabled people'. The empirical research that the findings I refer to are based on was conducted by myself and aimed at the exploration of the 'lived realities' of consensual 'SM' and its 'subjugated knowledges'.

One of the unexpected findings was that the Scene that developed around consensual 'SM' annually raises funds for a charity organization for people with disabilities called 'Outsiders' (with the staging of their annual 'Sex Maniacs Ball'). While this is obviously only a somewhat minor connection between consensual 'SM' and 'disabled' people, my field-observations revealed something far more crucial which points to a striking difference between so-called 'normal' clubs and Scene-clubs: the presence of people with disabilities as active participants. (Beckmann, 2001b, p. 93)

The 'conditions of domination' (Foucault, 1990) set by dominant discourses and ideologies of 'body'

For power to be self-sustaining, it must produce and reproduce definitions of reality which the objects of this power come to see as normal. Thus, the moulding and integration of 'the individual' is a central part of the production of power. (Broadhead and Howard, 1998, p. 2)

An existential part of this production of power is the moulding of bodies, both individual as well as social.

The notion of the 'body as project' is, according to Turner, closely associated with contemporary consumerism. Here the body is transformed into the site of 'hedonistic practices' which permanently seek to fulfil ever new desires.

The transformation of medical technology has made possible the construction of the human body as a personal project through cosmetic surgery, organ transplants, and transsexual surgery. In addition there is the whole panoply of dieting regimes, health farms, sports science and nutritional science which are focused on the development of the aesthetic, thin body . . . modern sensibility and subjectivity are focussed on the body as a representation of the self, such that the body is in contemporary society a mirror of the soul. (Turner, 1994, p. xii)

This relationship between body and soul originates in Hegel's philosophy, who saw in the body (and particularly in the face), a manifestation of the soul; the inner 'truth' of the person:

In the twentieth century, the twin beliefs that the face (and the body) mirror the soul, and that beauty and goodness are one, and are reflected in the face, still persist as they did in the past. (Synnott, 1993, p. 92)

Another signifier of 'body', in contemporary times, can be located in the transformation of statistical laws and probability claims into 'reality' that applies to discourses that focus on the body, both in the discipline of biology as well as in the media. In 'The Secret of Life: Informatics and the Popular Discourse of the Life Code', Janine Marchessault (1996) discusses the notion of 'the body as programme', which defines (ascribes) 'normality' as (to the) average and considers the implications:

> Evelyn Fox Keller maintains that the biological determinism and teleology at the heart of eugenics continues to thrive in genetics today. The problem we encounter in trying to situate the values and assumptions underlying genetics research is in establishing the norms upon which research is conducted, upon which notions of health and disease are being formulated. . . .
> Donna Haraway has traced a shift in the discourses of biochemistry at the end of the Second World War away from thinking about cellular relations between and inside organisms toward a more mechanistic and reductionist approach drawn from information theory: instructions, codes, messages, control and feedback mechanisms. (Marchessault, 1996, pp. 125–6)

Such shifts have an obvious impact on discourses and representations of bodies, in terms of 'disabled bodies'. Gordon and Rosenblum remarked: 'Most recently, hostility toward and devaluation of disabled people has materialized in the extreme: consider the "right to die" movement and a renewed interest in eugenics and bio-genetic engineering' (Gordon and Rosenblum, 2001, p. 12). A major influencing factor in such populist concerns is obviously the media.

Media representations

> In the posthuman world view, deliberate attempts to pursue perfection are seen as a complement to evolution, bringing the embodied self to a higher state of accomplishment. . . . Many have questioned the extent to which we are all being re-colonized by an American, and more specifically, a Californian 'body-beautiful' ideology. In so far as US corporations own the technology, they leave their cultural imprints upon the contemporary imaginary. (Braidotti, 1996, p. 13)

The stereotypes and assumptions of 'disability' are deeply ingrained in our western cultures and operate as a mere supplementation to the 'normal', the 'abled body'. Halperin explains: 'the very logic of supplementarity entails the unmarked term's dependence on the marked term: the unmarked term needs the marked term in order to generate itself as unmarked' (Halperin, 1995, p. 45). This is one similarity that the social construction of 'disability' has with so-called 'sadomasochism', as will be seen later.

Negative notions and images of disability are reinforced at various levels of society, not least within the public realm of media representations, which is hugely influenced by 'Americanisation'. These are significant to the continuation of discrimination and marginalisation of 'disabled people' within our society, and 'disability is typically constructed in social science and commonsense practices as "illness", despite the fact that most people with disabilities are healthy' (Gordon and Rosenblum, 2001, p. 14).

Several authors who have researched socio-cultural representations of disabled people within both the realm of the arts as well as the media found this to be valid (Darke, 1994; Davidson et al., 1994; Shakespeare, 1994; Shearer, 1981). The overwhelming presence of negative and/or one-dimensional representations and portrayals of 'disabled' people both in film and on television that were observed within these research projects was also highlighted by Shakespeare (1994).

This one-dimensional perspective on disability is reflected in charity telethons as well as in films that portray 'disability' as an essentially tragic and pitiable condition (Morris, 1991). Betsy Bayha, the director of the Technology Policy Division of the World Institute on Disability, remarked in 1999:

> With rare exception, the media use the same shopworn stereotypes to portray people with disabilities – the pitiable cripple; the courageous and inspiring hero; the broken person who'd be better off dead, unless, of course, there's a cure just around the corner. (Bayha, 1999, p. 1)

Pointing to an example of this notion of representation, Bayha remarked:

> Media coverage of Christopher Reeve provides abundant examples of how the media still gets disability coverage all wrong, focusing as it did on whether the former 'Super Man' would walk again. (Bayha, 1999, p. 2)

Morris (1991) observed that disabled people are absent from the realms of mainstream culture. However, an example of an extremely negative representation of 'disability' within mainstream culture can be found in the October 2000 print edition of a magazine called *Backpacker*, by the global company 'Nike'. This advert, for which Nike had to apologise to the 'crip community' (see: www.ragged-edge-mag.com/extra/nikead.htm), utilises notions of the traditional medico-moral discourse of the 'bad' body, in this case, the 'body disabled', to promote its running shoe 'Air Dri-Goat' (representing the 'good body', or at least its protection).

> Fortunately the Air Dri-Goat features a patented goat-like outer sole for increased traction, so you can taunt mortal injury without actually experiencing it. Right about now you're probably asking yourself, 'How can a trail running shoe with an outer sole designed like a goat's hoof help me avoid compressing my spinal cord into a Slinky® on the side of

some unsuspecting conifer, thereby rendering me a drooling, misshapen non-extreme-trail-running husk of my former self, forced to roam the earth in a motorized wheelchair with my name embossed on one of those cute little license plates you get at carnivals or state fairs, fastened to the back?'   (www.ragged-edge-mag.com/extra/nikead.htm pp. 1/2)

While rhetoricians usually focus on speech and written language, in the context of analysing advertisements that operate additionally with visual images, the study of persuasion can be very useful. While Nike does not use the image of a 'disabled body', 'its' absence as well as the image created by the text of the advert is very revealing.

A brief rhetorical analysis of the Nike advertisement that refers to some common principles of this form of analysis allows us to trace how 'Nike' attempted to use value-laden language and imagery to persuade consumers to buy their product. Nike's advert uses metonymic language (Berger, 1998) as it operates with the general association between a trainer or sports shoe and an 'able', fit, sportive 'body', which automatically appears to exclude the 'body disabled'. It further operates by using a verbal appeal, in suggesting that their trainer will prevent accidents and resulting death and/or 'disability', while at the same time it aims to target fears and anxieties about the potential 'risks' of life in general and sport-activities in specific.

This advert obviously reflects the contemporary obsession with 'risk'-taking from the comfort of a secure position (often using remote-control equipment) that allows for the quasi-experience of danger/death via simulation, but it further reveals a lot of information about the socio-cultural and political negativity and rejection of different embodiment.

The advert further operates through the use of oppositions (e.g. anxiety/security; 'ability'/'disability'). The 'former self' that this advert refers to is assumingly the 'good', the 'abled' body of medico-moral modernity and of the consumerist ideal of the 'body as project'. This is contrasted with 'a drooling, misshapen non-extreme-trail-running husk' of the aforementioned 'former self', a 'body' that, we are meant to perceive, is a signifier of the 'bad body', a 'body' that is wrongly programmed and thus 'out of order'. The life that so-called 'disabled' people lead is stereotyped here as a tragic, non-consensual ['forced' and 'fastened to the back'] and ridiculous [a 'license plate you get at carnivals or state fairs']; the complete opposite of the dream of the independent, 'rational man' of modernity, of the 'body beautiful' in pursuit of consumerist perfection.

It is crucial to go beyond the text *per se*, as every text has a socio-cultural and political context which, especially in advertising texts and images, is crucial to its effective functioning. Schwartz suggested that: 'Resonance takes place when the stimuli put into our communication evoke meaning in a listener or viewer'

(Schwartz, 1974, p. 24). In this example of the Nike advert, 'bodies' are clearly the bearers of powerful socio-cultural and moral meanings. Even the structuralist, semiotic tradition (e.g. Barthes, 1977; 1981) does not concern itself only with the analysis of existing images, but also with their place in a system of socio-cultural representations.

Here the notion of intertextuality becomes very important. It was first introduced by Kristeva (1980), who understands texts in terms of two axes (a horizontal axis connecting author and reader; a vertical axis which connects the text to other texts) that are united by shared codes. This implies that both the text and its reading are dependent on prior codes. It is thus of crucial importance to understand the 'structuration' (how the structure emerged) of a text. Despite the diversity of advertising messages, they all appear to take certain commonly held values, beliefs etc. for granted. In this advert by Nike, traditional western Enlightenment ideas and stereotypes of 'body' are evoked which are the 'prior codes' that determine both the text itself and the ways in which it is likely to be read.

The 'normalized body' in this advert (as in commonly held stereotypes) is constructed as closer to culture and 'in control', while the 'grotesque body' (Bakhtin, 1984) is associated with 'nature', an 'unruly body' (Foucault, 1977). This process of ascription has profound effects on the receptors of such advertisements, both 'abled' and 'disabled'. The representation of the 'good body', or of the 'self as project', is, in contrast, represented in Nike's advertising campaign with the slogan 'Just Do It', which operates like an imperative in that it: 'invokes a tension between spontaneity and calculated goal-orientation, and between will or self-control and the material of the body' (Bordo, 1998, p. 46; Cronin, 2000, p. 277).

This corresponds to Bordo's observations in 'Material Girl' (1998), which portray 'plasticity' as the postmodern paradigm for the capitalist, but essentially modern, consumer imagination of 'human freedom from bodily determination'. Bordo stated that:

> Popular culture does not apply any brakes [to the disdain for material limits of 'body' in pursuit of 'normalisation'] to these fantasies of rearrangement and self-transformation. Rather, we are constantly told that we can 'choose' our own bodies.

The immanent results of the promotion of normalising 'body-images' has become evident within the 'life-world':

> Medical science has now designated a new category of 'polysurgical addicts' (or, in more causal references, 'scalpel slaves') who return for operation after operation, in

perpetual quest of the elusive yet ruthlessly normalizing goal, the perfect body.   (Bordo, 1998, p. 46).

The operation and impact of such 'normalising' concepts, representations and practices of 'bodies' in terms of inclusion and exclusion within the parameters of capitalist consumerist societies is clearly biased towards 'individualist abled embodiment' as the only form of 'legitimised selfhood' and agency. The 'self as project' notion represented by Nike's advert aims to suggest a specific form of individuality as appropriate and legitimate, as Cronin (2000) elaborates:

> the will or self-control that threads through this process cannot be seen as a voluntaristic self-expression which calls the self into being. The ideal of the voluntaristic will of the individual is paradoxically framed through 'compulsory individuality'. . . . [T]his is compulsory in the sense that the expression of selfhood is framed as both a right and a duty, and the ambiguous terms of 'authentic individuality' within consumerist identity politics become one of the few ways to access a legitimised selfhood. Yet, . . . certain groups have suffered compulsory exclusion from these very terms of individuality.   (Cronin, 2000, p. 277)

In contrast to media representations that celebrate the 'good body', disabled bodies are mainly absent from the public arena of mainstream popular culture, in spite of at least (within the UK) 12% of the population being 'disabled', according to government data. Yet, disabled characters make up only a mere 1.5 % within TV films and dramas (Cumberbatch and Negrine, 1992) and if they are featuring within this context it is usually, in one way or another, in terms of misrepresentations and distortion of 'lived realities'.

Reports on disabled people on television usually emphasise extraordinary achievements and/or aim to generate pity. A combination of these two predominant modes of reporting is represented in the charity appeals for 'Children in Need', in which statements like 'These children have shown talent and determination in overcoming their disabilities' reinforce the images of 'disabled people' as victims, and of 'disability' as 'tragic fate' and as a state to be overcome.

Cumberbatch and Negrine's research (1992) showed that TV fiction programmes had a tendency to let their 'disabled' characters die at a three times higher rate than 'non-disabled' characters. Furthermore, in half of these fictional stories the 'disabled' characters represented 'criminals'. These sets of negative media representations are obviously extended in the area of horror and science fiction movies, which make use of the 'non-disabled' consumers' fascination with the 'body grotesque'.

This matches the still widespread characteristics ascribed to persons with impairment, as Gordon and Rosenblum (2001) state:

> such characterizations also draw on biblical liturgy, since disability was historically used to frighten people into 'moral' behavior and adherence to religious doctrine. Constructed as the punishment wrought by God on sinners, impairment became a metaphor for evil, immorality, and treachery.   (p. 13)

The obvious implication of this culturally sedimented belief is the association of physiological difference with social deficiency.

'Disability' is therefore really a complex form of social oppression and institutional discrimination that operates on various levels of contemporary society. Within the next section another social construction of the 'grotesque body' that has served to marginalise and subordinate human beings within western societies will be discussed, so-called 'sadomasochism'.

The societal non-consensual submission of 'bodies': parallels between 'disability' and 'sadomasochism'

The often negative or ridiculous but definitely dis-empowering discourses and practices observed in relationship to 'disability' can be seen to be paralleled by common beliefs and public representations of consensual 'SM' (see also, Beckmann, 2001a and 2001b). While commodities are often sold in 'sexual' packagings: for example, the curator of the 'Power of Erotic Design' exhibition at the Design Museum in 1997 said: 'I think erotica is back on the agenda,' the assistant curator added: 'Things have been sexed up a lot in the past four or five years,' and Bryan Appleyard calls the last decade of the twentieth century: 'the institutionally libidinous 1990s' (all quoted in the *Sunday Times*, 27 April 1997, pp. 6/7), the use of a diversity of 'sexualities' is still relatively rare.

The social construction of 'sadomasochism' medicalises and pathologises practitioners of this consensual 'bodily practice' in a way similar to how disabled people are regarded. As the construction of modern 'sexuality' is connected to 'truth'-production through discourses by legitimised experts, 'sadomasochism' had to be constructed alongside other 'peripheral sexualities' (Foucault, 1990) in order to serve the functional requirements of reason. The 'sadomasochist' is therefore a mere supplement functioning to define and stabilise the 'heterosexual' and his/her identity. Discourses of science in the realm of the thus constructed 'perversions' are based on the 'relational distance' that 'sexual' behaviour has in relation to 'normal coitus', the established norm of 'heterosexuality', as shown in the following example:

Non-coital sexual behaviour on the part of sexually mature individuals may be called abnormal only when it is practised not just as an introduction to or accompaniment of coitus but, despite opportunities for coitus, as the exclusive or preferred form of behaviour. Then only can we speak of sexual deviations. The further such behaviour is removed from normal coital behaviour, the more immature it is, the more rigid its performance, the more passionate dependence there is on it, the more justifiable it is to use the term perversion.   (Scharfetter, 1980, p. 257)

Traditional scientific accounts of 'sadomasochism' assume that practitioners cannot quite perform 'normal', defined as genital, intercourse (again parallel to the continuous 'asexualisation of disability'), and thus have to revert to an interaction of perceived violence-exchange. In this way, the social construction of both 'sadomasochism' and 'disability' suggests a lack of appropriate agency.

In his book *Thy Rod and Staff* (1995), Anthony focuses on 'flagellation', which is one of the most commonly used techniques of consensual 'SM'. Anthony points out that in contemporary western cultures the term serves as a representation: 'the impulses for which it stands are generally held to be embarrassing, incomprehensible, ludicrous, distasteful, bizarre, lunatic, criminal or irredeemably wicked' (Anthony, 1995, p. 15).

While 'SM' is used more frequently than 'disability' within media representations, its use is usually also negatively biased and sensationalising:

Fetish imagery has never been more common in music videos, haute couture, and mass media. S/M is a talk-show staple and a reliable staple of crime shows. While it's nice to have people admire our clothes and to hear jokes about handcuffs during prime time, these media references too often include damaging and dangerous stereotypes about us. When latex, leather, and metallic accessories are taken out of context, we get ripped off so the viewers at home can be titillated.   (Califia and Sweeney, 1996, p. xiv)

Even in media productions in which the stereotyping of alleged violence of the 'dominating' party, the 'S', is not the focus, the representation of the 'submissive' party, the 'M', as a weak, volitionless and ridiculous 'subhuman' still lingers on.

To give just one example: during *McCoist and MacAulay*, on BBC1 television (20 Nov. 1997 at 10p.m.), the hosts of the show interviewed a sex-model who had featured not only in what they stated were 'normal' sex movies but also in an 'SM' movie. She claimed to have undertaken some serious research within the 'fetish' scene in order to act her role and underlined that, in contrast to 'normal' clubs, the consensual atmosphere of the 'SM' and 'fetish' scene made it possible for women to wear exposing clothes and still be treated with respect and dignity. When she pointed out that she was taught by a professional 'Dominatrix' in 'how to dominate men', the interviewers asked for a performance.

The 'scene' that developed from there not only lacked any creative imagination, it also left out the most crucial elements of negotiation [about consensual inter-action] and a safety-word [that stops any action], *and* also portrayed the 'submis-sive' party, the 'M' (played by one of the interviewers), as mindless and weak. The 'submissive' was represented as a 'sad' person without agency and without pride and dignity. The audience of this 'stereotype-enforcement' feature obviously found their all-time stereotypes reflected and laughed immensely. Like 'disabil-ity', 'sadomasochism' is represented as not the 'real thing', as lacking, as 'unhealthy' by the dominant 'normalising' discourses of contemporary western countries:

> These effects of distortion that lead to a reinforcement of stereotypes of 'Sadomaso-chism' can also be seen in many 'SM' movies: 'Cinematic SM is twisted into the non-consenting, violent realm of the unhinged that we know it is not. Fetishism is used as an excuse for a bit of titillatory semi-nudity, or to identify the villain – the man in black leather. Horror films, in particular, will happily throw in a leather catsuit or a gratuitous bondage scene to spice up a mediocre script.   (Olley, 1993, p. 19)

Counter-discourses and representations that attempt to give a more authentic and positive view of consensual 'SM' practice are rare: examples are Nick Broomfield's *Fetishes*, which showed for two weeks in London during September 1997, as well as *Sick: The Life and Death of Bob Flanagan, Supermasochist*, a documentary by Kirby Dick, which provides an insight into consensual 'SM' as a possibility for a reclaiming of 'body', experienced and developed by a man who suffered from cystic fibrosis. Herein the agency and control of 'submissive' and 'dominant' consensual 'SM' practitioners is clearly reflected.

As movies and/or documentaries that do not operate with and thus reinforce negative, reductionist stereotypes about consensual 'SM' are very much in a minority and often are only shown in selected cinemas, the impact of distorting representations of consensual 'SM', like that, for example, in the movie *9 ½ Weeks*, will remain strong. Sensationalism is the common reaction to performances like the *Jim Rose Freak Show*, which annually features as part of the Edinburgh Festival and even advertises itself as a show of 'freaks'. Within this show 'bodily prac-tices' that are part of 'auto' and consensual 'SM' are performed for their 'shock value' (Beckmann, 2001a, p. 74).

As seen in the representation of 'disability' in the Nike advert above, as well as in the representation of 'sadomasochism' in the *McCoist and MacAulay* show, it appears to be the case that:

> people with impairments – just like those in stigmatised race, sex, and sexual orientation categories – are presumed to lack or be unable to realize the values and attributes the

culture esteems. They are not expected to be dominant, active, independent, competitive, adventurous, sexual, self-controlled, healthy, intelligent, attractive, or competent. (Gordon and Rosenblum, 2001, p. 14)

The potentially broad and destructive effects of such media representations can be appreciated with the help of *The Viewer Society*, by Thomas Mathiesen (1997). He suggests a supplementation of Foucault's concept of the process of 'panopticon' with its opposite the 'synopticon' which operates in a reciprocal relationship with each other. Mathiesen sees both processes as characteristic of our western societies. He argues that the situation in which masses of people focus on a selected few (embodied in the total system of modern mass media) represents the opposite of the 'Panopticon'. The 'synoptic space' performs its continuous power over masses of people through an active process of filtering and shaping the 'informations...within the context of a broader hidden agenda of political or economic interests' (Mathiesen, 1997, p. 226), while he elaborates on the functions of control and discipline performed by 'synoptic space' as shaping the broader enculturation of the population: 'synopticism, through the modern mass media in general and television in particular, first of all directs and controls or disciplines our consciousness' (Mathiesen, 1997, p. 230).

'Synopticon' thus functions in terms of social control through inducing people to aim for and define specific 'bodies' fit for the requirements of consumerism. Those who cannot 'fit' these parameters are feeling excluded and, in the worst case, internalise negative value judgements provided by the dominant culture. The following section will, in contrast to this, discuss the much more inclusive 'life-world' of consensual 'SM'.

The 'Scene' and 'bodily practices' of consensual 'SM' as a possible means to experience and live alternative 'bodies'

In contrast to this reductionist understanding, my presentation of consensual 'sadomasochism' is based on a critical criminological, methodologically mainly qualitative, social research project that I conducted in London's 'Scene' of consensual 'SM'. I conducted unstructured, focused interviews as well as participant observations within Scene-clubs, that aimed at exploring the 'lived realities' of consensual 'SM' and its 'subjugated knowledges'.

The empirical research into the 'life-worlds' of consensual 'SM' provided me with insights that stand in deep contrast to media representations of 'bodies' and 'sexuality'.

On the level of 'embodiment' the fieldwork within the consensual 'SM' Scene in London showed that notions of 'body image' in relationship to 'self' become relevant that are different from those dictated by the dominant consumerist society.

Within mainstream society specific interpretations and representations of 'gender', 'class', 'race', 'age', 'disability' etc. allocate 'bodies' in more powerful and/or powerless 'modes of being'. In contrast to this, the context of the 'Scene' of consensual 'SM' as well as the actual 'bodily practices' of consensual 'SM' detach 'lived bodies' from their socio-cultural position/limitation and foster an open, explorative and at the same time caring attitude towards one's 'self' and the other. The primacy of sensations and experience as opposed to mere 'body image' find expression in the 'spectacles of bodily practices' of consensual 'SM', which bring the tactile and existential dimensions of social existence to the foreground and indirectly invite participation. This sensual attitude prevalent in the Scene-clubs can be interpreted as providing a break from the representational distance created through the cult of 'body image'.

The 'paradigm of plasticity' (Bordo, 1998) fosters 'body practices' like 'body-sculpting' (e.g. body building, dieting) and elective cosmetic surgery procedures, thus promoting the achievement of normalising and homogenising 'body images'. The Scene, in contrast to this reductionism, promotes experimentation and exploration:

> somebody may start off in the Scene as a dominant or submissive in everybody else's eyes but we're all finding where we are in things. It's only ever by doing things that you can find out what works for you.   (Bordo, 1998, p. 12)

The 'Scene' of consensual 'SM' offers the practitioners disordered/deregulated spaces for the display, interaction and experiencing of 'lived bodies'. The creative use of 'lived bodies' is encouraged and thus stands in deep contrast to the alienating contemporary notion of the 'body plastic' (Bordo, 1998).

Consensual 'SM' can further be interpreted as disconnecting the fundamental philosophical pattern of the western world, which tied 'sexuality', 'subjectivity' and 'truth' together and in turn shaped human beings' relationship to themselves. In *The History of Sexuality* (1990), vol. 1, Foucault suggested that the only way to go beyond an identification of ourselves with our 'sex-drive' or 'genital desire' would be a return to 'bodies and pleasures'. Foucault's notion of 'desexualisation of pleasure', which he saw represented by consensual 'SM' play, implies not a complete rejection of all acts that might be conceived as sexual or genital but the detaching of sexual pleasure from its institutionalised genital dependence and thus its specifically constructed localisation in the individual body. This is obviously relevant in terms of its positive effects for 'disabled' people in particular, as some do not have the use of the genital region of the body for activities traditionally labelled 'sexual'.

Modernity did not only effect a redistribution of violence (Bauman, 1992) but also led to a limiting of legitimate pleasure to genital, 'sexual' pleasure. As consensual 'SM' aims at the production of pleasure through the empathetic 'play' with 'lived bodies' (Merleau-Ponty, 1969), which is not limited to 'sexual pleasure' and thus does not exclude people that are not 'genitally fixed', I consider the term 'body practice' and/or 'bodily practices' (Mauss, 1979) to be a more adequate term in order to describe this social phenomenon.

Contemporary representations of 'bodies' within the media also contain elements that amount to a 'compulsory [genital] sexuality'. 'In today's sexual climate, you are assumed to have a problem if you are not particularly into sex' (Litvinoff, 1997, p. 1). The 'field' of consensual 'SM' does offer a far more fluid and open understanding of the realm of the 'sexual'.

The practitioners of 'bodily practices' that I spoke to had very diverse backgrounds, were committed (Becker, 1960) to consensual 'SM' to different degrees and were thus not mere victims of a 'sexual compulsion' as often suggested in 'scientific' and/or media accounts. The motivations to engage in consensual 'SM' were also quite diverse:

1 as an alternative to 'normal' genital 'sexuality' (e.g. to enhance 'sex' within long-term relationships);
2 as a possible means to transgress gay and lesbian stereotypes of 'sexuality' (e.g. an alternative to mandatory penetrative 'sex' within gay culture and an alternative to the politically correct);
3 as a version of 'safe sex';
4 as a possible way of exploring the dimensions of 'lived body' (e.g. sensuality) and intimacy separate from the 'sexual' realm (e.g. gays 'playing' with women);
5 as a possible means to explore the transformative potentials of 'lived body' (e.g. tension release, relaxation and overcoming of traumatic experiences through appropriation);
6 as a possible way of experiencing 'transcendental' states.

All practitioners of consensual 'SM' emphasised that communication, trust, empathy, recognition of the other person, safety and reflection are far more pronounced and crucially important in consensual 'SM' than is practised in 'normal sex'.

This has specific relevance for people labelled as 'disabled', as a lot of research within the field of 'disability' has revealed that children as well as adults with 'disabilities' have to live with a much higher risk of becoming a victim of sexual abuse or assault than 'able-bodied' people (e.g. Sobsey et al., 1991). The framework provided by the Scene of consensual 'SM' as well as 'its' 'bodily practices' (Mauss, 1979) provide a different code of conduct and a different ethics in comparison with 'normal' social contexts and relationships, one that much more profoundly and effectively prevents the abuse of power. This explains also why 'disabled' people often feel more relaxed within the context of the 'Scene' than in other more mainstream club environments.

The 'Scene' of consensual 'SM' functions as an informally controlled learning-space for newcomers. As with any behaviour, consensual 'SM' 'body practices' have to be learned. The 'step' into the 'Scene' therefore, is the start of a learning process. Access to it does not merely imply access to tools, outfits, setting and atmosphere, but also the access to people. These 'significant others' teach new individuals specific scene-knowledges such as the appropriate rules of conduct of consensual 'SM', symbols and codes (language) with scene-specific meaning, as well as the importance of negotiation, consent and the use of safety-words and gestures (that stop any consensual 'SM' interaction).

The pleasure and limits of the 'bottom' (the 'submissive', receiving partner) always determine the actions of the 'top' (the 'dominating', giving partner). As the pleasure and safety of the partners engaged in consensual 'SM' 'play' are existentially interdependent, a 'good top' (the 'dominant' party) will not only rely on the beforehand negotiated safety-word or gesture but continuously care for and monitor the 'bottom' (the 'submissive' party). According to Anthony:

> if you are a 'top' you have to be aware of how your 'bottom' is feeling at every single stage. A 'top' has to take responsibility, like a 'bottom' has also to take responsibility. A 'top' has to be aware of how exactly his 'bottom' is feeling. Is he o.k., can he breath o.k. . . . is he mentally o.k. Sometimes a 'bottom' might say: 'Yes, I'm okay.' But they might not be o.k. as well. So it must be like a unit, you must have a sixth sense. You have to pick up on body-language, breathing. And you might say: 'Well, actually, I don't think you're okay.'   (Anthony, 1995, p. 7)

According to one of the informants in my study, Bette, communication and empathy are much more pronounced and practised in consensual 'SM' than in 'normal genital sexuality':

> I think that part of the thing is the difference between intercourse and beating somebody – with intercourse, man having intercourse with a woman, there's a very direct sexual path, there's a very sexually fixed pleasure. And therefore he has a motive for just getting what he wants.

But if what he does is not directly genital or sexual, I mean it may give immense satisfaction but the satisfaction it will give will be in the communication with the other person. The fact to get it right with the other person.

After reading the 'Hite report on male sexuality', Bette was astonished:

It's just so tragic in a way how limited what they appear to enjoy is. And how little use, you know, they are just so genitally orientated. It's just so terribly, terribly sad. You just think, what they are missing out on. You haven't explored your mind or other parts of the body. Have you not been taught about being fucked yourself or what about your nipples. I mean all you do is with your penises. It's so sad. I mean putting your penis in isn't much communication. And I mean sex doesn't have to be like that. And being a man doesn't have to be like that.   (Anthony, 1995, p. 7)

This comment shows clear parallels with Michel Foucault's criticism of the genital fixation of the concept of 'sexuality', which reduces pleasure to the genitals and further excludes people from the status of 'agency' who cannot engage, or choose to engage differently, in 'sex' (e.g. so-called 'disabled' or 'sadomasochists'). In consensual 'SM', 'bodily pleasure' is coded differently.

Since 1997, practitioners of consensual 'body practices' labelled 'sadomasochism' are now in danger of being prosecuted once their enacted 'plays' ('scenes') leave woundings that are not 'trifling or transient'. One of the main tools of discursive delegitimation of this form of 'sexual' interaction used by the courts was the accusation that consensual 'SM' would be 'uncivilised'. Based on the modern 'order of things' (Foucault, 1973), the dualism of 'civilisation', represented in 'its' highest form by the 'Enlightenment', and its supplementary construction of 'wilderness' serve as socio-political tools of regulation and control.

This becomes clear when reflecting on the 'lived experiences' of consensual 'SM'. The planning of interactions, the crucial importance of negotiations to establish consent as well as the amount of time invested in these private 'bodily practices', conventionally represented as 'perverse', do not really suggest a 'lack of civilisation' but rather a sophisticated application of one of 'its' assumed core-preconditions (the control of the 'sex-drive').

SM exhibits a high degree of theatricality; which belies the simplistic assertion that no one is able to control their desires. On the contrary, active SM is the perfect means by which one learns to do just that.   (Thompson, 1994, p. 160)

Last, but not least, the ambiguity of 'bodily existence' and its fundamental interdependence with its environment are acknowledged and explored in consensual 'SM', which is in stark contrast to mainstream representations and practices of 'body'.

Bette obtains relaxation from engaging in consensual 'SM' 'bodily practices':

'I mean I find that kind of sex [consensual SM] very relaxing. I've got a serious eye-condition and I had some laser-treatment in the hospital. Physically it's not that painful but very upsetting. I was very uptight. It's quite a nasty thing to have done. This woman X. came around and . . . she ended up beating me. And it was mainly unbelievably relaxing.'

Andrea: 'It can release you from tension?'

Bette: 'Yeah, absolutely. I just think physically if it's done well, you know it's very similar to being caressed.'

The access to the transformative potentials of 'body' is rarely facilitated in mainstream society, and especially useful for people labelled 'disabled', as tension-relief can often be helpful and does allow for a different perception of 'body'.

Conclusion

The constructed concepts of 'Otherness' associated with both the social construction of 'disability' as well as 'sadomasochism' prevent any genuine understanding that reflects the 'lived experiences' of the so-labelled and often publicly represented human beings, and lead to meaningless interpretations and discourses around constructed purities.

In this respect it is important to emphasise the bio-political (Foucault, 1990) connotations of the social construction of 'disability', as this term suggests that there are absolutes of 'ability'. However, every 'body' can only be really understood to be 'temporarily abled' (consider the experiences of hangovers, headaches etc.), and as Shildrick and Price (1996) suggest, the notion of TAB (temporarily abled bodies) captures the fragile embodiment of so-called 'abled bodies' far more appropriately and, at the same time, subverts the 'normalising' discourse that requires 'disability' as a supplementation (Halperin, 1995) to 'ability', which consequently assumes the status of being in control, coherent and 'normal'.

The goal of alternative representations should not be 'normalisation' but the acknowledgement of diverse experiences and of the complexity of 'lived experience' of human beings.

The associations of 'wilderness' and 'animality' in connection with both 'disability' and consensual 'SM' should thus be seen as mere strategical devices of power. In *Discourses of Sexuality*, Mae G. Henderson refers to Hayden

White's explanation of this strategic device; in his words it is a 'culturally self authenticating device' intended to 'confirm the value of [the] dialectical antithesis between "civilization"...and "humanity"' (Henderson, 1995, p. 324). These 'culturally self=authenticating devices' are elements of concepts of 'Otherness' that are often used as images of a form of subhumanity. These devices thus serve, through a process of negative self-identification on the side of the receiving individual, as a confirmation of a sense of superiority on the sender's side. Especially in consumerist societies that rely heavily on the proliferation of media images, these negative representations and inscriptions are dangerous and should be challenged as they operate as tools of 'bio-politics' (Foucault, 1990). In labelling the 'bodies' of 'disabled' people as well as the 'bodies' and associated 'bodily practices' of consensual 'SM' selectively 'uncivilised', the allegedly 'civilised' 'embodiment' and behaviour of mainstream society receives an indirect confirmation which points to the origin of these 'social censures' (Sumner, 1990).

REFERENCES

Anthony, E., *Thy Rod and Staff* (London: Little, Brown, 1995).

Appleyard, B., 'Sexiness for Sale', *Sunday Times*, 27 April 1997, pp. 6–7.

Bakhtin, M., *Rabelais and his World* (Bloomington: Indiana University Press, 1984).

Barilli, R., *Rhetoric* (Minneapolis: University of Minnesota Press, 1989).

Barthes, R., 'The Photographic Message', in R. Barthes, *Image, Music, Text* (London: Fontana, 1977).

Barthes, R., *Camera Lucida: Reflections on Photography* (New York: Hill & Wang, 1981).

Bauman, Z., *Intimations of Postmodernity* (London and New York: Routledge, 1992).

Bayha, B., 'Media's Crippling Coverage Misses Real Story of Disability Experience', in www.independentliving.org/docs1/bayha1999.html (1999), pp. 1–3.

Becker, H., *The Outsiders: Studies in the Sociology of Deviance* (New York: Free Press, 1960).

Beckmann, A., 'Deconstructing Myths: the Social Construction of "Sadomasochism" versus "subjugated knowledges" of practitioners of consensual "SM"', *Journal of Criminal Justice and Popular Culture*, 8:2 (2001a), pp. 66–95.

Beckmann, A., 'Researching Consensual "Sadomasochism", Perspectives on Power, Rights and Responsibilities – the Case of "Disability"', *Social Policy Review*, 13 (2001b), pp. 89–106.

Berger, A. A., *Media Research Techniques* (Thousand Oaks, CA: Sage, 1998).

Bordo, S., in D. Welton (ed.), *Body and Flesh* (Oxford: Blackwell Publishers, 1998).

Braidotti, R., 'New Formations', *Technoscience*, no. 29 (London: Lawrence & Wishart, 1996).

Broadhead, L. A. and Howard, S., '"The Art of Punishing": The Research Assessment Exercise and the Ritualisation of Power in Higher Education', in: electronic journal *Education Policy Analysis Archives*, 6:8 (19 April 1998).

Califia, P. and Sweeney, R. (ed.), *The Second Coming: A Leatherdyke Reader* (Los Angeles: Alyson Publication, 1996).

Cronin, A. M., in S. Ahmed, J. Kilby, C. Lury, M. McNeil and B. Skeggs (eds), *Transformations* (London and New York: Routledge, 2000).

Cumberbatch, Guy and Negrine, Ralph, *Images of Disability on Television* (London: Routledge, 1992).

Darke, P. A., 'The Elephant Man' (David Lynch, EMI Films, 1980): an Analysis from a Disabled Perspective', *Disability and Society*, 9:3 (1994), pp. 327–42.

Davidson, F. W. K., Woodill, G. and Bredberg, E., 'Images of Disability in Nineteenth-Century British Children's Literature', *Disability and Society*, 9:1 (1994), pp. 33–46.

Dixon, P., *Rhetoric* (London: Methuen, 1971).

Foucault, M., *The Order of Things: An Archaeology of the Human Sciences* (New York: Vintage Books, 1973).

Foucault, M., *Discipline and Punish* (London: Allen Lane, 1977).

Foucault, M., *The History of Sexuality*, vol. 1 (London: Penguin Books, 1990).

Gordon, B. Omansky and Rosenblum, K. E., 'Bringing Disability into the Sociological Frame: a Comparison of Disability with Race, Sex, and Sexual Orientation Statuses', *Disability and Society*, 16:1 (2001), pp. 5–19.

Halperin, D. M., *Saint Foucault: Towards a Gay Hagiography* (New York and Oxford: Oxford University Press, 1995).

Henderson, M. G., in D. Stanton (ed.), *Discourses of Sexuality* (Ann Arbor, MI: University of Michigan Press, 1995).

Knights, D. and Willmott, H., *The Re-engineering Revolution: Critical Studies of Corporate Change* (Thousand Oaks, CA: Sage, 1999).

Kristeva, J., *Desire in Language: A Semiotic Approach to Literature and Art* (New York: Columbia University Press, 1980).

Litvinoff, S., in H. Lacey, 'Are you Getting the Sex you Want?', *Independent on Sunday*, 'Real Life', 18 May 1997 (1997), p. 1.

Marchessault, J., 'The Secret of Life: Informatics and the Popular Discourse of the Life Code', *New Formations*, no. 29 (1996).

Mathiesen, T., 'The Viewer Society', in *Theoretical Criminology* (Thousand Oaks, CA: Sage, 1997).

Mauss, M., *Sociology and Psychology* (London: Routledge & Kegan Paul, 1979).

Merleau-Ponty, M., *The Visible and the Invisible* (Evanston: Northwestern University Press, 1969).

Morris, J., *Pride Against Prejudice: Transforming Attitudes to Disability* (London: Women's Press, 1991).

Olley, M., 'Pam Hogg – Warrior Queen of the Catwalk', in T. Woodward (ed.), *The Best of SKIN TWO* (New York: Richard Kasak Books, 1993).

Scharfetter, C., *General Psychopathology* (Cambridge: Cambridge University Press, 1980).

Schwartz, T., *The Responsive Chord* (Garden City, NY: Doubleday, 1974).

Shakespeare, T., 'Cultural Representation of Disabled People: Dustbins for Disavowal?' *Disability and Society*, 9:3 (1994), pp. 283–300.

Shearer, A., *Disability: Whose Handicap?* (Oxford: Basil Blackwell, 1981).

Shildrick, M. and Price, J., 'Breaking the Boundaries of the Broken Body', in J. Price and M. Shildrick, *Feminist Theory and the Body* (Edinburgh: Edinburgh University Press, 1996).

Sobsey, D., Gray, S., Wells, D., Pyper, D. and Reimer-Heck, B. (eds), *Disability, Sexuality, and Abuse: An Annotated Bibliography* (Baltimore, MD: Paul H. Brookes, 1991).

Sumner, C., *Censure, Politics and Criminal Justice* (Milton Keynes: Open University Press, 1990).

Synnott, A., *The Body Social* (London: Routledge, 1993).

Thompson, B., *Sadomasochism* (New York and London: Cassell, 1994).

Turner, B., in P. Falk, *The Consuming Body* (Thousand Oaks, CA: Sage, 1994).

Vickers, B., *In Defence of Rhetoric* (Oxford: Oxford University Press, 1988).

Vickers, B., 'The Recovery of Rhetoric: Petrarch, Erasmus and Perelman', *History of the Human Sciences*, 3:3 (1990), pp. 415–41.

Part IV

Morality and Health: Discourses of Good and Evil in Health Texts

This part examines morality discourses around health and illness. Brandt and Rozin (1997, p. 3) state:

> Rather than seeing health or disease as random and inevitable, societies have, throughout history, developed complex and sophisticated explanations for the causes and prevalence of disease. Embedded in these explanatory frames are deeply held, if often unstated, sensibilities about right and wrong, good and bad, responsibility and danger.

There is a growing body of work in this area, looking at the way in which media coverage of health issues is underpinned by discourses of judgementalism and morality. These include work on food (Belasco, 1997), teenage pregnancy (Gordon, 1997) and drug use (Courtwright, 1997). Perhaps the most obvious example involves coverage of HIV/AIDS and the constructions of 'innocent' and 'guilty' victims of the disease. Miller (1998), for example, has produced a study of television coverage of HIV/AIDS in the late 1980s which constantly uses this distinction in reporting the epidemic. This, though, is not only true in media coverage of health issues but also, through the content and tone of government social policy, the idea of 'good' and 'bad' health behaviour is reinforced.

There are two key issues at stake here. First, the expansion of public health discourses to further regulate individual lifestyle behaviours and deviant identities has been supported and encouraged: 'A strong underlying message in the discourses of health promotion is that the individual needs to take care of the self by adopting a certain kind of "lifestyle"' (Petersen, 1994, p. 36). And furthermore, that here is an escalating discourse about health as self-discipline 'and illness as a failure to regulate oneself' (p. 36). Howard Leichter makes this point in his excellent chapter, 'Lifestyle Correctness and the New Secular Morality' (1997), when he talks about the aims of what he calls the 'wellness movement' (the organised focus of a new 'secular morality'):

> The text of the wellness movement has been that adopting more healthy lifestyles will lead to longer, healthier, and more enriching lives. There is however, a subtext to the movement that has little to do with health and a great deal to do with social status. It is this dimension of the wellness movement that has infused it with a sense of moralism, or more appropriately, moral posturing, that I have chosen to call lifestyle correctness. . . . What I am suggesting is that what we are seeing today in the health and wellness movement is an analogous, if considerably less structured, effort to set and protect social boundaries by defining acceptable and unacceptable lifestyles . . . the notion of an 'elect' people who follow a behaviourally correct lifestyle is in my judgement especially invidious because it is a status that is all but inaccessible to the most vulnerable segments of society.   (Leichter, 1997, pp. 371–2)

The second issue points beyond the regulation of behaviour to the wider consequences of the increasing inseparability of 'health and lifestyle', to the promotion of the consumerist project through an unrelenting variety of media. The increasing number of products linked to the maintenance of a healthy lifestyle encourages mass consumption while further distancing the 'well wealthies' from the 'poorly-poors'. The costs of the 'wellness movement' are invariably high.

Morality discourses, we would argue, underpin the media's interest (maybe obsession) since the mid-1990s with health and lifestyle programming. This is most apparent through the medium of television but it is also true of the print media.

Elsewhere (King and Watson, 2001), we have outlined the potential of reconfiguring 'health' issues as 'lifestyle' issues and explored how the boundaries between the concepts of health, well-being and lifestyle have been blurred (Davidson et al., 1997; O'Brien, 1995).

This approach requires us to understand 'health' as something broader than an opposite to functional pathology and instead place it within its socio-political and cultural context. As Bunton et al. (1995, p. 2) state:

> In the 1960s a list of 'health related' commodities would have included items such as aspirins, TCP, Dettol and plasters. Today's, however, include: food and drink, myriad health promoting pills, private health, alternative medicines and videos . . . shampoo (for 'healthy looking hair'), sun oils, psychoanalysis, shell suits and so-on.

This broadening of definitions of health is, of course, reminiscent of Zola's (1975) observation that almost anything and everything 'when done too much or too little' can inevitably lead to certain ill-health and has been a central tenet of health promotion texts since the 1970s (Naidoo and Wills, 1994; Seedhouse, 1997; Tones et al., 1990). This blurring of the boundaries between lifestyle, consumption and health has been well documented, with some theorists arguing that 'health has been colonised in the name of "lifestyle"' (O'Brien, 1995, p. 203).

We would argue that while some people may object to health being colonised in this way, the concept of 'lifestyle' as presented in a variety of television programmes is similar to Seedhouse's (1997) idea of the foundations of health, which amalgamates medical, sociological, economic and psychological perspectives on the concept of health.

Moreover, a complex health matrix is inscribed in contemporary western societies' 'look better, feel better' obsession with lifestyle simulations, with the media invariably utilising (often moralistic) therapeutic discourse as a way of framing the action on the page/on screen. We witness our lives being (potentially) transformed from unhealthy/chaotic, to healthy/orderly (the before and after of *Home Front, Changing Rooms*, etc.) and in doing so we view the potential we have to live (morally, if not actually) healthy lives. John Ellis (1999), for example, has argued that television is a form of 'therapy' where we are helped to 'work through' the problems and chaos of our lives. Of course, this is the 'illusion of transformation' (Gripsrud, 2002), a televisual and temporally boundaried promise that for this time, in this space, we can experience emotions of change reminiscent of Seedhouse's (1997) foundations model of health and its ideas about individuals effecting change and moving towards better health. The increasingly popular chat show, either imported (*Oprah, Jenny, Ricki*) (Shattuc, 1997) or homegrown (*Kilroy, Trisha*), provides a prime example of morality discourses in action.

Why has there been this surge in the output of lifestyle programming? We would argue that this fairly recent obsession is an effect of a late capitalist, postmodern society's need to simulate order, combined with the powerful and often moralistic discourses of order, cleanliness and anti-infection characteristic of western societies, and possibly as a response to the threat of global contamination and disorder made (partially) visible through the very same media.

The roots of these ideas, however, could be traced to Enlightenment ideas of self-determination and a preoccupation with 'sorting ourselves out'. This, combined with the privatisation of 'family' and 'home' in the nineteenth century, the emergence of the concept of 'suburbs', and the separation of work from homelife (and consequently the institutionalisation of differential gender roles), all provided the groundwork for the emergence of magazines such as *Good*

Housekeeping (Bunton, 1997), which in turn provided the groundwork for a 'lifestyle' discourse. Dirt and disorder has been a recurring motif of public health discourses (see, for example, Anthony Pryce's chapter, elsewhere in this book) and is now manifest in the 'healthy lifestyle' programming in contemporary media – the modern version of 'now wash your hands' notices.

Whilst there are differences in the ways in which the lifestyle material is presented (for example, Alan Titchmarsh's conservative gazebos for elderly marrieds, compared with Diarmuid Gavin's postmodern designs for urban queers), the environments are still inevitably neo-liberal, largely privatised and reflecting 'worthy' recipients. These contemporary ideas can be traced to a time when the home acquired status as an inner sanctum set against the streets as threatening and dangerous:

> Domesticity is a social space that was first developed in what we might term the bourgeois period, in the early period of modernity, when the workplace and the home became separated.   (Gripsrud, 2002, p. 25)

The home in this version is 'celebrated and cherished more than ever as a safe haven for self-realisation and healthy experiences' (Gripsrud, 2002, p. 25) – the reality, as we know, is often somewhat different.

An interesting development however, has been the emergence of a 'discourse of shame', where victims are blamed for their 'poor taste in dress' (*What Not to Wear*), 'untidy homes' (*House Doctor*) or 'poor voices' (*Popstars*). In these programmes, a negation of the abject allows for the mainstreaming of bourgeois respectability.

We would argue that the mass media itself has the potential to create particular discourses, such as the discourse of 'lifestyle', through subtly reinforcing 'healthy' notions of living but which are themselves informed by the cultural prerequisites of a western capitalist society.

Philip Guy's chapter takes a historical perspective on the depiction of drug use in film. Guy argues that for many viewers it is the representations of drug use in films that form their opinion of drug use and drug users: 'for most of film history the audience has had very little experience of drug use. It has been cultural representations of drug use that have filled this void'.

The representation of drug users as 'other' (Hall, 1997) is examined, and parallels are drawn between morality discourses concerning drug use in cinematic representation and government policy in the US and UK (Courtwright, 1997; Furedi, 1997). Guy also draws on the work of Stevenson (1999), looking at issues of censorship and how morality discourses in cinema are reflective of discourses involving 'negative' health behaviours in society. Guy also draws attention to the ironic fact that despite these discourses of morality around drugs and drug users, the drug-film genre was so popular with cinema audiences at certain points in the twentieth century that it caused an upturn in the fortunes of an ailing film industry (Biskind, 1998).

Drawing on a variety of literary texts, Angela Kershaw explores how theoretorical, literary figures are located along a continuum. At one end, illness represents degeneracy, and at the other, a creative possibility. Kershaw explores this in relation to the notion of romanticism which shaped nineteenth-century literary ideas and provides us with an opportunity to see how illness is never just illness (Sontag, 1991) but is always constructed according to/against popular cultural and social epochs. The themes which emerge from her study include the notion of morality in relation to transgressive (homosexual) desires, and resultant punishment, discourses which link homosexuality, degeneracy and disease metaphors as well as examining the use of illness to represent social stigma in literary texts.

Kershaw also argues the case for the inclusion of the products associated with 'high' culture (Bourdieu, 1984) in a book about mass media:

> if cultural (and media) studies is convincingly to interrogate the problematic distinctions between 'high' and 'low' culture, its scope must, I think, be broad enough to embrace that which has traditionally been viewed as 'high' culture, if a simple substituting of the 'low' for the 'high' is to be avoided.

One key reason for this, she also argues, is that present-day constructions and representations of health and illness in the media have their roots in pre-twentieth-century media forms, such as the romantic novel.

REFERENCES

Belasco, W., 'Food, Morality and Social Reform', in A. M. Brandt and P. Rozin (eds), *Morality and Health* (London: Routledge, 1997), pp. 185–99.

Biskind, P., *Easy Riders, Raging Bulls* (London: Bloomsbury, 1998).

Bourdieu, P., *Distinction: A Social Critique of the Judgement of Taste* (London: Routledge, 1994).

Brandt, A. M. and Rozin, P. (eds), *Morality and Health* (London: Routledge, 1997).

Bunton, R., 'Popular Health, Advanced Liberalism and *Good Housekeeping* Magazine', in S. Peterson and R. Bunton (eds), *Foucault, Health and Medicine* (London: Routledge, 1997).

Bunton, R., Nettleton, S. and Burrows, R. (eds), *The Sociology of Health Promotion: Critical Analysis of Consumption, Lifestyle and Risk* (London: Routledge, 1995).

Courtwright, D. T., 'Mortality, Religion and Drug Use', in A. M. Brandt and P. Rozin (eds), *Mortality and Health* (London: Routledge, 1997), pp. 231–50.

Davidson, C., Frankel, S. and Davey-Smith, G., 'The Limits of Lifestyle: Reassessing "Fatalism" in the Popular Culture of Illness Presentation', in M. Siddell (ed.), *Debates and Dilemmas in Promoting Health: A Reader* (Buckingham: Open University Press, 1997), pp. 24–32.

Ellis, J., 'Television as Working Through', in J. Gripsrud (ed.), *Television and Common Knowledge* (London: Routledge, 1999), pp. 55–70.

Furedi, F., *Culture of Fear: Risk Taking and the Morality of Law Expectations* (London: Cassell, 1997).

Gordon, L., 'Teenage Pregnancy and Out of Wedlock Birth: Morals, Morality, Experts', in A. M. Brandt and P. Rozin (eds), *Morality and Health* (London: Routledge, 1997), pp. 251–70.

Gripsrud, J., *Understanding Media Culture* (London: Edward Arnold, 2002).

Hall, S., *Representation: Cultural Representations and Signifying Practices* (London: Sage, 1997).

King, M. and Watson, K., 'Transgressing Venues: Health Studies, Cultural Studies and the Media', *Health Care Analysis*, 9 (2001), pp. 401–16.

Leichter, H., 'Lifestyle Correctness and the New Secular Morality', in A. M. Brandt and P. Rozin (eds), *Morality and Health* (London: Routledge, 1997), pp. 359–78.

Naidoo, J. and Wills, J., *Health Promotion, Foundations for Practice* (London: Balliére Tindall, 1994).

O'Brien, M., 'Health and Lifestyle: a Critical Mess? Notes on the Differentiation of Health', in R. Bunton, S. Nettleton and R. Burrows (eds), *The Sociology of Health Promotion, Critical Analysis of Consumption, Lifestyle and Risk* (London: Routledge, 1995), pp. 191–205.

Petersen, A. R., 'Governing Images: Media Constructions of the "Normal" "Healthy" Subject', *Media Information Australia*, 72 (1994), pp. 32–40.

Seedhouse, D., *Health Promotion, Philosophy, Prejudice and Practice* (London: John Wiley, 1997).

Shattuc, J., *The Talking Cure* (London: Routledge, 1997).

Sontag, S., *Illness as Metaphor and AIDS as Metaphor* (Harmondsworth: Penguin, 1991).

Stevenson, J., 'Highway to Hell', in J. Stevenson (ed.), *Addicted: The Myth and Menace of Drugs on Film* (New York: Creation Books, 1999).

Tones, K., Tifford, S. and Robinson, Y., *Health Education: Effectiveness and Efficiency* (London: Chapman & Hall, 1990).

Zola, I., 'Medicine as an Instrument of Social Control', in C. Cox and A. Mead (eds), *The Sociology of Medical Practice* (Basingstoke: Macmillan, 1975).

Dope Fiends: the Myth and Menace of Drug Users in Film

10

Philip Guy

Introduction

Portrayals of drug use in film are as old as the film medium itself. Since 1894 when Thomas Edison commissioned *Chinese Opium Den*, a Kinetoscope loop or elaborate magic lantern show (Brownlow, 1990), more than a thousand films with storylines centred on drug use have been made. At times drug films have been central to the film industry. Even the very survival of the medium has been attributed to the drug film genre (Biskind, 1998).

Nevertheless, many of these films have been on the periphery of the film industry in terms of their distribution and impact on the public. They have also been on the periphery in terms of their impact on cinematography as an art or as a commercial enterprise. Some films, like *Assassin of Youth* (1935) and *Reefer Madness* (1936), are remembered for their notoriety. The sensational depictions of drug use in such films serve only to make later generations laugh with incredulity. Many more films are simply forgotten, probably deservedly so. There have also been films within this genre that have had a major impact on the public and on cinematography, influencing both the content and style of films and the public's perceptions of drug use. Drug films reflect the popular fears of their day. When these fears have had a strong racial form, the villain of the story is often black or at least foreign. These racial stereotypes work because for most of film history the audience has had very little experience of drug use. It has been cultural representations of drug use that have filled this void.

Drug use is a health issue and for much of their history drug films have depicted it as unhealthy. However, health itself is only indirectly addressed in most drug films. Even the best that the genre has to offer has tended to subsume health under a characterisation that focuses on deviance and morality. Generally drug use is represented culturally as deviant behaviour and drug stories draw a line between the law-abiding and the criminal as well as a line between the healthy, the sick and the immoral. Furedi (1997) outlines the discourses of fear at work in relation to these health issues, discourses which are also apparent in film representations of drugs and drug use:

> One of the most far-reaching consequences of these forms of thinking is to obscure the social causation of many of the problems people face.... Behind the people who are out of control is a society which has lost its way.... After all, a problem created by humans ought to be susceptible to effective intervention. The problem is caused by a moral flaw – and the only thing to be done is to punish and pray. (Furedi, 1997, p. 171)

Similarly, Courtwright (1997) argues that policy approaches to drug use and those who use drugs are driven by moral and religious beliefs – themes which are apparent in the 'them and us', 'good versus evil' discourses at work in films which represent drug use and drug users.

The aim of this chapter is to outline the lineage of many ideas about drugs and drug users. Using the storyline and style of three critically acclaimed films from three different decades, *The Man with the Golden Arm* (1955), *Easy Rider* (1969) and *Trainspotting* (1995), the continuity of many such themes within drug stories will then be drawn out and discussed.

The Lotus-eaters

The central plot-lines of drug stories and the characteristics of the principal participants were already established before the advent of cinema. In literature, drug storylines go back at least as far as Homer's *Odyssey* in 700BC. *The Odyssey* contains a story in which three innocent and unsuspecting members of a ship's crew are persuaded by a group of natives to imbibe the local drug. Their colleagues rescue the crew from their folly, against their will. Folly, in this case, seems to be no more than having found peace and contentment in convivial surroundings. This is something that, without explanation, the first drug warriors in the first drug war are unable to accept.

> Those who ate the honeyed fruit of the plant lost any wish to come back and bring us news. All they now wanted was to stay where they were with the Lotus-eaters, to browse on lotus, and forget all thoughts of return. I had to use force to bring them back to the hollow ships, and they wept on the way, but on board I tied them up and dragged them under the benches. I then commanded the rest of my loyal band to embark with all speed on their fast ships for fear that others of them might eat the lotus and think no more of home.   (Homer, 2003, p. 112)

There has been much speculation amongst scholars as to what the drug in this episode might be. The properties of hallucinogenic mushrooms and cacti have been known and understood since pre-history and have been suggested. Opium, cocaine and cannabis have also been placed in the frame. Such is the unanimity on drug users and how to deal with them that there has been much less discussion of the underlying message in Homer's tale.

At first sight it is reasonable to assume that this is a moral tale telling the reader that this kind of intoxication is wrong. However, Homer is not a disinterested player in the drama. He is the leader as well as the narrator and he has the practical issues of leadership to consider. If the crew do not return, or worse still, the rest of the expedition follow them, Homer's problem is that there would not be enough crew to sail the ship. This manpower problem is transferred into the Lotus-eater problem and intoxication. The separation of man from drugs is seen as the answer to the perceived problem. The action that is taken is not steeped in a sophisticated understanding of human motivation, even by the standards of 700BC, where we might have expected some reference to the soul as the driving force of mankind. This exclusively physical approach finds its contemporary parallel in the equally physical act of moving drug users away from the situational and emotional cues that precipitated their drug use and placing them in prison or residential rehabilitation.

Had he been morally neutral, Homer might have turned his story into an examination of conditions on board ship, the rigours of a long and arduous sea voyage, the way power is exercised or how praise, respect and status are accorded to the crew. Indeed any other aspect of the contribution made to the story by the actors involved and their environment could have been considered. Rather than looking inside his own social group or looking at his own actions for explanations and insights, Homer offers his readers one-dimensional characters whose only motivation seems to be intoxication. In doing so he provides a prototype of how many respond to drug use: by looking outside of their immediate social milieu. This is blame culture – but no one blames themselves. The Lotus-eaters could have been placed within a discourse that depicted them as hospitable people happy to share something of wonder and value with their visitors. Instead they are depicted as the cause of something that, although it is not death, is considered to be of equal magnitude.

The elements within this story are with us to this day. They can be seen in the elements that Monaco (2000) suggests as the focus for analysing film, the storyline, the imagery, soundtrack and syntax. All of these contribute to the message that drug use is bad for the user regardless of the user's view on the matter. Drug users are a threat to us and our way of life. Drug users cannot really help themselves and the pleasure they enjoy is a kind of corruption. Against this corruption it is legitimate to adopt severe means. Thomas (1997, p. 16) states:

> The stigma that in modern times attaches to those who indulge themselves at the expense of their health is the latest version of an age old association between illness and sin.

In America, Britain and many other countries, drug-possession offences carry prison sentences that are higher than those for rape. Drug-dealing offences often carry sentences that are higher than those for murder.

The fear of the outsider, whose guile and malevolence will corrupt the innocent, is a long-lived one within drug discourse. In the twentieth century, amongst other alien groups it has embraced communism, African-Caribbean and Asian immigration, and fears about Imperial Germany (Streatfield, 2001). Most recently, in our own time our drug problem has been blamed on the poppy growers of Afghanistan and their links to terrorism (Mowlam, 2002), as if drug problems did not exist before these concerns.

The Odyssey helps to establish the drug problem as one that is not home grown, and illustrates a general tendency towards one-dimensional characters whose actions are driven by drugs, rather than a multifaceted array of interests and motivations. This is not a politically neutral stance. It justifies the persecution of minority groups, serving to take the heat off the audience and the society they come from, and place blame safely on an out-group. The invention of cinema and its development as a mass medium followed, in its dealings with drugs and drug users, the path pioneered by *The Odyssey*.

Silent films: black and white stories

In Thomas Edison's *Chinese Opium Den* (1894) and many of the productions that have followed, the storyline presented to the audience has its origins in literature. Both the imagery and the storyline come from popular ideas about opium as they appear in the novels of celebrated authors such as Conan Doyle and Sax Rohmer, and the wave of anti-Oriental journalism typified by the output of the newspaper empire of William Randolph Hearst (Helmer, 1975). Courtwright (1997) describes how, in the USA in the 1870s, laws were passed to close down opium dens – a policy fuelled by moral outrage and racism:

> In pharmacological terms this policy was absurd. The morphine sold over the counter was ten times more powerful than the banned opium. Yet the legal distinction made moral and emotional sense, both because the Chinese labourers and white criminals who smoked opium were persona non grata and because they had acquired the habit through self indulgence.   (Courtwright, 1997, p. 237)

It may be said that this is art that is mirroring life. Here, however, life is also made to imitate art. This journalistic and artistic fantasy coalesced with a widespread distrust of Orientals. In some seaports populated by Chinese people, opium dens were opened specifically to conform to the depictions and attract curious tourists (Brownlow, 1990). It seems that the tendency to turn dockland areas into theme parks is not a new phenomenon.

However, Edison departs from reality in a number of other ways. The first widespread drug habit occurred on the Eastern Seaboard of North America, amongst cocaine-using, New Orleans stevedores in the late 1880s (Kohn, 1992). Edison's show does not reflect this reality. Cocaine at this time was a working man's drug, used to fuel long, arduous hours of physical effort. Edison's drug users, however, are the worst kind of well-to-do dilettante, well-heeled and foolish, characterisations that have endured to this day.

Edison and many who have followed are marking out a difference between the drug user and the audience. At this stage, film has yet to become the main cultural format for the discovery of personal identity that it was to become by 1920, and to remain until television became popular in the 1950s (Monaco, 2000). Nevertheless, judgements about normality are being made and corresponding messages are being given out in the service of the status quo, along the divide outlined by Foucault (1977): the audience would not enter an opium den because they are sane, sensible and law abiding; drug users enter an opium den because they are insane, perverted, desperate and criminals. They are clearly 'other' – not us (Hall, 1997) and this is another key theme in films about drug use or users.

In Chaplin's epic *Easy Street* (1917), the kind of person a drug user might be is driven closer to the image of the modern drug user, even though drugs are a minor aspect of the film. Drug use is linked with unpredictable and frightening behaviour, and crime; thus establishing a central characteristic of the drug user in films even before they had sound added to them. That Chaplin's drug user is an outcast would surprise few who regard alienation as a central attribute of drug users. This is a theme with a long life in literature and one that extends into films like *Trainspotting* (1995), almost eighty years later.

To view *Easy Street* means to catch a glimpse of a world where drug users are unpredictable and dangerous. Chaplin's drug user is a low-life, the scourge of the neighborhood, leaving few without a sense that drug users are a threat to ordinary people who may encounter them. Other films of the silent era were to add to the threat. In essence, the threat arises not just because of the actions of drug users as individuals, but also because behind them lies an alien, malevolent force. In contrast with their malevolence, drug users are also hapless, foolish, and their own worst enemy, and although drug use often involves individual tragedy, they are deserving of their fate.

That fate is simply dereliction, despair, death, and for females, seduction – a 'fate worse than death'? These are all attributes established in box office hits like *The Devil's Needle* (1916), *The Divided* (1916), *The Devil's Assistant* (1917), *A Romance of the Underworld* (1918) and *Human Wreckage* (1923). In adopting these characteristics the silent cinema is drawing directly from the self-disclosure genre of classic drug writing with its depictions of self-imposed pain and self-indulgent higher levels of consciousness, made notorious by nineteenth-century writers like De Quincey (1997).

The drug user as dangerous is paralleled and sometimes intersected by a depiction of drug users as hapless or easily misled. This contradiction only fails to move many drug plots down the scales of credibility because drug use is outside the experience of most of the audience. The hapless victim is most frequently female, gullible or easily led, someone who is sinned against as much as sinner. The hapless victim falls in with the bad crowd rather than being someone who is bad in themselves. In L. F. Baum's classic *The Wizard of Oz*, filmed in 1910, 1925 and, more famously, in 1939, the central character, Dorothy, encounters opium and falls under its influence through no fault of her own. Neither Dorothy nor her companions fully understand the power of the red poppies. Dorothy is thus a hapless victim, blameless for the state she drifts into.

> If the sleeper is not carried away from the flowers he sleeps on and on forever. But Dorothy did not know this, nor could she get away from the bright red flowers that were everywhere about; so presently her eyes grew heavy and she felt she must sit down and sleep. (Baum, 1998, p. 40)

Baum's story is an anti-adult fantasy, one in which it is the adults who are the real villains. Opium in this context is simply a product of the adult world.

This part of Baum's story has a long lineage. In *Othello*, filmed five times between 1922 and 1995, Shakespeare's only significant black character is sus-pected of using opium to seduce his innocent white victim before eventually murdering her (Hodgson, 2000). The connection between drugs, race, sex and racial defilement was common currency, even in apparently informed circles, for much of the twentieth century (Helmer, 1975; Morgan, 1982; Streatfield, 2001). The seduction of white females by oriental or black drug dealers or users has also been a consistent theme in cinema. The substantive elements of this plot were established in *The Divided* (1916) and *Human Wreckage* (1923). The former's depiction of white women in Chinese opium dens, it is suggested, fuelled the outrage of decent citizens (Hodgson, 2000).

Stevenson (1999a) provides an interesting example from Norwegian cinema, which suggests that there is something almost universal about the racist element in drug stories. In the film *Himmel Og Helvite* (1969), the main female character owes her seduction to the cannabis supplied to her and her boyfriend by a foreigner. The film's outsider group are the Norwegians' near neighbours the Danes, criticised at this time in Norway because of their liberal policies on sexuality and drug use. The character's eventual fate, as a prostitute, is sealed when she travels to the Danish capital Copenhagen to buy drugs. More recently the hapless victim, this time divorced from the original racist theme, can be found in *Traffic* (2002), a film that breaks the mould by calling into question many aspects of drug policy, but does so within a construction of the drug user that has been current for over a century.

In most depictions the 'bad crowd' or out-group reflect the contemporary fears of their times. Thus Black Americans take on the role pioneered by the Lotus-eaters in 1960s and 1990s America (*The Connection*, 1961; *Boyz 'n the Hood*, 1991). The Oriental is popularly attached to drug use in the early twentieth century in films like *The Secret Sin* (1915), *The Divided* (1916), *Human Wreckage* (1923) and *The Pace that Kills* (1928). Perhaps unsurprisingly given this lineage, it was communists who provided John Wayne with the archetype drug trafficker during the 1950s in *Big Jim Mclain* (1952). The storyline of *Big Jim Mclain* reflects the fears of Cold War America. John Wayne plays the part of a narcotics agent working for the House Un-American Activities Committee. The action takes place in Hawaii, a place that many Americans would, at the time, have regarded as the soft underbelly of their nation. The film ends the only way it could, given the prevailing political climate of its day, against a backdrop of Hollywood black-listings for anyone vaguely connected to left-wing politics. John Wayne successfully defeats an enemy that combines cannabis trafficking with communism and, lest anyone should be under any doubt as to the threat to the American way of life, terrorism as well.

The Man with the Golden Arm

By the 1950s the essential elements of the depiction of drug use were in place. It took an adaptation of *The Man with the Golden Arm* (Algren, 1990), to cement these elements into the contemporary junky stereotype. The central character of the story, Frankie Machine, begins as a hapless victim of a drug habit picked up as the result of a battle injury. He reaches rock bottom enslaved by heroin. Like *Easy Rider* (1969) and *Trainspotting* (1995), which followed, *The Man with the Golden Arm* achieved an influence that belied its relatively low budget. Directed by Otto Preminger, the film was nominated for three academy awards including one for its star, Frank Sinatra, for 'best actor'.

Frankie Machine is, while under the influence, driven, pathological, dangerous, ruthless and out of control. In adopting these characteristics, Algren is drawing on much that had passed for drug-user biography in cinema over the previous five decades. Frankie is the equivalent of Edison's dilettante, a well-heeled and foolish opium user. Here, however, his role as a jazz musician gives the character a 1950s sense of deviance. Frankie is cool and vicious. Nevertheless, change the name and the set and Frankie could be the tragic dope fiend in *Human Wreckage* (1923). However, it is the cementing of these elements together with the grisly specifics of a drug user's life that moulds the junky into contemporary form. The junky character is best summed up by William Burroughs (1993), in his seminal 1957 novel *The Naked Lunch*, adapted and filmed in 1991.

> You would lie, cheat, inform on your friends, steal, do anything to satisfy total need. Because you would be in a state of total sickness, total possession, and not in a position to act in any other way. Dope fiends are sick people who cannot act other than they do.   (Burroughs, 1993, p. 8)

Frankie Machine plays out the desperation outlined by Burroughs and survives as a character. Nevertheless, his story, like the rest of the genre it is part of, is meant to warn people not to take drugs. By the late 1960s, however, it was apparent that the anti-drug messages contained in many films were not being heeded, and to a drug-using audience they were not an enticement into the cinema.

Easy Rider

Easy Rider was made and released at a time when Hollywood's fortunes were at a low ebb (Biskind, 1998). The film became the second-highest grossing film in the year it was released (1969). *Easy Rider* combines the outsider as a source of danger; accurate representations of drug use; and, in order to counter depictions of pleasure, ultimately the death of the main characters.

This is a film *about* drugs, *by* the drug-using generation (Biskind, 1998). This generation would not accept crude portrayals of the drug experience that were out of kilter with the experience of themselves and their friends. The novelty in the storyline is that the central characters are murdered, rather than meeting their deaths directly through drug use. Thus a young audience that has largely forsaken cinema for a culture centred on pop music and fashion are attracted by characters they can identify with, and an older, more traditional audience are provided with an ending that is considered deserved and moral. Nevertheless, despite its adherence to the basic principle that no one is supposed to gain in a drug story, this film was seen as a counter-culture manifesto. It broke the formula for its genre and, in doing so, it was ground-breaking (Stevenson, 1999b).

The film opens with a scene in which the two central characters, played by Peter Fonda and Dennis Hopper, buy cocaine from a Mexican and thus play homage to the 'dangerous outsider' myth. The storyline of the film is concerned with a motorcycle journey across America. (in Figure 10.1). This links into a pre-existing notion with a long literary lineage that drug users are listless characters searching for a new reality; it also helps the film to claim its counter-culture credentials. After meeting up with a third character, played by Jack Nicholson, a scene takes place in which cannabis smoking is portrayed as a highly amusing and enjoyable activity.

A general rule of the drug genre then comes into play. Drug use always leads to personal disaster for those who are tempted, and no one is supposed to gain from it. In subsequent scenes the three characters are treated negatively by the locals in a town they visit, Jack Nicholson's character dies, and a bad experience is depicted as Fonda and Hopper take LSD in a cemetery. Fonda, Hopper and Nicholson do not die from drug use. They are, in fact, not portrayed as heavy drug users in the junky stereotype at all, but their deaths at the hands of reactionary rednecks is predictably within the rules of the genre.

The characters in *Easy Rider* are dark but generally there is no suggestion of complexity in their makeup. Nicholson's character actually owes much to the stereotypical hapless victim because if he had not joined Fonda and Hopper on their journey he would have survived. Any complexity behind their motivations and actions would, traditionally, within the drug genre be portrayed as chemically induced. Here, however, a new motivation, this time laced with 'laid back' hippy fatalism and 'let it be' stoned thinking, is apparent. Drugs are taken because they are anti-establishment and the characters are driven by a search for experience and sensation. *Easy Rider* thus catches the mood of its day.

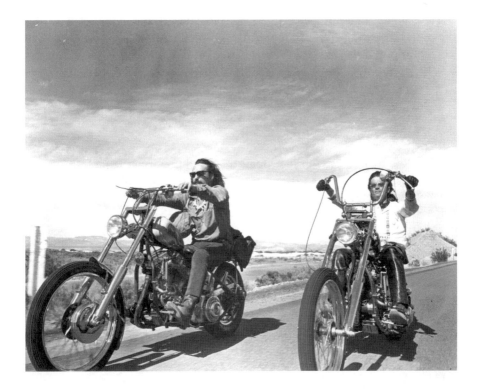

Figure 10.1   Dennis Hopper (*left*) and Peter Fonda (*right*) catch the mood of the day in
Easy Rider

Trainspotting

Trainspotting (1995) is yet another drug film based on a novel (Welsh, 1993).
Trainspotting is a bleak portrayal of drug use that places the drug user within
the contemporary 'inner city'/'urban deprivation' and 'troubled youth' discourse.
Like *The Man with the Golden Arm* and *Easy Rider*, the film's commercial success
as well as its critical acclaim have been influential. The fast 'in your face' pace
set by the narrative and the way the film was cut and edited have spawned many
imitators (Bracewell, 2003) and have become part of the 'mood music' of the
1990s in much the same way that *Easy Rider* underscored the 1960s. The film's
commercial success is also credited as having been pivotal in the revival of British
cinema, again inviting parallels with *Easy Rider*.

The central message of alienation that the film is based on is not novel; it is rather the post-Thatcher, acquisitive society that gives the film its contemporary feel. The central characters in *Trainspotting* are portrayed as having been let down by a society that has nothing of meaning to offer them. They thus reject conventional lifestyles and society's norms and values. The storyline appeals to a pre-existing discourse about drug users. It offers its audience what they would expect from a junky: underage sex, senseless violence, dole fiddling and casual theft, the stereotypical lifestyle attributes of the drug user.

This is a film that mocks the mainstream material aspirations and 'designer label' culture, particularly in the sound track and pop song 'Choose Life'. The voice of Mark Renton, the central character (see Figure 10.2), is played over a scene in which he is lying alone, drugged and unconscious on the floor of a seedy flat. The tone is sneering.

> Choose good health, low cholesterol and dental insurance. Choose fixed-interest mortgage repayments. Choose a starter home. Choose your friends.

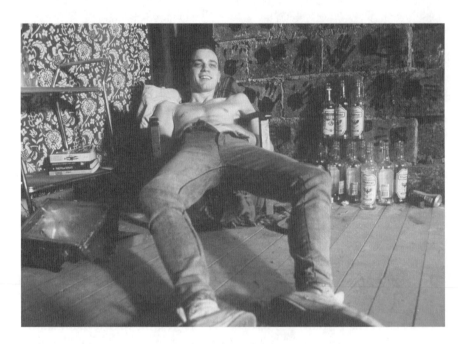

Figure 10.2 Ewan McGregor as Mark Renton fulfils societal expectations of young drug users in *Trainspotting*

The voiceover continues as the scene changes to a football match. Renton and the other main characters are mocking the national sport, the obsessional following it has and the value of competitiveness that it represents. At a deeper level they are also questioning the self-delusion of mainstream, everyday life and suggesting that it too is another form of intoxication.

> Choose leisurewear and matching luggage. Choose a three-piece suite on hire purchase in a range of fucking fabrics. Choose DIY and wondering who the fuck you are on a Sunday morning. Choose sitting on that couch watching mind-numbing, spirit-crushing game shows, stuffing fucking junk food into your mouth. Choose rotting away at the end of it all, pishing your last in a miserable home, nothing more than an embarrassment to the selfish, fucked-up brats you have spawned to replace yourself. Choose your future. Choose life.

Whilst appearing to portray and explore large-scale contemporary drug use and alluding to the working-class nature of the typical 1990s drug user, *Trainspotting* is actually another depiction, which has its genesis in the self-disclosure, pain and mind-expanding genre of drug writing that starts with De Quincy (1997) in the nineteenth century.

By the 1990s many drug films had departed even further from the everyday reality of drug use amongst the masses. Peel back the gritty realism and often characters were replicas of those created in the minds of the bohemian elite in their search for artistic and spiritual enlightenment. *Trainspotting* is an attempt at realism, but as such, it is a contradiction in its own terms, a classic drug story that is an attempt to get back to reality. The classic drug story is not about reality, it is rather, as Huxley (1954) would have put it, about opening the doors of perception.

Ultimately this discourse is rooted in the bohemian lifestyles of middle-class artists and writers – lives that the works of Huxley or Burroughs and other 'beat' writers of the fifties and sixties exemplify. The central tenet of this discourse is that drug use is an elitist and esoteric experience entered into to achieve greater understanding about reality, inner meaning and a higher state of consciousness. This depiction, however, is a world away from the ordinariness of the contemporary drug user.

Trainspotting uses alienation to suggest that drug users reject society. Mark Renton understands society, despises society and wants no part in it. Ironically, the bohemian elitists that originated the story's central theme, the search for meaning, would most certainly reject Mark Renton as too common, or just too much like 'every man'. De Quincy, Huxley and Burroughs, and others of their ilk, do not mock the commonplace and the ordinary, because the commonplace and the ordinary exist for the common man. This is a station in life they reject for themselves.

The possibility that those who have large drug habits may desire to be part of the mainstream, and use drugs to mask thoughts and feelings that would intrude on this possibility, is left unexplored. We are being given an old-established, esoteric and elitist message that does not fit in with a reality that may be down at heel and deeply troubled. We have to imagine, once we understand the archaeology of the story, that the bohemian elite have left the salons of nineteenth-century Soho, or the Parisian Left Bank, and are now on the dole and living on a run-down council estate.

For all of its novelty, in *Trainspotting* the discourse offered is the prevailing one, following in a long tradition. No one is suggesting that drug users really want to belong. The power of this morality discourse lies in its hidden message. If drug users are rejecting us, it is then easier for us to reject them. A discourse of 'otherness' underscores *Trainspotting* from start to finish.

Discussion

The aim of the filmmaker's art is to persuade the audience to suspend their disbelief and engage with the story. At some level the drug discourse is reflecting reality, but it is also arguably creating it. This can be seen in the ways in which *The Man with the Golden Arm* draws on the traditional strands of drug-taking stories, which are used to emphasise Frankie Machine's dangerousness.

In *Easy Rider*, it is the motorcycle journey that forms the locus for audience identification, running, as it does, in parallel with the American dream (Hill, 1996). Take away the drugs, the image of non-conformity and the experimentation, and replace the bikes with horses, and Hopper and Fonda could be going out, as many cinema heroes have done before them, to tame the Wild West. Ultimately, *Easy Rider* does not reject the American dream; despite its counter-culture credentials, it says, rather, the dream has yet to be achieved. The film is thus able to reach a young audience who can identify with the rebellious undercurrent to the main characters, and with the values of Middle America, who want the characters to fail. When the two hippies die in the final scene, few tears are shed. They didn't deserve to make it. Just like Homer's Lotus-eaters they took a short cut to happiness and paid the price.

Film depicts drug use in much the same way it treats alcohol problems, but with two crucial differences. The difference between the two depictions of intoxication goes to the heart of representations of drug use. Drug stories have many of the elements of Old Testament morality tales. Given the intention of teaching the audience a lesson, we are seldom invited to laugh at drug users; overall they are depicted as tragic figures. Charlie Chaplin's accidental lacing of food with cocaine in *Modern Times* (1936) and Woody Allen sneezing cocaine worth a small fortune into the air in *Annie Hall* (1977) are two rare exceptions, but in these cases drugs are peripheral to the story. The standard treatment of drug use is in direct contrast with the comic drinking antics of a W. C. Fields film or the slapstick plot-line of Charlie Chaplin's *The Cure* (1917). Dudley Moore's comic portrayal of a character with a chronic drinking problem, in *Arthur* (1981), is another example. The drunk is funny, the junky is not.

Many of the audience for *Easy Rider* and *Trainspotting* were young. They are, perhaps, the most important section of the audience in terms of its commercial success. These are people who were no longer prepared to experience their drug use vicariously through the actors' and the film crew's art. Parker et al. (1998) point to the normality of recreational drug use, both in the amounts being consumed in contemporary youth culture, and in the permissive attitudes of young non-drug users. *Trainspotting* recognised this new drug reality. The audience was invited to laugh at the central characters in a way they had not been before.

The second difference is that in depictions of alcohol problems the alcoholic often gets better (for example, *The Lost Weekend*, 1945, or *I'll Cry Tomorrow*, 1955). In drug films no one is supposed to be a winner and sobriety is less common than death in the final reckoning. *The Man with the Golden Arm*, for all of its reliance on pre-existing images of drug use and its role in shaping and packaging them further, changed that. Frankie Machine achieves this in a way few other drug characters do, by transforming his deviance into the sick role (Parsons, 1954).

The sick role requires of Frankie that he get better. This is what Frankie wants and this is what he achieves. The film is not morally ambiguous about drugs. Indeed, with a content drawn from the traditions of Hollywood drug stories, it is hard to see how it could be. Frankie goes through a tough time, one that few in the audience would wish for. However, the use of the sickness role is a chink in the armour of the moralists and it begins to make the film look like something it is not. *The Man with the Golden Arm* was released without a seal of approval from the censors and was originally only shown in independent film theatres. America's Legion of Decency dubbed the film 'morally objectionable' (Stevenson, 1999b, p. 39). The filmmaker is not free to make morally ambiguous films about drug use. The makers of *The Man with the Golden Arm, Easy Rider* and *Trainspotting* were all accused of doing so.

Conclusion

Drug stories have a long history and their transfer from print to film rests on a long lineage of ideas about drugs that are part of the common consciousness.

These ideas are essentially moral positions, which are drawn together and expressed in stories and representations of disapproval.

If representations of drug users have a ring of authenticity this may well be due to their longevity. The film industry's depiction of drug use suggests that drug users are not in control of themselves and so we should control them (Courtwright, 1997). Whilst they may, if they seek abstinence, be worthy of our sympathy, they are dangerous when intoxicated.

Attached to drug users are the fears that are contemporary to the film's time. When drug users are represented as hapless, weak or gullible they are also represented as the soft underbelly of society, easy prey for the enemy's drug-laden Trojan horse. The listless search for sensation and experience in *Easy Rider*, the danger portrayed in *The Man with the Golden Arm*, and the rejection of the mainstream in *Trainspotting* offer a challenge to the viewer. The idea that there are those who reject the viewer's norms, values and political landscape is an uncomfortable one for any audience. Discomfort is eased, however, if the villain of the story has a different nationality or skin colour. Then drug use becomes much more intelligible as a threat from outside that can and must be resisted.

Drug films thus rarely provide a depiction of health need or one that might elicit empathy. All too often in film, the drug user is given the attributes of an enemy who should be resisted and ultimately defeated. Drug users have been scripted along these lines for over a century. This does not seem to have led to a greater understanding of drug use. If it has made any difference at all, it has been in making the drug users easier to reject and making their lives more marginalised and punitive than they would otherwise have been.

Film depictions of drug use are interesting for what they say but also for what they do not bring into focus. If people are portrayed as driven to take drugs, this obviously serves a purpose for those who claim this predicament for themselves. Emotionally damaged users can hold themselves in limbo by invoking the power of drugs, and thus not face the pain of self-discovery. The notion of the all-powerful drug that enslaves its user also explains the drug users' actions, even in the face of persistent attempts to get them to stop. For those whose task it is to solve drug problems the notion of all-powerful, enslaving drugs, or the user who rejects the mainstream, provides a ready-made answer to the accusation that they have failed.

Depictions that are one-dimensional, using only a need to take drugs as a motivational factor, deny the possibility of complexity. They also deny the possibility of a deeper reality waiting to be understood. This deeper reality may be one in which people take drugs not to escape from society, but rather, to mask personal feeling and experiences so that they can feel 'normal'. This could be the real story. The challenge would be to make a film as acceptable to its audience, as free of an underlying moral discourse, and as entertaining as drug films have been hitherto.

REFERENCES

Algren, N., *The Man with the Golden Arm* (London: Pan, 1990).

Baum, L. F., 'The Wizard of Oz', in J. Zipes (ed.), *The Wonderful World of Oz* (London: Penguin, 1998).

Biskind, P., *Easy Riders, Raging Bulls: How the Sex 'n' Drugs 'n' Rock 'n' Roll Generation Saved Hollywood* (London: Bloomsbury, 1998).

Bracewell, M., *The Nineties: When Surface was Depth* (London: Flamingo, 2003).

Brownlow, K., *Behind the Mask of Innocence: Sex, Violence, Prejudice, Crime – Films of Social Conscience in the Silent Era* (Berkeley: University of California Press, 1990).

Burroughs, W. S., *The Naked Lunch* (London: Flamingo, 1993).

Courtwright, D. T., 'Morality, Religion and Drug Use', in A. M. Brandt and P. Rozin (eds), *Morality and Health* (New York: Routledge, 1997), pp. 231–50.

De Quincey, T., *Confessions of an English Opium Eater* (London: Penguin, 1997).

Foucault, M., *Discipline and Punishment: The Birth of the Prison* (London: Allen Lane, 1977).

Furedi, F., *Culture of Fear: Risk Taking and the Morality of Law Expectations* (London: Cassell, 1997).

Hall, S., *Representation: Cultural Representations and Signifying Practices* (London: Sage, 1997).

Helmer, J., *Drugs and Minority Oppression* (New York: Seabury Press, 1975).

Hill, L., *Easy Rider* (London: British Film Institute, 1996).

Hodgson, B., *Opium: A Portrait of a Heavenly Demon* (London: Souvenir Press, 2000).

Homer, *The Odyssey* (London: Penguin, 2003).

Huxley, A., *The Doors of Perception* (London: Chatto & Windus, 1954).

Kohn, M., *Dope Girls: The Birth of the British Drug Underground* (London: Lawrence & Wishart, 1992).

Monaco, J., *How to Read a Film* (Oxford: Oxford University Press, 2000).

Morgan, H. W., *Drugs in America: A Social History, 1800–1980* (New York: Syracuse University Press, 1982).

Mowlam, M., 'Fight Terror: Legalise the Drug Trade', *Guardian*, 19 September (2002).

Parker, H., Aldridge, J. and Measham, F., *Illegal Leisure: The Normalisation of Adolescent Recreational Drug Use* (London: Routledge, 1998).

Parsons, T., *Essays in Sociological Theory* (London: Free Press of Glencoe, 1954).

Stevenson, J., 'Norwegian Drug Cinema: "Heaven and Hell" ', in J. Stevenson (ed.), *Addicted: The Myth and Menace of Drugs in Film* (New York: Creation Books, 1999a).

Stevenson, J., 'Highway to Hell', in J. Stevenson (ed.), *Addicted: The Myth and Menace of Drugs in Film* (New York: Creation Books, 1999b).

Streatfield, D., *Cocaine: An Unauthorised Biography* (London: Virgin, 2001).

Thomas, K., 'Health and Morality in Early Modern England', in A. M. Brandt and P. Rozin (eds), *Morality and Health* (New York: Routledge, 1997), pp. 15–34.

Welsh, I., *Trainspotting* (London: Secker & Warburg, 1993).

FILMS IN DATE ORDER

Chinese Opium Den (1894)
The Wizard of Oz (1910)
The Secret Sin (1915)
The Devil's Needle (1916)
The Divided (1916)
The Cure (1917)
Easy Street (1917)
The Devil's Assistant (1917)
A Romance of the Underworld (1918)
Othello (1922)
Human Wreckage (1923)
The Wizard of Oz (1925)
The Pace that Kills (1928)
Assassin of Youth (1935)
Modern Times (1936)
Reefer Madness (1936)
The Wizard of Oz (1939)
The Lost Weekend (1945)
Big Jim Mclain (1952)
I'll Cry Tomorrow (1955)
The Man with the Golden Arm (1955)
The Connection (1961)
Easy Rider (1969)

Himmel Og Helvite (1969)
Annie Hall (1977)
Arthur (1981)
The Naked Lunch (1991)
Boyz 'n the Hood (1991)
Trainspotting (1995)
Traffic (2002)

Disease, Decay and Dread: Literary Constructions of Illness

11

Angela Kershaw

Introduction

The convergences between illness and literature are many and various. That the myth of the consumptive poet is as ubiquitous as the myth of the consumptive heroine implies (at least) two possible points of departure for a study of literary constructions of health and illness. On the one hand, the literary trope of the sick artist (Keats, Shelley, Proust, Schiller, Chopin, Chekov...the list goes on) suggests the existence of a positive link between illness and creativity. On the other hand, Verdi's Violetta, Puccini's Mimi, and a host of other consumptive heroines, prove that illness is a metaphor teeming with significances.

Freud's theory of creativity offers one obvious point of entry for an analysis of the sick artist. For Freud, the relationship between artist and art mirrors that between any subject and phantasy: the artist uses creativity to overcome mental trauma (Freud, 1956).[1] This approach could, by extension, serve to investigate the artist's psychological and aesthetic responses to physical trauma. Such analyses are, however, the province of psychoanalysts and biographers.

The present chapter focuses instead on the symbolic possibilities of illness, which is appropriate in the context of a book seeking primarily to examine representation. Some readers may be surprised to find a chapter on literature in a book which declares itself to be a study of 'the media'. Yet if cultural (and media) studies are convincingly to interrogate the problematic distinctions between 'high' and 'low' culture, its scope must, I think, be broad enough to embrace that which has traditionally been viewed as 'high' culture, if a simple substitution of the 'low' for the 'high' is to be avoided. Literature has always been a vehicle (medium) for the transmission of particular messages, and still has a part to play in the construction of discourses, which are adopted and/or resisted by subjects in the real world. The literature of the past underpins many received ideas which remain current today and of whose origins we may often be unaware. This chapter suggests that this might be the case as regards some of our ideas about illness.

The texts: approaches

My approach to the texts I analyse in this chapter will, then, be primarily rhetorical, rather than biographical or psychoanalytical. I do not seek out authorial motivations, but attempt to understand the effect of images of illness in a given text on the reader's interpretation of that text and its messages. To do this, I apply an analytical grid to the works in question: I should like to propose a schema according to which illness images might be located along a continuum between two poles. At the 'negative' pole, illness represents some sort of degeneracy (individual or collective); at the 'positive' pole, illness represents some sort of creative (not necessarily aesthetic) possibility.[2] This reading method will allow us to discern the thematic and interpretive significance of the images. Are they used, for example, to enhance and develop the characterisation of an individual protagonist in the story? Or do they characterise a group: perhaps a society, or a nation? Do they have a moral or a political significance? Do they function as a warning? Or do they, on the contrary, serve to recommend or validate a particular course of action or mode of behaviour? I proceed, then, first by identifying examples of illness images, and secondly by analysing their function in relation to the text's overall 'message', thus deconstructing the text's internal functioning.

Any literary text is composed of a multifaceted network of images and other writing strategies, each conveying segments of meaning which go to make up a coherent whole. The task of the literary critic is to extract, temporarily, some of the pieces of the puzzle in order the better to understand the literary edifice we call a 'text'. In this chapter, I extract the pieces marked 'illness' and hold them up to the light, then evaluate them according to the positive/negative continuum before replacing them and looking afresh at the text as a whole.

Before examining some examples of illness images in literary texts, let us pause to consider the two poles of our analytical framework in a little more detail. I should perhaps make clear from the outset that I wish to make no judgements about the appropriateness or otherwise of illness images. Susan Sontag (1991) prefaces her seminal 1978 essay *Illness as Metaphor* by rejecting metaphor as an unhelpful way of understanding illness; since my aim here is to understand representation, not illness, my judgements must be aesthetic rather than moral. The reader should not therefore attach too much significance to my designation of the polarity as positive/negative: a metaphorical construction employed to designate moral degeneracy clearly has a negative content, but this does not imply any condemnation of the writer who adopts that image, nor indeed of the existence of that image in our discursive systems. An analysis of the effect of illness images on actual patients and sufferers is beyond my competences as a literary critic and beyond the scope of the present chapter.

At the 'negative' pole, one might begin by citing the plagues of classical antiquity and Biblical narratives. The allegorical use of plagues is common throughout western literature: illness stands for the sins of a culpable society, on whom the plague is visited as a punishment. Plague is transmitted not only by 'divine wrath' (Sontag, 1991, p. 41), but also by an infected individual: pestilence implies contagion. Illness, then, can stand for any evil that carries the potential for transmission around a group of people. Perhaps the most famous modern 'negative' illness image relating to a collectivity is the 1947 novel *The Plague*, by Albert Camus (who was himself tubercular). Here the plague acquires an overtly political significance: in Camus's allegorical representation of the Nazi occupation of France, the plague symbolises not only National Socialism, but all totalitarian systems and their multifarious implications. Such uses of illness images in a political context are common and can be said to derive their relevance from the image of the body politic: 'if it is plausible to compare the polis to an organism, then it is plausible to compare civil disorder to an illness' (Sontag, 1991, p. 77).

Of course, illness images also function to characterise individuals. For example, individual guilt is communicated via illness images in Biblical stories, where faithful characters are cured of leprosy, blindness, and a range of other afflictions. According to a physiognomical logic, many nineteenth-century literary texts portray morally suspect characters in terms of some physical ailment or deformity. Illness images relating to the individual can designate social as well as moral stigma: tuberculosis, for example, is the archetypal 'disease of poverty and deprivation', conjuring up images of 'thin garments, thin bodies, unheated rooms, poor hygiene, inadequate food' (Sontag, 1991, p. 15). Sontag has argued that it is mysterious diseases – such as tuberculosis in the nineteenth and early twentieth centuries – that offer the greatest negative metaphorical possibilities, and characterises the process of the creation of such metaphors as follows:

> Any important disease whose causality is murky, and for which treatment is ineffectual, tends to be awash in significance. First, the subjects of deepest dread (corruption, decay, pollution, anomie, weakness) are identified with the disease. The disease itself becomes a metaphor. Then, in the name of the disease (that is, using the metaphor), that horror is imposed on other things. The disease becomes adjectival. Something is said to be disease-like, meaning that it is disgusting or ugly.   (Sontag, 1991, pp. 59–60)

A more recent analysis, by Sander L. Gilman, presents a convincing account of our psychological motivations for the creation of such metaphors. For Gilman:

> It is the fear of collapse, the sense of dissolution, which contaminates the Western image of all diseases.... But the fear we have of our own collapse does not remain internalized. Rather, we project this fear onto the world in order to localize it and, indeed, to domesticate it. For once we locate it, the fear of our own dissolution is removed.   (Gilman, 1988, p. 1)

In other words, we create illness metaphors in order to manage the generalised fear of dissolution of the self and loss of control, which is what real illness is to us, since metaphors allow us to define and specify, and therefore neutralise, our fears.

At the other end of the scale, 'positive' illness images also abound in literary texts. Here, it is Romanticism that provides us with the archetype. Romanticism offers the image of the consumptive poet (Keats, Shelley), producing poetry which is (potentially) inspired by illness and which also ascribes a multiplicity of positive values to illness. In his history of tuberculosis, Thomas Dormandy points to 'the acutely heightened awareness of many tubercular patients' (Dormandy, 1999, p. 14), citing Keats's long letters to his sister at the height of his illness as an example; indeed, Keats (like Katherine Mansfield) wrote much of his best known and loved work while suffering from the disease which was ultimately to claim his life. These medical and biographical facts have been mythologised and transformed into the figure of the suffering, superior, creative individual. Sontag cites Shelley consoling Keats that 'this consumption is a disease particularly fond of people who write such good verses as you have done...', and remarks that

> So well established was the cliché which connected TB and creativity that at the end of the century one critic suggested that it was the progressive disappearance of TB which accounted for the current decline of literature and the arts.   (Sontag, 1991, p. 33)

The Romantic vision of tuberculosis was of a disease which 'etherialized the personality, expanded consciousness' (Sontag, 1991, p. 20), of a disease which 'speeds up life, highlights it, spiritualizes it' (Sontag, 1991, pp. 14–15). Disease, as Gian-Paolo Biasin has noted, can function as a metaphor for introspection (Biasin, 1967). The Romantic is nothing if not introspective. Furthermore, for the Romantic who 'sought superiority by desiring, and by desiring to desire, more intensely than others do' (Sontag, 1991, p. 46), tuberculosis, 'thought to produce spells of euphoria, increased appetite, exacerbated sexual desire' (Sontag, 1991, p. 13), became emblematic.

Illness and Romanticism

A second trope connecting illness with Romanticism is that of the beauty of pain and suffering. 'The dying tubercular is pictured as made more beautiful and more soulful' (Sontag, 1991, p. 17), and the pale, emaciated 'tubercular look' (Sontag, 1991, p. 30) was quite the fashion for the living. Sontag describes how, in much nineteenth-century literature, the reality of the symptoms of tuberculosis were ignored as the disease was adopted by writers seeking to give their heroes and heroines a beautiful death:

> Agony became romantic in a stylized account of the disease's preliminary symptoms (for example, debility is transformed into languor) and the actual agony was simply suppressed. Wan, hollow-chested young women and pallid, rachitic young men vied with each other as candidates for this mostly (at that time) incurable, disabling, really awful disease. (Sontag, 1991, p. 30)

Tubercular death was not only aesthetically beautiful, but was also indicative of moral beauty. 'Nineteenth-century literature is stocked with descriptions of almost symptomless, beatific deaths from TB' (Sontag, 1991, p. 16), deaths which are generally characterised by resignation and serenity (Sontag, 1991).

Finally, the Romantic had a tendency to believe that pain, in one form or another, was a precondition for creativity. In the context of an account of Keats's notion of indolence, Alethea Hayter isolates in some of Keats's letters 'a conviction that pains and troubles were necessary to school the intelligence into a soul' (Hayter, 1968, p. 321) and points to 'the wakeful anguish which was a needful condition of creative response' (Hayter, 1968, p. 323). I am straying here into that territory best reserved for biographers and psychoanalysts. It is, however, important to contextualise the Romantic mythologisation of illness within the Romantic understanding of the possible effects of pain on the suffering individual.

The Romantics enjoy an emblematic status in a discussion of positive illness metaphors, but they are not the only source. For example, more recent writers have added another positive value to illness metaphors in their association of pathology and protest. Biasin, reading Auerbach and Lukàcs, finds in early twentieth-century literature 'an escape into the pathological as "a moral protest against capitalism", a protest which, however, often lacks "a sense of direction" and expresses only "nausea, or discomfort, or longing"' (Biasin, 1967, p. 89) – a variation on the *mal du siècle*.[3] The pathology–protest theme was variously adopted by French feminist writers in the 1960s and 1970s: in texts such as Simone de Beauvoir's *Les Belles images*, Marie Cardinal's *The Words to Say It* and Christiane Rochefort's *Les Stances à Sophie*, female characters express their protest against capitalism and against patriarchy via somatic dysfunctions. Biasin concludes that in twentieth-century literature, disease

> becomes subtly emblematic of a particular *vision du monde*...which is concerned with the inadequacy of reality to give a significance and a transcendence to man as a social and as a metaphysical animal. Disease is used...as a particularly effective means of expressing such inadequacy and of presenting a hard, problematic ontology.... Disease...above all appears to be an ontological category of twentieth century man.   (Biasin, 1967, pp. 101–2)

Afflicted by the alienations of the new century, 'twentieth-century man' uses illness metaphors to express his newly problematic human condition, and thus reflects the metaphorical strategies of his brothers at the turn of the previous century. Here, the dividing line between the 'positive' and the 'negative' is blurred: whilst the ontological introspection undertaken by 'twentieth-century man' makes him a 'superior being' in the Romantic sense (consider Jean-Paul Sartre's nauseous Roquentin), none the less his alienation is anything but positive.

Literary texts of the early twentieth century, then, provide particularly fertile ground for an examination of illness images. Whilst their authors were susceptible to the 'nouveau mal du siècle' (Hewitt, 1988) which afflicted 'twentieth-century man' (to say nothing of twentieth-century woman), their cultural environment had not yet let go of nineteenth-century clichés – positive and negative – about illness. The texts of Edith Thomas, Katherine Mansfield and Thomas Mann use illness in various ways and for various ends.

Edith Thomas (1909–70) was a French writer whose works have now all but passed into oblivion. Thomas, a communist fellow-traveller in the 1930s, made her literary debut in 1934 with a novel entitled *La Mort de Marie* (*The Death of Marie*), which recounts the death of a young girl from tuberculosis. Thomas herself suffered from the disease, but, unlike Katherine Mansfield (1888–1923), recovered. Mansfield is a much better known landmark on the literary horizon.

She published her first collection of stories, *In a German Pension*, in 1911, drawing on her experience of a miscarriage in 1909 in Bavaria, where she had been sent by her mother on account of her illegitimate pregnancy. However, she produced most of her best known work after the First World War, and after the diagnosis of her tuberculosis in 1918. Thomas Mann (1875–1955) is, of course, one of the great giants of modern European literature. Mann is the author of a large number of well-known short stories as well as of magisterial novels such as *Buddenbrooks* (1901), *The Magic Mountain* (1924) and *Doctor Faustus* (1947).

Edith Thomas

Edith Thomas adopts illness – specifically, tuberculosis – as the mainstay of the plot of *La Mort de Marie*. The novel recounts Marie's arrival at the home of her grandmother, where she is diagnosed as tubercular, is confined to bed and eventually dies. The second half of the text is devoted to the grandmother's neurotic response to that death. In this novel, illness functions thematically rather than metaphorically: Thomas investigates (and condemns) the social stigma attached to tuberculosis, the exaggerated fear of contagion, which leads to the isolation of the patient, and the cruelty of the 'carer'. In her fourth novel, *Le Refus* (*The Refusal*, 1936), Thomas returns to the illness motif, but here, illness has a symbolic function that is rather more complex. *Le Refus* is a female apprenticeship novel (Suleiman, 1983) which tells the story of Brigitte's journey towards communist commitment. As in *La Mort de Marie* (1934), the central female protagonist is tubercular. The novel begins with her return to her family after a spell in a sanatorium, which seems to have cured her. Thomas has not abandoned her commentary on the social contexts of tuberculosis; indeed, in this later novel, her critique of the inscription of illness in bourgeois discourse is more successfully integrated into the text's political subtext and its strategies of characterisation. The reader learns that Brigitte's departure for the sanatorium was delayed to allow her to attend her sister's wedding because, her father points out:

> Nous n'avons pas besoin, je suppose, de faire savoir à tout le monde qu'elle doit se reposer. [I presume that there is no need to tell everyone that she has to rest.] (Thomas, 1936, p. 32)

As we have seen, tuberculosis was considered to be a disease of the poor: Brigitte's bourgeois, patriarchal father will no more accept this chance coincidence of his daughter's body with that of the proletariat than he will the coincidence of her political perspective with theirs. His denial of her illness is echoed at the end of the novel when Brigitte's political pilgrimage to England to escape her class of origin and to achieve solidarity with the workers is represented by her family as a young lady's study trip to learn the English language. It appears that the disruptive body, like disruptive political opinions, was not admitted by the inter-war bourgeoisie.

Within the context of this socio-political critique, illness functions as a symbol for Brigitte's opposition to bourgeois ideology. Since the text's political message is explicitly anti-bourgeois, the illness image can be read as a positive one. Disease is a positive beginning: Brigitte's illness is represented as a time of solitude and confinement that allows for profound reflection and therefore for intellectual and political development. The reader is given to understand that it is her period of exile in the sanatorium which has permitted the development of a critical perspective on the bourgeois values of her family, which is the root of her subsequent politicisation and eventual conversion to communism. Just as, for the Romantics, illness was generative of writing, so for Brigitte, illness is generative of positive political commitment.

Brigitte's political commitment is not her only transgression against bourgeois values. The novel establishes a link between Brigitte's commitment and her sexualised relationship with her friend Anna, in that both communist commitment and homosexuality represent an attempt to disrupt the bourgeois value system. Furthermore, Brigitte's potential for disruptive sexuality is associated with her tubercular body. At the start of the text, Brigitte presents her exile as

> le châtiment du péché contre l'esprit, celui dont on ne parle pas, celui de n'avoir jamais rien aimé [the punishment for sins against the spirit, the one that remains unspoken, of never having loved anything].   (Thomas, 1936, p. 11)

The choice of vocabulary here ('celui dont on ne parle pas') suggests that Brigitte might have been exiled as much for her homosexual desire – unspoken desire, desire that dare not speak its name – as for her diseased lung. Tuberculosis and homoeroticism appear to coincide again a few pages later in a brief episode in which Brigitte's sister Annie wants to get into Brigitte's bed: does Brigitte refuse because of her lungs or because of her transgressive desire? The episode remains inconclusive, but serves at least to reinforce the link between homosexuality and illness already evoked.

In *Le Refus*, then, the sick body is privileged as a site of politicisation, albeit temporarily, since the possibility for action is of course predicated upon successful recovery. None the less, it is possible to locate Thomas's text within the twentieth-century tradition cited by Biasin of representing pathology as protest. In *Le Refus*, tuberculosis is associated with transgression against the bourgeosie, which is valued positively by the narrative. Illness is also presented as ontologically beneficial, since it offers the possibility for introspection – Brigitte has time to think when she is ill – and for separation from one's milieu; it is precisely separation and introspection which allow Brigitte to construct for herself a new subjectivity that is better, according to the text's value system.

Katherine Mansfield

Biographers have interpreted the relationship between Katherine Mansfield's illness and her writing in various ways.[4] In his introduction to the Oxford World's Classics collection of Mansfield's stories, D. M. Davin reads her as a highly self-critical author, suggesting that,

> [t]o defeat the disease and to write in spite of it, these were her most urgent purposes and in time she came to see them as one: the flaw in her health and the flaw in her writing she began to think of as radiating outwards from a flaw central to herself. (Mansfield, 1981, p. x)

The vocabulary chosen here suggests a complex relationship on the part of Mansfield, both to her illness and to her writing self: whilst the notion of a 'flaw' indicates a negative relationship, the vocabulary of struggle ('defeat') suggests a heightened desire both to get better and (therefore) to write better, which might ultimately be creatively enabling. In her full-length study of the ways in which Mansfield's illness grounded her writing, Mary Burgan acknowledges that Mansfield's physical debility must have impeded her writing. Virginia Woolf recalled that Mansfield felt that 'illness . . . breaks down one's privacy so that one can't write' (Burgan, 1994, p. 118). However, Burgan also shows that Mansfield's knowledge that she was writing against time drove her to create (Burgan, 1994). In her journal, she wrote

> I don't want to find this is real consumption, perhaps it's going to gallop – who knows? – and I shan't have my work written. *That's what matters.* How unbearable it would be to die – leave 'scraps', 'bits' . . . nothing real finished. (Burgan, 1994, p. 126)

Burgan argues that writing functioned as a kind of therapy for Mansfield: writing physical detail into her stories was a way of examining the body; her stories were a means of expressing a diagnosis (Burgan, 1994, p. xiv). Burgan concludes that Mansfield's writing allowed a (temporary, imagined) restoration of the self which enabled Mansfield to live (Burgan, 1994, pp. 174–5). Burgan's conclusion echoes Gilman's theory of our motivations for the creation of illness metaphors:

the self, which illness threatens to fragment and ultimately to destroy, can be reunited and reasserted via writing.

In the collection *In a German Pension* (2001), the first-person narrator is, along with most of the other inhabitants of the pension, undergoing a *cure* for an unspecified illness.[5] The significance of her illness is, as in Thomas's *La Mort de Marie* (1934), primarily structural, in that it provides a context in which the acerbic narrator can comment on the people she meets and their interactions, and on her situation as a foreigner. Occasionally illness crops up as a metaphor, for example in 'A Birthday', where an expectant father expresses his disgust with his servant, the town where he lives, and even the doctor, via metaphors of contagion and disease (Mansfield, 2001). However, it would not be true to say that illness is a defining textual motif in Mansfield's *œuvre*, either symbolically, structurally or thematically.

This supports biographical theories of Mansfield as an author writing *against* illness. When she does create sick characters, they tend to appear as burdensome. For example, 'The Man Without a Temperament' has been robbed of his temperament by his wife's illness, which has exiled them both to a Continental hotel. His life now consists only of the observation of the minutiae of hotel society, of the fetching and carrying of shawls and capes, in short, of inactivity. His enforced inertia is thrown into relief by the euphoric playfulness of the honeymoon couple, and by his memories of their own younger, active selves. 'The Daughters of the Late Colonel' have devoted their entire lives to caring for their invalid father and have thus been deprived of the opportunity to marry, to live as women. In 'This Flower', the subject's relationship to her own illness – or possibly pregnancy, the story is characteristically ambiguous – is examined, as the narrative is focalised through the patient rather than the carer. Here, illness itself is a burden: so much so, that its reality remains a guilty secret between doctor and patient that must not be revealed to the patient's lover. This story also thematises the social stigma of illness. A discreet doctor has been chosen 'just in case it's – well, what we don't either of us want it to be' (pregnancy? tuberculosis? since the nature of her ailment is undisclosed, the story conflates the social stigma of the unmarried mother with that of the tubercular), and since '[o]ne can't be too careful in affairs of this sort' (Mansfield, 2001, p. 661). It is difficult then to distil any positive messages out of Mansfield's thematisation of illness.

Two elements of Mansfield's writing are particularly interesting as regards the symbolic use of illness: the representations of sexuality and of poverty. Burgan shows how, in her journal and letters, Mansfield designated her lesbianism via a vocabulary of illness, thus repeating contemporary discourses of homosexuality as disease and degeneracy. She suggests that Mansfield used such discourses to deny responsibility for her own lesbianism (Burgan, 1994). An example of this strategy in Mansfield's fiction is to be found in 'At the Bay', where lesbianism appears as contagion, transmitted from the racy Mrs Harry Kember to the sexually frustrated Beryl:

> 'I believe in pretty girls having a good time', said Mrs Harry Kember. 'Why not? Don't you make a mistake, my dear. Enjoy yourself.' And suddenly she turned turtle, disappeared, and swam away quickly, quickly, like a rat. Then she flicked round and began swimming back. She was going to say something else. Beryl felt that she was being poisoned by this cold woman, but she longed to hear. But oh, how strange, how horrible! As Mrs Harry Kember came up close she looked, in her black waterproof bathing-cap, with her sleepy face lifted above the water, just her chin touching, like a horrible caricature of her husband. (Mansfield, 2001, p. 220)

Mansfield's appropriation of the illness trope in the context of homosexuality is diametrically opposed to Thomas's: whilst Thomas links tuberculosis and lesbianism positively in the context of her opposition to bourgeois codes of behaviour, Mansfield uses disease negatively to reinforce the homophobia of her time. Mansfield's tendency to conflate pregnancy with disease is another facet of the metaphorical web that links sexuality and illness in Mansfield's writing (Burgan, 1994). There is a political element here: referring to *In a German Pension* (although the analysis could be extended to other texts), Burgan suggests that the imagery in Mansfield's childbirth stories:

> evokes anger against the woman's destiny to suffer the yoke of physical pain and engages an impulse to find a justification for acceptance of such pain which might transcend blind submission to sexual convention and patriarchal ideology. (Burgan, 1994, p. 75)

Again, illness conveys what for Mansfield is a negative aspect of female experience. Pregnancy is represented by Mansfield as a central element in the deterioration of the working-class woman's body. It is in 'Life of Ma Parker' that the pregnancy–poverty–disease association is most fully explored. Ma Parker, who 'had thirteen little ones and buried seven of them' (Mansfield, 2001, p. 304), lives in a body whose very mode of existence is pain:

> To take off her boots or to put them on was an agony to her, but it had been an agony for years. In fact, she was so accustomed to the pain that her face was drawn and screwed up ready for the twinge before she'd so much as untied the laces. That over, she sat back with a sigh and softly rubbed her knees … (Mansfield, 2001, p. 302)

Her story is one of an entire family blighted by illness. The death of her husband, a baker, from 'consumption' gives Mansfield the opportunity to ironise contemporary medical diagnoses, whilst also hinting at the environmental causes of disease amongst the poor:

> It was flour on the lungs, the doctor told her at the time. . . . Her husband sat up in bed with his shirt pulled over his head, and the doctor's finger drew a circle on his back. . . . 'Now, if we were to cut him open *here*, Mrs Parker,' said the doctor, 'you'd find his lungs chock-a-block with white powder. Breathe, my good fellow!' And Mrs Parker never knew for certain whether she saw or whether she fancied she saw a great fan of white dust come out of her poor dear husband's lips . . . (Mansfield, 2001, p. 305)

Tuberculosis also scotches the next generation: the reader learns at the start of the story that Ma Parker has just buried her grandson Lennie:

> From Lennie's little box of a chest there came a sound as though something was boiling. There was a great lump of something bubbling in his chest that he couldn't get rid of. When he coughed, the sweat sprang out on his head; his eyes bulged, his hands waved, and the great lump bubbled as a potato knocks in a saucepan. But what was more awful than all was when he didn't cough he sat against the pillow and never spoke or answered, or even made as if he heard. Only he looked offended. (Mansfield, 2001, p. 307)

It is clear that Mansfield is writing against the Romantic mythologisation of the disease when she writes the social and physical realities of tuberculosis. When disease is used in this way in literary texts, it is more correct to speak of metonymy, since the part comes to stand for the whole: physical illness is a real aspect of the lives of the poor that stands for working-class oppression and misery in general.

Mary Burgan's excellent biographical and textual study shows the relationship between Katherine Mansfield's illness and her creativity in all its complexity, positive and negative. On a textual level however, it is fair to conclude that Mansfield's use of illness is overwhelmingly negative. Mansfield's sick characters experience their illness as ontologically negative. Illness expresses Mansfield's homophobia. And, in opposition to the Romantic stereotype of tuberculosis, Mansfield represents disease in all its unpleasant reality, in stories of poverty such as 'Life of Ma Parker'.

Thomas Mann

As Stephen C. Meredith has pointed out, Thomas Mann's work is densely populated with sick characters:

> Mann had a lifelong interest – some would say obsession – with illness. We may note, en passant and in a partial list, that Christian Buddenbrook suffered from a nervous disorder;

Thomas Buddenbrook, like many of Mann's characters, had weak teeth, from which, somewhat ludicrously, he dies; Frau Klöterjahn and Herr Spinell, in *Tristan*, had tuberculosis; von Aschenbach succumbs, in Venice, to the plague; Rosalie von Tümmler, in *The Black Swan*, dies of cancer; the scabs on Müller-Rosé's back (*Felix Krull*) are from secondary syphilis; and Adrian Leverkühn (*Doctor Faustus*) goes Müller-Rosé one better by developing a florid case, described in painstaking detail, of tertiary syphilis. (Meredith, 1999, pp. 110–11)

Taking into account also the story of Hans Castorp's seven-year spell in a tuberculosis sanatorium, in *The Magic Mountain* (1924), it will be clear to the reader that I cannot hope here to provide a comprehensive account of Mann's literary uses of illness. I focus on Mann's 1912 story 'Death in Venice', because it illustrates concisely some of the ways in which Mann makes use of the motif of disease in his fiction. 'Death in Venice' tells the story of Gustav von Aschenbach, famous man of letters, who becomes infatuated with the beautiful young boy Tadzio during a trip to Venice. Like Mansfield and Thomas, Mann integrates disease into the plot structure of his text: Venice becomes infected with Asiatic cholera, and Aschenbach catches it and dies. Disease also plays a complex role in the symbolic structures of the story.

Of the three authors in question, Mann provides the most overt and self-conscious re-writing of Romantic constructions of illness in terms of superiority, beauty and creativity. We learn that 'Aschenbach's native constitution was by no means robust' and that as a child, his precarious health had 'necessitated a private education' (Mann, 1998, p. 203). Aschenbach personifies the coincidence of physical and intellectual delicacy. Tadzio embodies the Romantic stereotype of Beauty:

Was he in poor health? For his complexion was white as ivory against the dark gold of the surrounding curls. (Mann, 1998, p. 220)

He had also had the impression that the way Tadzio from time to time drew himself up with an intake of breath was like a kind of sighing, as if from a constriction of the chest. 'He's sickly, he'll probably not live long', he thought again, with that sober objectivity into which the drunken ecstasy of desire sometimes strangely escapes; and his heart was filled at one and the same time with pure concern on the boy's behalf and with a certain wild satisfaction. (Mann, 1998, p. 255)

Writing, according to Mann's narrator, is an 'act of begetting between a mind and a body' (Mann, 1998, p. 240): creativity is a physical activity. Like Mansfield, Aschenbach is motivated by intimations of mortality, or 'his artist's fear of not finishing his task – the apprehension that his time might run out before he had given the whole of himself by doing what he had it in him to do' (Mann, 1998, p. 200). However, whilst Mansfield's deteriorating health threatened her ability to produce, Aschenbach's impulse to create threatens his body, because '[b]y art one is more deeply satisfied and more rapidly used up' (Mann, 1998, p. 209).

So for Mansfield, ill health threatens creativity, whilst for Aschenbach, creativity threatens health. Mansfield and Mann thus suggest, in opposite ways, that since creativity is so much imbricated with the body, physical change – such as that produced by illness – must have an effect on writing. Aschenbach defines that effect positively when he represents cholera in terms of creative possibility:

> But at the same time his heart filled with elation at the thought of the adventure in which the outside world was about to be involved. For to passion, as to crime, the assured everyday order and stability of things is not opportune, and any weakening of the civil structure, any chaos and disaster afflicting the world, must be welcome to it, as offering a vague hope of turning such circumstances to its advantage. (Mann, 1998, p. 246)[6]

Here we encounter a variation on the theme of tuberculosis as a heightened state of existence propitious to the artist: the artist's passion will be awakened by the cholera crisis.

Aschenbach gradually emerges as a superior, sickly individual, infatuated with the sickly beauty of Tadzio, and aware of the profound links between his creative and his physical selves. However, like many of Mann's artists, he is an ambivalent figure, demonic as well as superior. His story is that of a man's descent into corruption. The textual vehicles for the expression of that corruption are homosexuality and disease. Mann turns the symbolic tables on the reader as the illness motif which initially signifies beauty and superiority comes to stand for ugly immorality.

Mann's negative association of illness with homosexuality takes various forms. As in much of Mansfield's work, homosexuality is portrayed as contagion: Tadzio is kept away from Aschenbach by his family in case the boy is 'infected' (Mann, 1998, p. 252). Aschenbach's pederastic desire is represented as a 'guilty secret' via its association with the cholera epidemic, which the authorities are afraid to acknowledge:

> Thus Aschenbach felt an obscure sense of satisfaction at what was going on in the dirty alleyways of Venice, cloaked in official secrecy – this guilty secret of the city, which merged with his own innermost secret. (Mann, 1998, p. 246)

> . . . that adventure of the outside world which darkly mingled with the adventure of his heart. (Mann, 1998, p. 250)

Aschenbach's satisfaction at Tadzio's sickly appearance and at the onset of the plague is then over-determined, for both indicate the potential availability of the boy: Aschenbach hopes Tadzio shares his own 'sickness'; he hopes the circumstances of the epidemic might demolish the normal social barriers which separate them. Tadzio is equated with the now dangerous city: Venice threatens Aschenbach's health just as Tadzio threatens his sexuality. Pederasty is ultimately designated as the source of Aschenbach's immorality when he takes the indefensible decision not to warn Tadzio's family of the imminent danger presented by cholera, because he cannot bear the resultant separation from the boy. Thus the symbolic association between pederasty and disease already established threatens to become a reality.

Mann gives free expression to the physical and social realities of cholera, so as to indicate the extent of the threat posed by Aschenbach to Tadzio. By juxtaposing the horror of the plague with Romantic myths of illness, Mann supplies the dark underside of Aschenbach's understanding of the epidemic as pregnant with creative and sexual possibilities. The narrator describes the 'emaciated and blackened corpses of a ship's hand and of a woman who sold greengroceries, the dehydration, suffocation and fatal convulsions of the victims' (Mann, 1998, p. 257), and suggests that, far from inducing creativity, the plague

> led at the lower social levels to a certain breakdown of moral standards, to an activation of the dark, antisocial forces, which manifested itself in intemperance, shameless licence and growing criminality, including robberies and murders.   (Mann, 1998, p. 258)

Thus illness has a contradictory symbolic function in the text, designating not only the creative and aesthetic superiority of Aschenbach and Tadzio, but also the base corruption of Aschenbach. For by the end of the story, we feel that Aschenbach's death from cholera is a just punishment.

As readers, we must condemn Aschenbach's moral sickness – how could true love fail to warn its object of such a danger? But we are at the same time sympathetic to the intensity of Aschenbach's emotion, and to his superior sensitivity. 'Death in Venice' is a fundamentally equivocal text, and it is the motif of illness that expresses that equivocation. The text's defining concepts – pederasty, Venice, cholera – are connoted both positively and negatively. We have seen that Aschenbach's pederasty is 'diseased', that is, morally suspect, but it is also creatively productive:

> He shaped upon Tadzio's beauty his brief essay – that page and a half of exquisite prose which with its limpid nobility and vibrant controlled passion was soon to win the admiration of many. (Mann, 1998, p. 239)

The same is true of Venice:

> This was Venice, the flattering and suspect beauty – this city, half fairy tale and half tourist trap, in whose insalubrious air the arts once rankly and voluptuously blossomed, where composers have been inspired to lulling tones of somniferous eroticism. (Mann, 1998, p. 248)

Disturbingly, cholera itself is portrayed as voluptuous and exotic as well as threatening and ugly:

> Originating in the sultry morasses of the Ganges delta, rising with the mephitic exhalations of that wilderness of rank useless luxuriance, that primitive island jungle shunned by man, where tigers crouch in the bamboo thickets, the pestilence had raged with unusual and prolonged virulence all over northern India... (Mann, 1998, p. 256)

This ambivalent representation of cholera gives the lie to a simplistic conclusion suggesting that it is the tuberculosis-like symptoms that characterise Aschenbach and Tadzio, that are encoded positively, whilst cholera, according to the tradition of literary plagues, is encoded negatively. In the final analysis, Aschenbach is right – that cholera is creatively productive is proved by the very existence of the text. It is a testament both to Mann's art and to the flexibility of illness as a symbol, that these multiple significances can be contained in so satisfying a fashion within such a short text.

Conclusion

In Mann's 'Death in Venice' then, illness continually crosses over the positive/ negative polarity, contributing to the reader's sense of moral and aesthetic disorientation which is ultimately the text's great triumph. In Mansfield's stories, illness is attracted to the negative pole, expressing some of the more problematic aspects of female experience. In Thomas's *Le Refus*, illness gravitates towards the positive pole, clarifying and texturing the novel's political messages. In all three texts, illness is an extremely productive symbolic resource. On the evidence of these very different texts, we must conclude that illness as a literary motif means what the writer wants it to mean, since illness as a symbol floats between the 'positive' and 'negative' poles, even within a single text. It is an ambivalent signifier: there are, no doubt, as many different modes of representing illness in literature as there are subjective responses to the actual experience of illness. And so, for those interested in the inscription of illness and health in discourse, 'literature', understood as an example of 'high' culture, offers a particularly rich resource.

In the context of the potential need for a contestation of dominant discourses on health and illness in a given cultural, social and historical context (discourses which might, for example, be seen to disempower specific groups of people such as the sick or disabled), the literary text presents various advantages. Whilst literature cannot of course be said to escape commercial demands, it is, none the less, arguably less defined by its commercial context than genres which fall into the category of 'mass media', since the 'literary' author does not necessarily write in order to make money, and since the worth of the literary text is not defined by its saleability. The literary text – seen by some theorists as by definition an example of protest – is therefore less constrained by criteria such as norms of acceptability, and is more free to explore the whole range of possibilities for the cultural inscription of illness. Furthermore, the literature of the past and of other cultures is readily accessible to readers of a given culture in the present, offering insights into the huge variety of discursive constructions of illness that have been imagined at other times and in other places. Thus, in a particular cultural context in which dominant discourses about illness might be deemed inappropriate or unhelpful, literature offers an inexhaustible bank of alternative representations. It is, then, precisely in the indeterminacy of the literary metaphor of illness that its power lies. Sontag's characterisation of the metaphor of tuberculosis can be applied to the reception of literary illness images in general. They are, '[l]ike all really successful metaphors...rich enough to provide for two contradictory applications' (Sontag, 1991, p. 26).

NOTES

1. For a study of psychoanalytic theories of creativity, see Andrew Brink, *The Creative Matrix: Anxiety and the Origin of Creativity* (New York: Peter Lang, 2000).
2. I would not, of course, wish to suggest that this is the only possible model for an analysis of the relationship between illness and literature: I simply offer it here as one productive way of conceptualising that relationship.
3. On the *nouveau mal du siècle*, see Hewitt (1988).
4. Claire Tomalin's biography of Mansfield, *Katherine Mansfield: A Secret Life* (New York: Knopf, 1988), is a good source on the facts of Mansfield's illnesses.
5. Or it is possible that, like the author, the narrator has been sent away because of an inconvenient pregnancy. Mansfield tends to conflate pregnancy and illness in her stories, frequently expressing, via her characters, an extreme hostility

towards childbearing. A biographical explanation of this feature of her stories might be her inability to have a child with John Middleton Murray.

6. Meredith (1999) examines the links between creativity, illness and crime in Mann's work.

REFERENCES

Biasin, G. P., 'Literary Diseases: From Pathology to Ontology', *Modern Language Notes*, 82 (1967), pp. 79–102.

Burgan, M., *Illness, Gender and Writing: The Case of Katherine Mansfield* (Baltimore, MD: Johns Hopkins University Press, 1994).

Camus, A., *The Plague* (Harmondsworth: Penguin, 1947).

Dormandy, T., *The White Death: A History of Tuberculosis* (London: Hambledon Press, 1999).

Freud, S., 'The Relation of the Poet to Day-Dreaming', in S. Freud (ed.), *Collected Papers*, vol. IV (London: Hogarth Press, 1956), pp. 173–83.

Gilman, S. L., *Disease and Representation: Images of Illness from Madness to AIDS* (Ithaca, NY: Cornell University Press, 1988).

Hayter, A., *Opium and the Romantic Imagination* (London: Faber & Faber, 1968).

Hewitt, N., '*Les Maladies du siècle*': *The Image of Malaise in French Fiction and Thought of the Inter-War Years* (Hull: Hull University Press, 1988).

Mann, T., *Death in Venice, and Other Stories* (London: Vintage Classics, 1998).

Mansfield, K., *Selected Stories*, with an introduction by D. M. Davin, World's Classics Series (Oxford: Oxford University Press, 1981).

Mansfield, K., *The Collected Stories* (London: Penguin Classics, 2001).

Meredith, S. C., 'Moral Illness on the Magic Mountain', in S. D. Dowden (ed.), *A Companion to Thomas Mann's 'The Magic Mountain'* (Columbia: Camden House, 1999), pp. 109–40.

Sontag, S., *Illness as Metaphor and AIDS as Metaphor* (Harmondsworth: Penguin, 1991).

Suleiman, S., *Authoritarian Fictions: The Ideological Novel as a Literary Genre* (New York: Columbia University Press, 1983).

Thomas, E., *La Mort de Marie* (Paris: Gallimard, 1934).

Thomas, E., *Le Refus* (Paris: Éditions Sociales Internationales, 1936).

Glossary

Audience   Of critical importance to the film industry, now an important area of research for media and cultural studies, with work focused on reception theory (i.e. how audiences interact with texts such as film/television and how they 'read' or make sense of such texts), and the spectator as subject.

Beat writers   Generally used to refer to a set of young American writers in the 1950s, notably Jack Kerouac and William Burroughs, writing about bohemian lifestyles and developing notions of counterculture, later taken up in the 1960s. Kerouac's *On the Road* is viewed by many as the seminal 'beat' novel.

Censorship   Censorship of film and television varies between nations. In some countries it is limited to rating systems, in others films are banned in their entirety or cuts are made. Sex, violence and politics tend to be the main areas of censorship. Lobbying groups, such as the National Viewers' and Listeners' Association, often raise the profile of these issues, leading to debate between public and government about power and control over media products.

Commodification   A process associated with capitalism whereby things are turned into commodities to be bought and sold, often obscuring the origin of those products (i.e. the use value is obscured by the exchange value). Commodities also denote and confer social value and status and thus many argue that most areas of (post)modern life have been commodified by major corporations, transforming individuals into mass consumers.

Consumerism   Relates to the mass consumption of goods by individuals and groups through a process of capitalist commodification. Consumerism is the generic theory of consumption, whose constitutive influences include mass global economies, global media (especially advertising) and aestheticisation (marketing).

270

Content analysis Method of analysing texts by describing (usually quantitatively) the content. The purpose of content analysis is to examine a group of texts (selected according to the research question/design), classifying their content and analysing the results according to a thematic and theoretical framework.

Disability Contested definitions between the biomedical model (i.e. disability as a feature of the individual – the impairment thus disables the individual from normal functioning) and the social model (i.e. that disability is a social construct – it is society which disables the individual with an impairment). Disability studies has become a field in its own right, with many theorists analysing the ways in which cultural texts position a range of individuals living with impairments.

Discourse analysis An attempt to identify the ways in which discourses – regulated ways of speaking about the world and the ways in which knowledge is produced – operate within texts.

Documentary research A generic term to describe the use of textual material for research (as opposed to primary data) in a variety of disciplines.

Genre Originally seen as a way of organising film according to type, especially in the Hollywood system of the early twentieth century, e.g. Western, Musical, Romantic Comedy, etc. Later introduced as a key concept in film theory in the 1960s.

Globalisation Concept used to describe the ways in which modern developments in communication, travel, industry and economy have allowed for greater knowledge of the world and greater communication across time/space. The sharing of media texts has been a central feature of globalisation.

Governmentality Refers to a form of regulation through which populations are subject to top–down bureaucratic discipline. The way in which government produces discourses, particularly around health and social issues, which then inform social policy. Many commentators have argued that the media have a key role in this process.

Health promotion A term which refers to an overall concept – a mixture of educational, legislative and economic measures designed to improve the health of groups/nations – but also a profession, established in the 1960s. The term 'health promotion' came into being in the mid-1980s and has sparked a huge body of academic research and competing models.

Heteronormativity A term used to describe the everyday naturalization of heterosexuality in speech, action and structure (policies, laws, expectations etc.) reliant on gendered performances and the exclusion of 'deviant' sexualities.

High/low culture Authors as diverse as Bourdieu (writing in relation to good taste and judgement), and Hunt, writing about British low culture in the 1970s, have outlined the ways in which a distinction between high and low culture operates in society. High culture was always associated with good taste, status and (often) class; low culture with popular, slapstick, 'trash'. Theorists such as Lyotard saw the collapse of the distinction between high and low culture as a central feature of postmodern society. Elsewhere (M. King and K. Watson, 'Transgressing Venues: Health Studies, Cultural Studies and the Media', *Health Care Analysis*, 2001) we have discussed this distinction and its parallels in academia.

Image In cinematic terms the image refers to the smallest unit of meaning, i.e. a single shot. However, in film theory, and media and cultural studies, the concept of image is generally debated in relation to the preferred meaning or the iconography of the image, i.e., what connotations does a particular image have?

Individualisation Relates to the idea that we are all bound into the processes of individualisation in late-capitalist/postmodern society. Individualisation refers to the inevitable decline of collective experience, whereby individuals become polarised even when experiencing 'common troubles'. Linked to notions of risk and responsibility in that the individual is positioned as the author of his/her own fate.

Moral panic Emerged as a way of understanding the reaction of a 'consensual' group, or the eliciting of a reaction, to a range of issues deemed to be of threat to the moral order. Contemporary examples of subjects of moral panics have been: HIV/AIDS; paedophilia; BSE; Islam. In media terms, theorists have explored the ways in which moral panics are framed by media reporting.

Morality Generally taken to mean the distinction between good and bad in relation to human behaviour. A body of work has recently developed looking at the ways

in which morality discourses operate in media coverage of health issues and how they underpin much social policy.

Narrative   The construction of a meaningful sequence out of events/experiences etc. In recent years, the idea that life is 'narratively enacted' has become popular – that is, that we make sense of our lives and experiences through the construction of narrative. In media terms, the idea of narrative has been used to make sense of the stories and characters of texts (see Vladimir Propp and Lévi-Strauss, for example). In film, for instance, the narrative moves through a number of expected or disrupted conventions (i.e. the plot-line 'maps' a narrative shape of beginning, middle and end according to the genre, and characters have roles, etc.). Even news/documentary is narratively enacted – it constructs/shapes a set of stories that indicate a preferred reading.

Panopticon   Nineteenth-century design for a prison, with one central tower overlooking all the cells (prisoners could not see each other but could all be seen by one guard), used by Foucault (*Discipline and Punish*, London: Tavistock, 1977) as a way of understanding the concepts of surveillance and governmentality particular to enlightenment and 'modern' thinking. Links into the idea that populations can be surveyed and controlled not through force, but through an internalising of the 'gaze' (i.e. people monitor their own behviour, as in the case of health-promotion strategies which rely on individuals looking after their own health).

Polysemic   Originally meaning the existence of several meanings in a single word, this term is applied to media texts to mean that there can be several meanings/interpretations of a single text. This idea has generated a great deal of debate within the field of media and cultural studies and film theory.

Postmodernism   Concerned with a set of philosophical and epistemological positions (i.e. notions of what constitutes knowledge and truth). An anti-essentialist position which challenges the Grand Narratives associated with 'modernist' thinking (modernism is associated with the Enlightenment ideas of progress, 'truth'-finding, etc.). Postmodernist writers (such as Lyotard) highlighted the fractured, transitory and simulated nature of contemporary society, where knowledge is perspectival and partial (i.e., contesting the modernist idea that 'reality' is 'out there' waiting to be discovered; instead, 'realities' are constantly

socially constructed through such things as narrative). In media terms, this can be applied to a variety of positions, from audience (i.e. perspectival 'readings' of texts) to the actual construction of texts (i.e. characters being flawed, complex, and narrative reflecting heterogeneous and layered societies).

Sick role Theory developed by Talcott Parsons in the 1960s to describe the roles of patient and doctor and the function of the sick role. The sick role functions (according to Parsons) as a regulating mechanism to ensure that people are given the incentive to return to health as soon as possible, and is characterised by sets of expectations and obligations for both the doctor and the patient.

Soap opera Particular media genre with multiple characters and plot-lines, episodic in nature. Originally developed in the US on radio (known as 'soap operas' because they were originally sponsored by detergent companies), now associated mainly with television. UK examples include *Coronation Street*, which has been running since the early 1960s. Imported Australian 'soaps' such as *Neighbours* became popular in the UK in the 1980s.

Structuralism This originates from the study of language. Structuralism uses the concept of signifying practices, which generate meaning as an outcome of structures that lie outside of any given person. Structuralism favours a form of analysis in which phenomena only have meaning in relation to each other – systems of relations – rather than emanating from a particular source.

Surveillance The monitoring and collection of information about populations. Linked to the concept of governmentality – the aims of surveillance are to supervise and regulate. In a media and cultural studies context, surveillance is often used to mean the way in which discourses operate to regulate behaviours.

Viewing pleasures Linked to audience research and associated with the journal *Screen* in the 1970s, this concept relates to different readings of texts by audiences and a debate about whose 'gaze' predominates. Feminist film theorists, such as Laura Mulvey in the 1970s, argued that visual texts are always viewed from a male spectator position, but this has since been contested.

Index

Page references in *italics* refer to figures and tables